# DEMENTIA AND OLD AGE MENTAL HEALTH

## A History of Services in Australia

# DEMENTIA AND OLD AGE MENTAL HEALTH

## A History of Services in Australia

## BRIAN DRAPER

Australian Scholarly

First published 2022 by
Australian Scholarly Publishing Ltd
7 Lt Lothian St Nth, North Melbourne, Vic 3051
Tel: 03 9329 6963
enquiry@scholarly.info / www.scholarly.info

ISBN 978-1-922669-90-2

Cover design: Sarah Anderson

# Contents

# Preface

The background to this book is embedded in my early career experiences. In the early 1980s when I was training in Sydney to become a psychiatrist, a combination of an enjoyment of working with older people and an awareness that Australia was beginning to experience the impact of population ageing influenced me in deciding on a career in old age psychiatry, or psychogeriatrics as it was known in that era. There was no formalised old age psychiatry training program in Australia and few hospitals or community services provided specialised care for older people with mental disorders or dementia. Lidcombe Hospital was one of the few hospitals in NSW that provided services and training in old age mental health. I completed my last year of psychiatry training there in 1985 under the supervision of Sid Williams learning the ropes about dementia assessment and management as well as other mental disorders of late life.

During that year it became clear that the combination of increasing numbers of older people with dementia and mental disorders but with limited health and community service options for treatment and care meant that there was an opportunity to develop specialised services for older people with dementia and mental disorders in Australia. The UK experience during the 1970s in developing psychogeriatric service models as espoused by Tom Arie, who was a frequent visitor to Australia in the 1980s, provided a template for service development that at the outset was a 'do it yourself' approach that brought together interested clinicians and administrators to meet the needs of older people without additional resources. Thus when I commenced as a consultant psychiatrist at St George Hospital, Kogarah in late 1985 I decided to follow a similar path and fortuitously met Andrew Cole who had just been appointed as the Director of the St George Community Rehabilitation and Geriatric Service. Together we decided to develop a community based dementia assessment and management service within our existing commitments. At the time there was no clinic in the area for assessment of dementia.

The timing of this 'do it yourself' dementia service could not have been better. In 1986 the Hawke Government commenced an Aged Care Reform Strategy based on the 1982 McLeay Report that recommended the introduction of standardised assessment procedures prior to admission to a nursing home, reform of nursing home funding to control growth and expenditure, and an expansion of community-based aged care services. It was this report that first focused attention on the problem of dementia in nursing homes even though it had been a mounting issue for decades. With the Aged Care Reform Strategy came the development of Geriatric Assessment Teams (later renamed Aged Care Assessment Teams) and the funding for community services that was released in annual enhancements over the late 1980s and early 1990s. Our efforts in the year or so before the enhancements placed the St George service in a good position to receive enhancements and build a dementia service. These changes also signaled the more formal recognition that dementia care was primarily a Commonwealth responsibility thus to a large extent separating it from the rest of old age mental disorders that remained a State responsibility.

The same could not be said for the NSW State public mental health services that in the mid-1980s were commencing reforms based on the Richmond Report that had largely ignored older people but set in train the policy for older people's mental health to be located in aged care. The only new development was for a different model of long-term residential care for older people with serious mental illness – the Confused and Disturbed Elderly (CADE) units. No plans had been made for the needs of older people with acute mental disorders either in the community or in hospital. Only Victoria of the other states was showing promise of developing comprehensive services. In this period I had an informal meeting with Des Nasser who was the Acting NSW Director of Mental Health who suggested that service developments for older people required evidence that they would be effective to sway decision-makers in mental health policy. This led to the commencement of my academic career and research interest in old age mental health and dementia services as I decided to undertake an evidence-based systematic review that examined the effectiveness of treatments and services for older people with mental disorders. An early version appeared in the 1988 *Barclay Report* to the NSW Minister for Health, the final version in the *Australian and New Zealand Journal of Psychiatry* in 1990. After I moved to join Henry Brodaty at Prince Henry Hospital in 1992, an important thread in my research career was the development and evaluation of older people's mental health and dementia services that has included numerous empirical studies, systematic reviews, books, guidelines (including contributions to the Clinical Guidelines for Dementia in Australia), and a report on old age mental health services for WHO. It has also encompassed the training of old age psychiatrists and during the 1990s I was responsible for developing and implementing a two-year old age psychiatry advanced training program within the Royal Australian and New Zealand College of Psychiatrists and involved in establishing its Faculty of Psychiatry of Old Age. This work paralleled the major developments that occurred around the country in both the Commonwealth led development of services for people with dementia and their carers, the more varied State-based older people's mental health services in the 1990s and 2000s, the establishment of professional specialist groups in nursing and psychology and the advocacy organisation, Dementia Australia. I was both a participant and an observer of these changes.

In all of this work I was struck by the limited information available for the period before the 1970s in Australia. For example, in their paper examining dementia policy in Australia, Cecily Hunter and Colleen Doyle focus on the period from the late 1970s onwards. Similarly, Samantha Loi and Anne Hassett focused their description of the history of aged mental health services in Victoria from the 1980s with only brief mention of what happened before then. Australian historical research about mental health, such as the works of Stephen Garton, Milton Lewis, Catharine Coleborne, James Dunk and Eric Cunningham Dax have included limited reference to older people or dementia despite using archival material. Similarly, works by Stephen Garton, Pat Jalland, Brian Dickey and Joan Brown that have focused on benevolence, poverty and ageing have had little mention of dementia and other old age mental disorders. The numerous Royal Commissions and Government inquiries are well documented albeit without a specific consideration of older people with mental disorders and dementia. One exception is the study by Anthea Vreugdenhil of dementia and older admissions to New Norfolk Lunatic Asylum in nineteenth century Tasmania using the admission registers. It provides some insights into the plight of older people with mental disorders, their families and the limited care options available.

This book aims to fill this gap by initially examining the eighteenth and nineteenth century international influences on the understanding of mental disorders, dementia and ageing. Commencing with the arrival of the First Fleet, there is an examination of the first 60 years of colonisation and the mental disorders noted in older European and Aboriginal people using a range of data sources across the country from the nineteenth century onwards. It examines over three hundred archival mental health casebooks of older people aged 60 years and over admitted to lunatic asylums in the nineteenth century in NSW and Tasmania to better understand the reasons older people were admitted, the types of mental problems they faced, and the outcomes of their admissions. Mental health diagnoses in this period were often different to those used today, for example dementia was diagnosed in people with chronic psychoses, and thus as far as possible with the information available a contemporary diagnosis was made and the extent to which a nineteenth century diagnosis would receive such a diagnosis today was estimated. This is facilitated by my experience in numerous research studies in deriving clinical diagnoses from medical records. Lunatic asylum admission registers from Victoria in the nineteenth century and Western Australia in the early twentieth century provide further insights into the types of problems faced by older people including the ageing of long-stay patients admitted as young or middle-aged adults. Annual reports from the Inspector General of the Insane (or equivalent) of each colony/state that were provided to their governments, but mainly those from NSW, Victoria and Queensland from the late nineteenth to mid-twentieth centuries contain reasonably detailed statistical information about older people in mental health services from the second half of the nineteenth century through to the early 1970s. Together these reports document the disproportionate admissions, deaths, and accumulation of older people in the nineteenth century lunatic asylums which became the twentieth century mental hospitals. Indeed the earliest data about patients in an Australian lunatic asylum that was recorded in the 1828 NSW muster demonstrated that the proportion of older people in the Liverpool Lunatic

Asylum was much higher than in the general population and this observation regarding mental hospital remained the case for about 150 years. The biographies of some famous older Australians such as John Macarthur, Gregory Blaxland, Hamilton Hume and Alfred Deakin from the nineteenth and early twentieth century who had late life mental disorders or dementia are included.

But why did older people require disproportionate admission to lunatic asylums in the nineteenth century and mental hospitals in the twentieth century? It was not just due to an ageing population as older people did not want to live in institutions. The examination of mental health casebooks found that the vast majority of admissions had serious mental disorders or moderate to severe dementia. While the appropriateness of admissions of people with dementia to lunatic asylums and mental hospitals was frequently raised by the Inspector Generals around the country, there was a lack of viable alternatives for those whose dementia resulted in behavioural change such as wandering, aggression or poor cooperation with carers. The extent to which dementia in the community was placing pressure for admission to the asylums was gleaned by determining estimates of dementia prevalence in the nineteenth century colonies. These graphically illustrate the likely dementia prevalence in each colony for each decade from 1861 onwards and showing, for example, how Tasmania had the highest rates of dementia in the country in the nineteenth century due to its ageing convicts. The impact on institutions was magnified by the lack of family and community supports in most of the colonies.

Despite a steadily ageing population, until the 1960s there was little change in what community or institutional services were available for older people with dementia and mental disorders. The Stoller Report in 1955 described the poor conditions in the overcrowded mental hospitals in Australia, which remained the main location of long-term care for people with moderate to severe dementia although other State run facilities were also playing a role particularly when there was significant physical debility. It took the advent of Commonwealth funding for nursing homes in 1963 to lead to them eventually becoming the main location of long-term residential dementia care by the 1980s. It was the work of Herbert Bower and G. Vernon Davies in Victoria from 1956 onwards that led the way in moving towards a comprehensive older people's mental health service structure with acute assessment, rehabilitation and various elements of community care.

The eventual split of dementia care from mental health services gained momentum in the 1980s and has never looked back. Most service developments for people with dementia post-diagnosis are funded by the Commonwealth, while the States fund large elements of dementia assessment as well as mental health services which are responsible for other mental disorders in old age. There has been marked variability between the States and Territories on service developments since the 1980s. There has also been a variability in the terms used to describe mental health services for older people including psychogeriatric services, older people's mental health services, aged persons mental health services, specialist mental health services for older people are some examples. While I have used the terminology reflected in various reports and jurisdictions in the different time periods, where no term is specified I have used the term 'older people's mental health services'.

The Commonwealth-funded dementia services that initially were guided by the 1982 Macleay Report, the 1986 Aged Care Reform Strategy, the 1992 National Action Plan for Dementia Care and the 2005 Dementia Initiative are described along with the various contemporary issues that shaped developments.

The extended historical focus demonstrates that the challenges of the care of older people with dementia and mental disorders are not new. In the absence of community services, mental hospital and nursing home admissions increase at a disproportionate rate to population growth. Repeated Royal Commissions and Inquiries into mental health and aged care institutions for over 150 years have shown that there are ongoing problems in providing quality care with the repeated themes of inadequate staff training, staff numbers and remuneration, inadequate funding, poor physical conditions, and lack of adequate recreational resources being mentioned in recommendations. The repeated failure for recommendations to be adequately addressed provides warning for the current Aged Care Royal Commission's recommendations that are at risk of receiving the same fate in the wake of COVID budgetary pressures. Recent mental health reports including that from the Productivity Commission are striking in the near absence of consideration of older people.

Why has there been so little change? A number of themes emerge which include ageism and mental health stigma which have both been apparent since the early nineteenth century. Older people with mental disorders and dementia have the double whammy. Within the mental hospitals and asylums, it was the wards that provided care for mainly older people that usually had the worst conditions; there was a hierarchy of neglect. While funding deficiencies are insufficient explanation of neglect, inadequate financing has contributed to deficiencies in care for older people with dementia and mental disorders, whether it be in institutions or community settings. Without proposing a preferred alternative funding mechanism, it is suggested that unless Australia accepts that quality care of older people with dementia and mental disorders requires more funds to pay for more community care and institutional options, better trained and remunerated staff, and a reorientation towards a dementia-friendly approach to services (which would also be good for other mental disorders) that is person-centred, improvements will be hindered.

The future of old age mental health and dementia care is likely to be affected by other issues as well which include international influences, technological developments, such as the use of robotics and information technology, more effective prevention and treatments of dementia and mental disorders, increased involvement of consumers and carers in service provision, and better integration of care across many domains. The historical perspective on how developments in treatment and care have led to change over time is a theme considered throughout. Another theme which has become more apparent post Second World War relates to the challenges of providing quality care to diverse populations and specific chapters are devoted to Aboriginal and Torres Strait Islander and Culturally and Linguistically Diverse populations.

# Chapter 1

# Mental Health and Dementia in Old Age: A Brief Overview of International Influences on Colonial Australia

## Ageing in Eighteenth-century England

In the eighteenth century, the proportion of people in the English population aged 60 years and over had been largely unchanged from the periods of Ancient Rome, Medieval Europe and seventeenth-century England, fluctuating at between 6 and 8 per cent.[1] By the end of the eighteenth century, at the time of the first European settlement in Australia, rapid population growth driven by increased fertility and economic hardship were beginning to have an impact on English society.[2, 3] Families were having difficulty in supporting their older relatives and more impoverished older people turned to their community for relief. Under the Poor Laws, the infirm aged, which included those who were senile with dementia, were deemed as the most deserving of parochial poverty relief and by the late eighteenth-century persons aged 60 years and over accounted for 34 per cent of parish pensioners.[4, 5] By the last decade of the eighteenth century the Poor Laws were in crisis due to a number of factors that coincided which included rapid population growth, rapid inflation, unemployment, the decay of cottage industries, the growing impact of the 1773 Enclosure Act that forced many landowners off the land, and harvest failures.[6] Yet the proportion of older people in the population was at a historically low level of around 7 per cent, but according to Pat Thane, the aged became a focus of concern in part because efforts were made to identify factors that were contributing to poverty.[7] Poor relief to the aged was only paid to those who were infirm but there were increasing numbers needing it. How many of these had dementia or other late life mental disorders is not known. Susannah Ottaway, in her history of old age in eighteenth-century England, focuses on physical debility as the main reason for late life decline and dependency, barely mentioning mental or cognitive health issues.[8]

## Classification and Phenomenology of Dementia in the Nineteenth Century

By the late eighteenth century there was already a considerable body of work that addressed the classification of the various types of mental disorders, particularly in the writings of Philippe Pinel and William Cullen. While many of the diagnostic categories or labels have evolved over the last two centuries, the concepts behind them have changed much less. This is particularly the case with the use of the word 'dementia', which from an old age perspective is of the greatest interest. Psychiatric historian Germán Berrios noted that the term 'dementia' can be traced back to the second-century Greek philosopher Celsus with evidence that it entered into western vernaculars in the final decades of the seventeenth century. Similarly the concept of dementia started to form in the seventeenth century and in the eighteenth century six conceptual strands came together to shape the nineteenth-century concept of dementia. In the early nineteenth century, dementia was a disorder of cognition affecting any age group, caused behavioural incompetence, was chronic but not necessarily irreversible, could complicate any type of psychiatric disorder, and was congenital or acquired.[9] It was a diagnosis frequently used across the age range and applied to individuals whose mental disorder impaired their intellectual function, with poor attention and ability to reflect, and often being described as 'incoherent' or 'imbecile'.[10] Dementia in old age due to 'senile decay' or 'dotage' had been recognised in the mid-eighteenth century as one type of primary dementia and was already believed to be due to anatomical changes in the brain, although the term 'senile dementia' did not appear in English until James Cowles Prichard's 1835 *A Treatise on Insanity and Other Disorders Affecting the Mind*.[11,12] Perhaps the first detailed description of what would be clearly recognised in the twenty-first century as an older person with dementia complicated by psychosis was published as a case study in 1785 in the German medical journal *Gnothi Sauton*, the first journal to specialise

2

in psychological and psychiatric issues. The anonymous authors described a 75-year-old man Johann Christoph Becker who had a fifteen-year history of gradual cognitive decline complicated by delusions of being persecuted by a tall black man who wanted to kill him and use his flesh in sausages.[13] One unusual aspect of this case study is that the person being described was identified but the authors were not, quite the opposite of modern case studies.

In the first half of the nineteenth century, dementia occurring in old age was well recognised but represented a relatively low proportion of people diagnosed with dementia as most cases were in younger people which would in the most part be psychoses in which disordered thinking and incoherence were the prominent features. Prichard's *Treatise on Insanity* influenced clinicians about the causes, nosology and treatment of insanity in the English-speaking world, particularly England and its Australian colonies. His work was in the form of an accessible and clear synthesis of the existing literature and very openly acknowledged the work upon which his treatise was based. European scholars and clinicians, particularly those from France such as Pinel, Jean-Étienne Esquirol, Étienne-Jean Georget and Louis-Florentin Calmeil, were regularly cited but he also included the work of British authorities such as Cullen, John Locke and Samuel Tuke. On the topic of dementia, his treatise was largely based on the works of Pinel, Esquirol and Calmeil. Prichard described dementia as one of his four types of insanity and, drawing on the work of the French psychiatrist Esquirol, recognised that it was different to idiocy which was due to congenital intellectual impairment. He also recognised that dementia had primary and secondary causes, the latter including protracted mania, epilepsy, and severe delirium. Prichard's description of senile dementia makes a number of important observations. First, there are degrees of cognitive impairment with the first stage being 'forgetfulness or loss of memory', the second being 'irrationality or loss of reason', the third being 'incomprehension', and the fourth being 'loss of instinct or volition'. He gave detailed descriptions of these stages, noting for example, that the loss of memory affected recent memories rather than past memories of earlier life.[14] His second observation was that senile dementia was not universal in older people and that lifestyle influenced it, although he felt that a 'life of too much activity and excitement, of mental exertion beyond what the constitutional strength of the individual is capable of supporting without

3

constant effort' had a deleterious effect.[15] His third observation was that alcohol abuse could cause senile dementia; while modern research certainly confirms it as a cause of dementia, it tends to occur in midlife rather than late life.[16] Finally he importantly observed that senile dementia is quite distinct from moral insanity that can occur in old age; indeed here he was anticipating the modern clinical dementia assessment where mental disorders such as severe depression need to be excluded, although he believed that a person with senile dementia was unlikely to have other severe psychological symptoms causing anxiety, morbidity or unhappiness, an observation not supported by current research.[17] Amentia, a term derived from the work of Cullen in the eighteenth century, was also used in the first half of the nineteenth century to describe a similar range of disorders with cognitive impairment as the main feature, though by the latter part of the century it gave way to the term dementia.[18]

In his 1843 book on mental hygiene that featured in Australian newspaper articles of the period, the American William Sweetser had a view about the cause of senile dementia that still, in some respects, rings true today.[19] He stated 'elderly persons who all at once give up their accustomed occupations and consequently their mental activity and retire to enjoy their ease and leisure, will not rarely, especially if they have been previously free livers, experience a rapid breaking up of their mental and perhaps bodily powers passing sometimes into a more or less complete state of what has been termed senile dementia'.[20] The sense conveyed is that older people need to remain active to prevent dementia.

By the end of the nineteenth century, the concept of dementia was essentially that which is used in the twenty-first century. The two main changes over the century were that dementia is acquired and not congenital, that is, a person is not born with dementia but acquires the disorder during life even if there is a genetic cause such as with Familial Alzheimer's disease or Huntington's disease. Those who are born with a cognitive disorder are classified as having an intellectual disability. The second is that dementia is an organic disorder and that the cognitive changes commonly found in people with functional psychiatric disorders such as chronic schizophrenia are not part of a dementia syndrome. In contemporary psychiatric diagnostic systems such as DSM 5, if cognitive deficits are better explained by a psychiatric disorder, then the diagnosis of dementia (or Major Neurocognitive Disorder as it has been renamed) is not supported.[21] Of course some people with a psychiatric disorder will develop dementia later due to another disease such as vascular dementia, which is regarded as comorbidity, that is, the person has two disorders. These two differences contribute to the observation that when using the contemporary diagnostic criteria for dementia it becomes age-related with the number of cases increasing exponentially with age. While dementia can occur in the young, it is uncommon.[22]

## General Paralysis of the Insane (Dementia Paralytica) in the Nineteenth Century

But one type of dementia that became prominent in younger people in the nineteenth century was dementia paralytica or General Paralysis of the Insane (GPI) which largely afflicted men in their 30s to 50s, although it could occur in old age.[23] By the late nineteenth century up to 20 per cent of males admitted to British asylums received this diagnosis;[24] Australian asylums had similar experiences.[25] Although syphilis was postulated as being the cause of GPI in the nineteenth century, this was not established until the early twentieth century. GPI led a chronic and inevitably fatal course generally passing through three stages over one to five years but with some surviving much longer. The first stage involved speech defects, eye irregularities and poor coordination of facial muscles accompanied by mental exaltation; the second was characterised by paralysis, worsening muscle coordination and mental enfeeblement; while the final stage had widespread paralysis and complete loss of intellectual function before death through exhaustion or seizures.[26] Post mortems demonstrated that there was chronic inflammation of the arachnoid lining of the brain,[27] and by mid-century was one of the key factors influencing the emergence of the view that insanity was caused by physical medical disorders (championed by alienists, the term used in the nineteenth century to describe psychiatrists) as opposed to moral issues.[28] The use of the word 'moral' in the nineteenth century was different to current usage and was reflecting psychological rather than ethical issues.[29,30] As is noted in later chapters, this move away from psychological to physical understandings of insanity was reflected in Australia in the management of asylums in the second half of the nineteenth century with the move from non-medical to medical management.

# Classification and Phenomenology of
## Other Mental Disorders in the Nineteenth Century

In the early nineteenth century, 'insanity' was used to describe individuals who in contemporary language would be described as being 'psychotic'. The term 'psychosis' was not introduced until the late nineteenth century.[31] Prichard, drawing on the earlier work of Pinel, categorised the forms of insanity into four broad groups – moral insanity, mania, monomania, and incoherence (dementia). Prichard's diagnostic categories were not age-related and each of the broad categories could appear in older people. He introduced the term 'moral insanity' which was the English version of Pinel's *'manie sans delire'* (madness without delirium). Moral insanity was, according to Prichard, 'a morbid perversion of the feelings, affections, and active powers, without any illusion or erroneous conviction impressed upon the understanding'.[32] In other words, this was what is described in modern psychiatry as a mood disorder without psychosis, particularly depression, but also mild forms of mania (hypomania).

According to Prichard, the 'Mania' category was equivalent to 'raving madness, in which the understanding is generally deranged.'[33] This is not the equivalent to the modern day concept of mania which is regarded as one of the mood states in bipolar mood disorder.[34] Rather, it is a broader psychotic illness with prominent disorder of the order, flow and content of speech, with associated mental and physical excitement which might manifest as agitation or aggression. The person might become preoccupied with various delusions and talk incessantly (or rave) about them without let up. The individual's reason was disordered and often seemed unaware that they spoke nonsense.[35]

Another deviation from modern day usage involved the term 'melancholia' which was regarded as a subtype of mania involving reduced behavioural output, for example, the person might become bedridden. It was not regarded as being the polar opposite of mania, and pathological affect, such as profound sadness, was not part of the concept although it was not excluded from it.[36] Melancholia in old age was largely regarded as a prelude to dementia and thus those diagnosed with senile melancholia were expected to eventually dement. Many nineteenth century alienists regarded late life melancholia as a sign of impending dementia and believed that it was otherwise rare in older people who no longer had the passions that caused melancholia in younger people.[37] By the mid-twentieth century it was well established that a severe episode of depression could cause reversible cognitive impairment and mimic dementia, so-called 'depressive pseudodementia' with the key issues of importance being its relatively short course and reversibility with treatment of the depression. Although not restricted to older people, nor to severe mood disorders, it is more likely to occur in melancholic depression in late life.[38] What is less well known is that in 1883 Albert Mairet described a case series of 21 patients (mean age 41 years) with 'melancholic dementia', that had a short course before onset of cognitive impairment, anxious or depressed mood, and good prognosis with long lasting remissions. His work had little impact at the time, but was part of a growing recognition that was emerging in the late nineteenth century that dementia associated with functional psychoses in younger people was likely to be different to the organic dementia changes found in senile dementia.[39] As will be noted in later chapters, mania was a common diagnosis in older people in nineteenth-century Australian lunatic asylums from the 1850s onward, while melancholia appeared from the 1870s onwards and was mainly in people who were depressed.

From a legal perspective, by the early nineteenth century lawyers had recognised that individuals could be 'partially insane', in other words, while having evidence of insanity (psychosis) they retained competence to manage their affairs. This was legitimised by the diagnostic category of monomania that Esquirol introduced in around 1810 and which appeared as the fourth broad diagnostic category of insanity in Prichard's *Treatise on Insanity*.[40] As a diagnosis, monomania lost favour in the second half of the century, although the recognition that individuals could have a psychosis and retain competence to manage their affairs remained.

Delirium is a common mental disorder in older people with the modern understanding being that it is an acute change in mental state over a few days characterised by fluctuating attention and wakefulness, impaired cognition, and perceptual changes (illusions or hallucinations) caused by a physical illness.[41] There are a number of factors that increase an individual's vulnerability to delirium which include old age, severe medical illness, dementia, sensory impairments, and depression. Thus, from an old age mental health perspective, delirium is a very important diagnosis to make as it might be indicative of an underlying life-threatening emergency.[42] By the early nineteenth century the diagnosis of delirium, which from antiquity was recognised as a cluster of mental and behavioural symptoms associated with physical illness, was already regarded as a separate mental state to conventional madness with the distinguishing feature being the presence of fever.[43] Incoherent, hallucinating afebrile individuals who in contemporary medicine would be diagnosed with delirium due to, for example, an acute stroke or cardiac failure, would in the early nineteenth century have been diagnosed with a form of insanity albeit associated with the physical illness. By the mid-nineteenth century the Austrian Ernst von Feuchtersleben was proposing that the presence or absence of fever to differentiate delirium from insanity was unsatisfactory and that demarcation should be based on natural history, symptoms, and aetiology.[44] Not all agreed and the debate continued throughout the rest of the nineteenth century and this nosological uncertainty is likely to have influenced decisions about admissions to lunatic asylums. Oddly, one interesting finding in the later chapters is that delirium was not diagnosed in nineteenth-century Australian lunatic asylums.

## Nineteenth Century views on the impact of Age on Mental Disorders

Prichard discussed the impact of age on recovery from insanity and quotes the work of Esquirol where few were reported to recover after the age of 50. However, Prichard adds a note of optimism by pointing out that there were twenty recoveries in this age group and that four out of the twelve aged over 70 recovered. He also cites work by Georget on the age profile of admissions of lunatics to hospitals in England and France where 209 out of 4409 admissions were aged 60 years and over. While noting that most admissions occurred in individuals aged 30 to 40 years, he cautions that although there were fewer older admissions, without knowing the numbers of people in the community in each age group, the relative proportion of admissions in different age groups cannot be determined. He quotes Esquirol as telling him in a personal communication that there is a 'proportionately increased frequency of mental disease with the advancement of age' and that after the age of 70 most of this could be attributed to senile dementia.[45] Historian Emily Andrews notes that David Skae, who was the Medical Superintendent of Morningside Asylum in Edinburgh from 1846 until 1873, was the seminal exponent of somato-aetiological classification of mental disorders that recognised the various impacts of life course issues on the diagnoses of mania and melancholia in addition to the existent senile dementia. This resulted in the introduction of the diagnoses 'senile mania' and 'senile melancholia' to describe older people with these disorders in which age was believed to be a factor in causality, with senile mania diagnosed in NSW asylums from the 1850s onwards and senile melancholia from the 1880s onwards. Thomas Clouston, Skae's successor at Morningside, continued this life course approach in his textbook *Clinical Lectures on Mental Diseases*.[46]

## The Asylum Movement and the Impact of an Ageing Population in Britain

The nineteenth century witnessed the development of asylums as the focus of treatment of the mentally ill. From the eighteenth century, there were repeated reports of appalling conditions for institutionalised lunatics (the term used to describe the mentally ill in that era),[47] and the elderly in poorhouses and workhouses managed by parishes. No special provisions were made for lunatics and indeed they were not specifically the responsibility of the parish until 1744. In general, these were individuals with chronic serious mental disorders who were often vagrants and unable to hold down employment. Those who were acutely insane would more likely be cared for in a lunatic hospital such as Bethlem (Bedlam) or Bethel which were privately run and placed a limit on the duration of admission, cured or not.[48] The workhouses were based on the moral principle that social uselessness was sinful and therefore the poor should be made to work and this required discipline.[49] Unsupervised and untrained keepers used a custodial approach that was conducive to abuses and brutality. Troublesome individuals were chained and manacled; they were often filthy, without clothes, and sleeping on dirty straw.[50]

British philosophers of this Enlightenment period, such as David Hume and John Locke, were emphasising that bad experiences could have a deleterious impact on a person's mind and lead to, or exacerbate, madness. A natural follow-on from this philosophy was that by education it could be possible to undo the damage done. This became the basis of the 'moral treatment' movement and reintroduced the perception that the mentally ill were blameless, their mental derangement was caused by external disturbances of the laws of human nature, with the Frenchman Pinel being the influential advocate. Perhaps the best example of this moral treatment model of care was epitomised by layman Samuel Tuke's York Retreat, a family-owned private asylum. The York Retreat was founded in 1792 for mentally disordered brethren of the Society for Quakers and very quickly glowing reports featured in the press and medical journals across Britain, Europe and North America. There were no physical restraints as the Tuke family created a moral environment involving respect and dignity. Patients were fed well, wore good clothes, and joined the Tuke family for tea parties as their guests. Although many of the elements in the York Retreat model of care were not replicated elsewhere, this was the beginning of the asylum movement in psychiatry that lasted for over 150 years from about 1800. This movement spread to the English colonies and was highly influential on developments in Australia.[51]

Population ageing driven by a combination of lower fertility and increased life expectancy impacted on the asylums in the second half of nineteenth-century Britain.[52] The 1845 Lunacy and County Asylums Acts had provided the legal basis for including older people with senile dementia amongst the insane. Initial uncertainty about this was resolved when the Lunacy Commissioners wrote to the Lord Chancellor in 1848 that while people who were regarded as imbecile from senility were not 'ordinary lunatics', because they were incapable of managing their own affairs, they should be offered the same protection under the Act. In this period, the Lunacy Commissioners were extremely critical of the standard of care of the aged and incurable lunatics in workhouse lunatic wards and were seeking a better alternative in the county asylums. In the same year, a separate communication to the Lord Chancellor indicated that the key issue for admission to a county asylum was whether the person was of unsound mind, and whether or not the person was regarded as dangerous.[53]

Over the second half of the nineteenth-century asylums in Britain became overcrowded as the number of people declared insane increased each year. This increase was across all age groups and mental disorders. For example, a study of admissions to two Oxford Asylums (Warneford and Littlemore) between 1826 and 1900 found that the proportion of admissions aged 60 years and over remained fairly constant over the period and was higher than the proportion of older people in the general population.[54] In 1850, there were seven thousand people in county asylums in England and Wales, by 1890 there were 53 thousand and the size of the average asylum had increased from 300 to 800 patients.[55] Older people with senile dementia represented a component of the increase. Senile dementia in the nineteenth century was believed to be due to the effects of ageing rather than disease of the brain. Patrick Fox, in his overview of the history of Alzheimer's disease, observes that in the mid-nineteenth century it was believed that the aged were unable to efficiently replace dying brain cells and quotes Carole Haber in saying that this 'constituted the pathological state known as old age'.[56] From the 1870s this influenced lunatic asylum administrators in Britain to argue that this 'natural decay' of ageing should not be regarded as an active form of lunacy and should exclude older people with senile dementia from admission. But this approach had little effect. In 1880, when diagnostic records were first kept, there were 509 people admitted to lunatic asylums in England and Wales with a diagnosis of senile dementia and this increased to 906 in 1900 despite the efforts to curtail such admissions. The workhouses remained the main alternative form of institutional care for older people in Britain and had a main focus on physical disability. Those with senile dementia who were quietly confused could be tolerated but once significant behavioural disturbances occurred, admission to a lunatic asylum was often sought. This frequently led to disagreements between institutions over a patient – the lunatic asylums focusing on the inappropriateness of admissions due to physical health and natural decay, the workhouses focusing on the mental infirmity and behavioural disruption. Emily Andrews comments that people with dementia were not welcome in either type of institution 'but their presence reveals one of the key functions which these institutions performed: absorbing and containing unmanageable and undesirable behaviour, preserving the order of the outside world, and providing care (often in a very minimal sense) to people whose needs had transcended the financial, practical and emotional capacity of the people around them'.[57]

These issues related to the appropriateness of mental hospitals for people with dementia and where best to care for older people with significant physical disability or health concerns also played out in Australia and remain as influential in the organisation of care for older people in the twenty-first century as they were in the late nineteenth century. As will become clearer over the rest of this book, they have been influential factors in the development of old age mental health and dementia services in Australia over the last 50 years.

## Emil Kraepelin and the Classification of Mental Disorders

The classification of mental disorders evolved over the second half of the nineteenth century with an increasing focus on symptoms and disease groups. Before the groundbreaking work of Emil Kraepelin towards the end of the century, the classification of mental disorders was chaotic. Examination of Australian mid-nineteenth-century lunatic asylum casebooks described in later chapters is testimony to that. In the late nineteenth century the classification system that had the greatest impact in New South Wales (NSW) was devised by Britain's Medico-Psychological Association in 1882 with its 'Form of Insanity' Classification, which was published in a report of its thirty-seventh annual meeting and was used in the Inspector General of the Insane Annual Reports from 1883 until 1931 with minor revisions over the period. This classification had the broad categories of congenital or infantile mental deficiency, epilepsy, GPI, mania, melancholia, and dementia, with the latter three having sub-classifications that included 'senile'.[58] Roger Blashfield in his review of pre-Kraepelinian classificatory systems, identified 16 different systems that had very low concordance with on average 15 per cent of the diagnoses in one system matching the same name in another. Despite the inconsistencies, it is noteworthy that there were broad consistencies which included the recognition that classification based on aetiology would be optimal but the state of scientific knowledge did not allow that and so classificatory systems were based on symptoms. One diagnosis that appeared most reliably across systems was senile dementia, which appeared in over half of the classifications.[59] In later chapters I present information about the diagnoses of older admissions to nineteenth-century Australian asylums and clearly this implies that they have to be interpreted with caution.

In the 1899 sixth edition of his textbook of psychiatry *Ein Lehrbuch der Psychiatrie*, Kraepelin proposed a nosology of mental disorders based on course and outcomes which included dichotomising the major psychoses into manic-depressive psychosis (now bipolar disorder) and dementia praecox (now schizophrenia). This classification system was the basis of psychiatric diagnosis throughout the twentieth century and remains influential today.[60] The diagnosis 'paraphrenia' appeared in Kraepelin's nosology as a paranoid psychosis with attenuated hallucinatory experiences. In 1863 Karl Kahlbaum had used the term 'paraphrenia' to refer to refer to insanities that appeared at the transitions of life with a senile form. In the twentieth century, with the ageing population and the influence of the English Newcastle group in the 1950s, the diagnosis 'late paraphrenia' came into fashion though this had lost favour by the end of the century.[61]

# Chapter 2

# The Early Colonial Days and First Asylums in NSW

Little is known about the pre-European contact Australian Aboriginal population demographics in the eighteenth and early nineteenth centuries. Estimates of the number of Aboriginal people on the Australian continent in 1788 range from 300,000 to one million, with one estimate for south-eastern Australia being 250,000.[1] In January 1788 there were around fifteen hundred Aboriginal people in coastal Sydney.[2] The age profile of the population is unknown.

Less than one per cent of those on the First Fleet was aged 60 years and over, which is understandable given the need to establish a new colony.[3] Within days of landing, a tent hospital was established on the west side of Sydney Cove by Principal Surgeon John White.[4] Despite the First Fleet being regarded as a relatively healthy one, the first three months after arrival found many to become debilitated, particularly from the effects of scurvy and dysentery.[5]

The colony endured a famine over the next two years. David Collins records that 'labour stood nearly suspended for want of energy to proceed; and the countenances of the people plainly bespoke the hardships they underwent'.[6] With the arrival of the Second Fleet in June 1790, the poor health of its convicts necessitated the construction of a portable hospital that by mid-July had 488 persons receiving treatment mainly for scurvy, dysentery and malnutrition. As with the First Fleet, less than one per cent of convicts were aged 60 years and over.[7]

Indeed, this did not change much over the next 60 years. By examining the ages of a random sample of over 6600 convicts out of the 162,000 convicts transported to Australia, Lloyd Robson estimated that only about 0.5 per cent were aged 60 years and over and only a further 0.6 per cent were aged 55 to 59 years.[8] In common with other 'new world' colonies such as the United States, the colonists were predominantly younger males.[9] There were approximately six times more males than females and this changed very little in the first 50 years of colonisation.[10, 11] There were relatively few grandparents. Immigrants, whether by transportation or free settlement, severed ties with the older generation and it has been argued that the Australian family was 'born modern' with the nuclear family shorn of extended family of grandparents, uncles, aunts and cousins.[12, 13] Even by 1846, the NSW census showed only two per cent of the population was aged 60 years and over, with two-thirds being male.[14]

David Collins and Watkin Tench reported the impact of the harsh conditions in the first years of the colony on the health and wellbeing of the colonists, with the high mortality and the large number of convicts deemed unfit for labour.[15, 16] It is also likely that the long periods of reduced rations and periods of famine, poor living conditions, extremes of weather, and the psychological impact of being distant from family in Britain contributed to chronic ill health in some free colonists who resigned their positions. Augustus Alt, a soldier and land surveyor from the First Fleet, drew up the first plans for Sydney town with wide avenues and room for expansion. In November 1791, at the age of 60, he requested relief as surveyor general due to ill health but continued to act as magistrate. He was fully invalided in 1801 on half-pay pension and aged 83, died at Parramatta.[17] Governor Phillip's health had been failing from the effects of hard work, privation and exposure since 1790 and he made several requests to be relieved before his permanent departure in December 1792 at the age of 54. He eventually recovered, returned to sea duty in 1796, before his retirement at the age of 67 and death at 75.[18] Henry Brewer, an eccentric man, was rated a midshipman on the *Sirius* but largely performed clerical duties for Phillip. On arrival, he was appointed provost-marshal and his duties became more demanding as the settlement grew. These duties included directing the convict constabulary, for maintaining good order in the community, and court duties. Towards the end of 1795, through failing health, he became incapable of carrying out his duties and died in March 1796 at the age of 57 'worn with old age and infirmities'.[19, 20]

In his journal, Collins repeatedly mentioned that general melancholy pervaded the colony for periods from 1790 to mid-1792. There are a number of reports about impacts on the older convicts.[21] In *The Fatal Shore*, Robert Hughes claims that the first recorded suicide in the colony occurred in 1789 when Dorothy Handland, who was probably in her early 60s, hung herself in 'a fit of befuddled despair' from a gum tree in Sydney Cove.[22] However, this seems unlikely as she was recorded by Collins to have departed the colony on the *Kitty* in June 1793.[23] The first recorded episode of self-harm in the colony occurred in April 1788 when Collins reported that an unidentified elderly female convict hung herself to the ridge-pole of her tent after being accused of stealing a flat-iron. She was discovered and cut down before it was too late.[24]

When the colony was established, the Colonial Medical Service was not responsible for the administration of lunacy which was regarded as a matter of benevolence derived from the 'old Poor Law' practice in England. In the first decade of the nineteenth century the mentally deranged who required confinement were incarcerated at Parramatta Gaol in harsh and unrelenting conditions, likely to be preyed on and abused by other inmates and the gaolers. Some of these were older people but there are no details available.[25,26] Examples of the types of mental derangement that afflicted older people in this period can be gleaned from the *Sydney Gazette*. In 1808, John Gold a 72-year-old labourer twice attempted suicide by hanging and then by jumping into a well. The cause was attributed to jealousy of a woman.[27] In 1809, George Padbill an old settler was 'in tolerable circumstances' but it was conjectured that a 'temporary embarrassment of a pecuniary nature' precipitated his act.[28] The twin themes of relationships and money that were regarded as being the causes of these events were indeed fundamental to the lives of ageing colonists. Without someone to provide informal caregiving support and the finances to live on, an older person, particularly if at all physically or mentally disabled, would struggle. Older infirm convicts and emancipists were especially vulnerable as the few government pensions were directed to former government employees.[29] The extent to which these issues contributed to the suicides of five First Fleet convicts when aged in their 50s during the early nineteenth century is not known.[30] Alcohol misuse was a factor likely to contribute to premature ageing with rum being the currency of the period.[31] Apart from contributing to an individual's debts, the impact of alcoholism on mental and physical well-being was already understood in that era. From the First Fleet, 61-year-old Zachariah Clark died of an alcohol-related death on Norfolk Island in 1805.[32]

Governor Lachlan Macquarie arrived in the colony in December 1809. Among the many challenges he faced, the needs of the mentally ill, physically ill, and the aged and infirm were priorities. An early achievement was the opening of the 200-bed two-storey general hospital in 1811 that was the forerunner of Sydney Hospital in Macquarie Street, although building was not completed until 1814. It was colloquially named the Rum Hospital after the controversial method of financing the building by the grant to the tenderers of a monopoly to import 45,000 gallons of rum over a period of three years, provided that construction was at no cost to the Government. This development addressed the needs of those who had acute physical illnesses.[33]

There was a need to provide more appropriate containment than Parramatta Gaol for those who were too mentally deranged to live in the community.[34] Each of the colony's Governors had been charged with the care and custody of 'lunatics and idiots' (in modern parlance, the mentally ill and those with intellectual disability) and their estates. There was no definition of what constituted being a 'lunatic' or an 'idiot' and no requirement for a medical examination before commitment, although most often that occurred.[35] In 1811 Macquarie ordered that the former convict stone barracks on part of the Castle Hill Agricultural Settlement that had been abandoned in 1810 should be converted into an asylum for the mentally deranged.[36, 37] The first six patients were transferred from Parramatta Gaol in May 1811 along with a keeper and a cook. The Reverend Samuel Marsden was put in charge but he was largely absent establishing churches in New Zealand and was replaced by George Suttor as asylum superintendent in 1814.[38] In his instructions Macquarie insisted that the facility should be clean, food properly issued, activities provided for the patients, force and fraud avoided, and for there to be regular reports.[39] Macquarie's instructions were consistent with the model of care known as 'moral treatment' that was popular in Europe at the time. Despite being lauded in the *Sydney Gazette* that 'every provision that humanity could suggest has been made for their accommodation and comfort',[40] the building was in disrepair throughout the life of the asylum, beds were infested with vermin and there was an inadequate, irregular supply of clothes with many dressed in rags, almost naked, and without shoes.[41] There was often in excess of forty patients and the untrained staff comprised only two male assistants and a female nurse until 1821 when two more staff were added.[42]

The running of the asylum was not smooth with conflicts between Suttor and the resident surgeons William Bland, until he resigned in 1815, and Thomas Parmeter until 1819 when both Suttor and Parmeter were dismissed by Macquarie. The appointment of William Bennett as superintendent and the abolition of the position of resident surgeon seemed to settle matters.[43, 44] Few details of the patients have survived but some were aged and most were convicts. There were problems with violent behaviour, including one murder, and in 1821 Superintendent Bennett reported that 'one violent male patient had beaten an elderly patient unmercifully'. In February 1826, when there were 36 patients, two were aged over 70. There is little information about the nature of the mental disorders. Treatments used included blistering, emetics, wine & bark (quinine), head shaving, cupping and bleeding. Flogging was used as punishment for stealing. Restraints and strait waistcoats were used for the violent.[45] Following adverse findings by a Grand Jury on the standard of care and adequacy of buildings at Castle Hill, the asylum was closed in 1826 with patients being transferred to Liverpool Asylum.[46]

The aged and infirm also received attention during Macquarie's term and it was private benevolence that took the lead. The NSW Society for Promoting Christian Knowledge and Benevolence was formed in 1813 and provided outdoor relief, mainly with food and beverages, and some limited financial support. Of nine cases listed in its first annual report, five were aged with some degree of disability or destitution such as 'an old helpless man aged 85' and 'an aged woman, a cripple'.[47] In 1818 it was reformed as the Benevolent Society of NSW due to debts incurred.[48] In the last year of Macquarie's governorship in 1821 the Benevolent Society acquired an asylum that was built at Government expense to accommodate 50 to 60 people. Problems with discipline usually involved alcohol which was banned.[49] Severe moral and religious standards were enforced and inmates were not allowed to leave the premises without permission.

Beverley Earnshaw comments that it was unlikely that ex-convicts would have been in the Benevolent Asylum by choice, as having survived the convict system, the charity system was another form of restraint and it was regarded as a last resort for those who were senile, dying or incapacitated. During the convict's sentence the Government supplied their material needs, but often there was a gap between the expiration of a sentence and their requiring care in the

Benevolent Asylum. Aged convicts were expected to work and this continued after the expiration of their sentence. It was those who were infirm who were more likely to become paupers unable to support themselves and their family that were reliant on charity, which was conditional, and had to eke out a living in whatever way they could, for example, by fishing or gathering oysters. Although infirmity was frequently acquired during the convict's term, Beverley Earnshaw reports that in the 1820s and 30s, four to five per cent of convicts had some type of physical or mental impairment when transported.[50]

Once the Benevolent Asylum was established, the Benevolent Society focused its efforts on providing indoor relief, with outdoor relief of goods and food mainly provided to families. By 1825, the asylum was overcrowded with 93 residents, many requiring medical attention that was provided on an honorary basis by Dr William Bland. Inmates were forced to sleep on the floor, there was a lack of privacy, with quarrels and fights frequently occurring. By 1830, the Benevolent Society's annual report notes that there were now 144 residents of whom 98 were aged 60 years and over.[51] How many of the older residents had significant mental impairment, particularly dementia, is unknown. But there were certainly some, as witnessed by Second Fleeter William Priest who was admitted to the Benevolent Asylum on 18 December 1821 at around the age of 60. His condition was recorded as 'paralytic, very feeble and loss of intellect' which may have been describing vascular dementia. He died in 1826.[52]

Grace Karskens studied older people living in the Rocks area of Sydney between 1822 and 1828. Twenty-five were aged over 65, almost all were convicts or ex-convicts and most had arrived twenty to thirty years earlier. Relationships and families remained important for economic security, support and to avoid loneliness. Many had multiple marriages and it was not uncommon for there to be large age differences between partners. Ownership of property and other material comforts were lures to find companions to care for them in their old age. Less than a quarter of those over the age of 65 were living with their spouse and overall 43 per cent were with family. The majority were either living alone independently or in a dependent relationship as servants, lodgers, or in the Benevolent Asylum. Contrary to popular depiction of older people, most were property owners and still working. Older people did their best to continue their work and lifestyle for as long as their health allowed. A few retired, but only if they were unable to work and were able to secure a pension.[53]

Karskens points out that ageist attitudes were rife in early Sydney as witnessed by articles in the *Sydney Gazette* and *The Australian*. The behaviour of older people was often depicted as ridiculous or unbecoming when similar behaviour in younger people passed without comment. Older women were lampooned for drinking, older men for having an interest in sexual relations. Descriptions of older people often included emotive terms such as 'tottering', 'feeble', and 'worn-out'. An example provided by Karskens is ex-convict Andrew Frazier, who by his 60s had become a wealthy baker and publican, made an unfortunate marriage to a 20-year-old convict woman Eleanor Hatton who frequently got drunk and absconded. He took her to a magistrate in 1825 and the reporting by William Charles Wentworth (the former explorer who crossed the Blue Mountains in 1813) in *The Australian* is a prime example of these ageist attitudes in the press. He not only identified Frazier in his article, but by way of puns and demeaning descriptions, held him up to ridicule. Subsequently Frazier's relationship with his wife continued to deteriorate, he started to drink heavily and died an alcohol-related death in 1827.[54]

By the 1820s NSW had a lower mortality rate than England which was likely due to a better diet and healthier environment that would be mainly enjoyed by those who were financially secure.[55] A copy of an anonymous letter in *The Sydney Gazette* in July 1830 from 'a Gentleman in Sydney' written to someone in England and most likely published to encourage free settlers to come to the colonies, claimed that conditions were so good that 'the women begin again to have families, and old men appear to take a new lease of life. Crutches, blindness, and other deformities are rarely seen'.[56] Hyperbole but with a grain of truth in it. Alcohol abuse, however, remained an issue for older people. William Clarke, who had a long history of alcoholism, died in 1822 'a very infirm old man' at the age of 57.[57] Second Fleeter Michael Connor, at the age of 82, was dismissed as a constable in 1826 due to 'outrageous behaviour and drunkenness'.[58]

Between 1827 and 1831, a spate of suicides occurred that was regarded by the editors of the *Monitor* and *The Australian* as representative of collective madness related to the autocratic Governorship of Sir Ralph Darling, who had become deeply unpopular during the drought and economic downturn of 1826–1829. As James Dunk has described, they were regarded as 'Darling's suicides' and one of these in February 1828 was of the 62-year-old George Galway Mills.[59] Mills had a colourful background. He was born on the island of St Kitts in the Caribbean to a fourth-generation planter family and although he inherited his father's plantations, he spent most of his time in England. He secured a seat in the House of Commons in 1804, which he resigned on the expectation of being appointed to accompany Lord Douglas on a mission to Russia but this fell through and as recompense he was offered the place of fifth commissioner to the West Indies in January 1807. He was in debt due to a combination of a decline in trade to the West Indies, war, and his lifestyle and was confined in King's Bench for debts of over £43,000 and was unable to take up the appointment. He managed to free himself from debt by claiming parliamentary privilege in questionable circumstances after getting another seat in Parliament in July 1807. He immediately resigned and was employed as a Government spy in Prussia. He remained in Europe in various roles until 1818 when he was returned to Parliament. His wife died in 1820 and he lost his seat.[60] He was appointed as the Registrar of the Supreme Court of NSW in 1824 in an appointment felt by Chief Justice Forbes to be a sinecure. He soon joined the social set at the Turf Club becoming friendly with sheriff John Mackaness. In late 1827 Darling dismissed Mackaness and a number of other crown appointments for indiscretions at the Turf Club in which he perceived that they had defamed the Government.[61] Mills believed that he was soon to be dismissed and became suicidally preoccupied, seeking advice from Dr William Bland about the use of laudanum before shooting himself two days later in February 1828. At the inquest it was reported that he had been depressed for a month since resigning as Secretary of the Turf Club and after he received bad news in a letter. Bland reported that Mills had been disturbed for two weeks, agitated, anxious, depressed and suicidal although calmer on the morning of his death.[62] Mills had again been in debt and had also stood security to Mackaness, a situation that Darling described in his report to Under Secretary Hay, 'with the impossibility of extricating himself from the difficulties which immediately surrounded him, he appears to have been driven to desperation'.[63] The inquest determined that he shot himself in 'a fit of insanity'.[64] From a modern psychological autopsy perspective, Mills appears to have developed a severe major depression as a consequence of his life stressors, a common finding in late life suicide.

With the closing of Castle Hill Asylum in 1826, Liverpool Lunatic Asylum was a temporary solution located in the parsonage of St Luke's Church in Liverpool which was being used as a temporary court house at the time. The two-storey brick building surrounded by a paling fence had been erected during Macquarie's governorship and was designed by colonial architect Francis Greenway. By 1828, Thomas Plunkett had been appointed superintendent and in January 1829 Dr Patrick Hill became 'head surgeon' for the town of Liverpool which included responsibility for the lunatic asylum.[65] It soon became overcrowded and by 1828 there were 36 patients as recorded in the census in November of that year. Of these patients, fifty per cent were aged 50 and over with eleven aged 60 and over,[66] the oldest being 84-year-old John Mortlock who was described by Dr Hill as 'debilitated with confirmed insanity'. Mortlock had been working as an assigned servant to prominent colonist John Macarthur as late as 1825.[67] The oldest woman was First Fleet ex-convict 78-year-old Elizabeth Hall who had arrived on the *Lady Penrhyn* and had been in Castle Hill Asylum since at least 1822.[68] The 1828 Census demonstrated for the first time in Australia that older people were being disproportionately admitted and cared for in lunatic asylums, which remained the case for the next 150 years. The census indicated 3.8 per cent were aged 60 years and over in the colony but over 30 per cent of those in the asylum were aged 60 years and over,[69] although by 1838 the last year of operation of the Liverpool Asylum, this had dropped to around 10 per cent, this was still more than double the proportion of older people in the colony at that time.[70] A contextual issue that was to arise again in the 1890s was the economic slump in the colony.[71] In such times, the burden of caring for disabled older people at home is likely to have contributed to greater use of lunatic and benevolent asylums for relief.

There is insufficient information about the cases to know the precise reasons for admission. The case descriptions of the period use terms such as 'confirmed insanity', 'idiot', and 'deranged' with added descriptors indicating the severity, fatuousness, the presence of epilepsy, or a physical component ('cripple', 'paralytic').[72] Over the thirteen years of its operation, the overcrowding at Liverpool steadily worsened. Staffing was minimalist. In September 1838 when there were 87 patients, in addition to superintendent Plunkett, there was an overseer, a cook, a gatekeeper, two keepers and a night watchman. Only Plunkett and overseer Gillespie were free men and paid – the rest were unpaid convicts. However, there was also a convict female attendant, elsewhere described as a nurse, paid a gratuity of eight pence per day.[73, 74] Efforts were made to follow moral treatment principles by engaging as many patients as possible in work in the kitchen, garden or pulling carts. Compared with its predecessor at Castle Hill, the Liverpool Asylum was much less conflicted and there were fewer episodes of patient violence.[75]

Of course in all eras most people with mental disorders are not in asylums or hospitals. They live in the community with family, friends, alone, or in some type of lodging and this was undoubtedly the case in the first half of the nineteenth century. Biographies of prominent older citizens of that time give an indication of the types of mental health issues that were present.

James Birnie was a sea captain by profession, a merchant and ship owner. He arrived in NSW with his wife Martha in 1809 when he was in his 40s and engaged in local sealing and whaling, as well as carrying merchandise from England to Sydney before going to the fishing grounds. He became an active member of colonial society moving in the company of the Reverend Samuel Marsden and becoming involved with the Missionary Society and NSW Philanthropic Society. He received several land grants from Governor Macquarie. By the mid-1820s, when he was in his mid-60s, his alcohol abuse had become problem and was impacting upon his ability to manage his financial affairs. His wife took him to the Commission of Lunacy to have him declared insane in order to have his estate managed appropriately. In her evidence Martha testified that he was frequently intoxicated for weeks at a time and showed 'such imbecility and wandering of mind' to the extent that he was unable to manage their affairs. She noted that this was the case whether he was drunk or sober – which would suggest from a modern day perspective that he might have developed alcohol-related brain damage.[76, 77] His affairs were placed in the care of a fellow merchant Richard Jones. Despite his history of alcohol abuse, he was recorded in the 1828 census as being resident in the Benevolent Asylum,[78] although he apparently lived out his life with his wife at home until his 1844 death.[79]

Philip Schaeffer, a German widower who had fought on the British side in the American War of Independence, arrived on the Second Fleet on the *Lady Juliana* in June 1790 with his 10-year-old daughter Elizabeth as a civilian superintendent of convicts. They had originally been on board HMS *Guardian* and had survived its sinking in December 1789. Due to his poor English, he did not last long in his role as a superintendent and gave up his appointment in April 1791, taking up a land grant of 140 acres at Parramatta making him one of the first free settlers in the colony. He named his farm 'The Vineyard' and in addition to the 29 acres of maize and wheat he had sown, by October 1791 he had one acre of grape vines. These were the first privately grown vines in Australia as at the time the only other vines were in the Governor's garden at Parramatta. He was said to have been a prolific vine grower and in 1795 he produced 90 gallons of wine.[80,81] In 1797 he sold The Vineyard having taken up another land grant at Field of Mars in 1794. He made little progress with his farming over the next 15 years. He married Margaret Mackinnon in 1811 and despite further land grants at Long Reef and Broken Bay, by 1825 they were petitioning for a further 100 acres due to being 'poor and infirm and upwards of seventy years of age'. Although this petition seems to have been granted, according to Reverend J.D. Lang, Schaeffer sold off the land piecemeal due to 'old age, poverty and intemperance'.[82] Indeed it is alleged that his fondness of alcohol was behind his loss of fortunes.[83] He was later admitted to the Benevolent Asylum where he died before November 1828. His wife Margaret was admitted to the Benevolent Asylum in December 1831.[84]

Irishman Nicholas Divine arrived with the Second Fleet on the *Lady Juliana* in 1790 at about the age of 50 to become the principal superintendent of convicts in Sydney. He was dismissed from his post by Lieutenant Governor Foveaux in 1808 and applied to be reinstated by Governor Macquarie who refused and pensioned him off as he was old, infirm and deaf.[85] He retired to his farm where he grew apples and oranges on two adjoining land grants that he named Burrin after his birthplace. These covered most of the current suburb of Erskineville and almost all of Newtown east of King Street.[86] In 1824 Divine was assaulted and robbed by four ruffians when he was returning from town. He was severely and brutally treated being kicked while on the ground.[87] After the beating he was unable to communicate, dress or feed himself and dribbled incessantly.[88] He gradually lapsed into imbecility.[89] His wife died in 1827 and two months later Divine allegedly conveyed his property to his assigned convict servant Bernard Rochford, who had been transported for administering illegal oaths.[90] Under the agreement Rochford was to gain all of Divine's landed property provided he met all Divine's needs until his death.[91] After Divine died in May 1830, according to newspaper reports at the age of 104 but more likely in his 90s, Rochford sold the property and by 1833 the area was becoming known as New Town. Divine's Irish relatives became aware of the sale, they eventually sent out a representative John Devine who laid a claim to the property in 1846 in part on the grounds that Divine had been of unsound mind. By this time there were thirty owners.[92, 93] The case became known as the Newtown Ejectment Case and was the longest civil court case in Australian history up to that time with proceedings lasting over nine years including an appeal to the Privy Council. Eventually a compromise out of court settlement was reached.[94]

John Macarthur enlisted in the New South Wales Corps in 1789 and travelled with his wife Elizabeth and infant son Edward on the Second Fleet. At Cape Town he developed a near fatal illness involving fevers and lumbago. He was insensible for a long time clinging precariously to life and was expected to die. His recovery was gradual and left him afflicted with bouts of 'flying gout accompanied by nervous depression' for the rest of his life. He was in almost constant pain and dyspepsia which destroyed his taste for wine and food.[95] A somewhat arrogant and haughty man, when in pain Macarthur was prone to poor judgement and temper. His querulous, argumentative, litigious behaviour became a pattern of interaction with Governors and others in administrative positions. Governor King described him as 'this perturbator' and the label stuck.[96] His energy and entrepreneurial spirit in establishing Elizabeth Farm from land and stock grants soon had him as one of the major landholders in the colony. He was the main instigator of developing the wool industry in Australia using Spanish merino sheep and through this achieved great acclaim. He was full of grand plans to develop a great chartered corporation to further the wool industry but found little support from Governor Macquarie. In September 1818, he wrote that his state of depression was 'so much increased that I often pass weeks without one cheerful moment, and I am seldom relieved from this dreadful gloom, except by the return of an acute attack of pain'.[97]

In his fifty-eighth year in 1825 he was one of three unofficial nominated members of the newly-created Legislative Council but his increasingly erratic and temperamental behaviour was eroding his authority. His moods fluctuated from periods of intense gloom and anguish to times when he drove himself to a fury and pounced on new fads and enterprises. As Governor Darling wrote 'In a former letter, I mentioned some of the thousand projects he had to view for the aggrandisement of the Australian Agricultural Company. They *all* seem to have vanished, as the excitement, in which they were engendered, subsided'.[98]

His son John died in 1831 and this precipitated a deterioration in his mental state with his grief spurring frenzied action. He was agitated, not sleeping well and felt very low. At times he had trouble getting out of bed, at other times he was in an over excited state of anxiety setting numerous plans into motion like 'steam engine power' but changing his mind all the time. In mid-1832 he deteriorated further and in his deep fits of melancholia he became morbidly jealous and had delusions that his wife Elizabeth was unfaithful to him, that he was being poisoned, and that his daughters had robbed him.[99] A formal writ of *de lunatic inquirendo* was issued with Dr Wardell giving medical evidence and the Attorney-General being present. The declaration of his lunacy reads: 'John Macarthur ... for these three months last past, (has) been so depressed of his reason and understanding that he is altogether unfit and unable to govern himself or to manage his own affairs.' Officials observed there was 'little hope of restoration'.[100] His feelings of persecution became so violent that he could not bear to see his wife and daughters who sought refuge in Sydney while he remained at his Elizabeth Farm property. They lived the last few years of his life in virtual separation. For a period he recovered and lived quietly to the extent that there were malicious rumours of a family plot against him. He was transferred to his Camden Park estate to avoid these rumours. In March 1834 an episode of violence when he was in recurring pain made it necessary to restrain him and he was moved to a cottage that had been built for him fourteen years earlier where he died at the age of 67 in April 1834.[101] The nature of Macarthur's mood swings would suggest that he had a severe form of bipolar disorder, formerly known as manic-depressive psychosis, that worsened with age. The periods of hectic overactivity and numerous grand projects, a few of which succeeded but many of which disappeared without a trace, interspersed with intense periods of depression is well documented by contemporary observations and his own correspondence.

By the 1830s NSW was a flourishing colonial society with large profits from wool, whaling and land revenue[102], which allowed Governor Bourke to plan infrastructure development that included a new asylum to replace the Liverpool Asylum.[103] The site chosen was Bedlam Point on Parramatta River and here the Tarban Creek Asylum (later to be renamed Gladesville Hospital) was constructed between 1836 and 1838 to the designs of Colonial Architect Mortimer Lewis.[104,105] The Secretary of State for the Colonies appointed Joseph Digby, who had experience in a London asylum, as keeper and his wife was appointed matron.[106] Digby believed in the philosophy of the day that insanity was caused by moral issues in the context of social and psychological stresses. Therapies aimed to keep the patient occupied with purposeful activities such as gardening or domestic work while providing a friendly milieu to enable the patient to talk about their concerns. The medical staff held similar views but believed that it was only with medical control that such outcomes could be achieved.[107]

Tarban Creek Asylum opened in November 1838 with the transfer of female patients from the female factory in Parramatta and then in 1839 with male patients from Liverpool Asylum which then closed.[108] While the precise number of older patients at this time is unknown, it would not have differed much from the around 10 per cent aged 60 years and over recorded at Liverpool Asylum in September 1838. In October 1838, John Blaxland had protested in the Legislative Council about various costs incurred by the colony, one of which was against £3000 allocated to support paupers at Tarban Creek, a cost he felt should be part subsidised by the British government 'who send *aged infirm* convicts to the colony'.[109]

There were still many people of all ages with serious mental illnesses who remained in the community. Francis Oakes was a former chief constable of the colony and former missionary who was said to have 'dishonoured his calling by moral defection'. He had made his mark in the colony by lodging the deposition that led to the prosecution of John Macarthur after the overthrow of Governor Bligh. Oakes had been dismissed from office during the 'Rum Rebellion'. He went to England with Bligh in 1810 as a witness in George Johnston's court martial. Upon return to Australia he became the superintendent of the Female Factory at Parramatta until 1822.[110] A Commission of Lunacy was requested by his wife and two sons in 1840 when he was 70, with supportive evidence from two doctors and two clerics. The Commission found that he had been insane, with lucid intervals, for nine years. He died in 1844.[111]

By 1839 the Benevolent Asylum was also feeling the strain and it was extended with the building of a south wing. In June 1839 there were 281 asylum residents of whom 132 were aged 60 years and over.[112] It was clear that the asylum was increasingly providing permanent domicile for the aged and chronically infirm. An informal agreement was in place with the general hospital regarding the division between acute disorders that were the province of the general hospital and chronic infirmity to the Benevolent Asylum. Thus the Benevolent Asylum had become the nursing home of the colony.

By 1844 Digby was concerned about overcrowding at Tarban Creek and requested that the 'chronic, old and harmless cases' be transferred to another establishment to reduce the risk of accidents occurring through violent and dangerous patients needing to be accommodated in the same cell, although he stressed that there had been no incidents to date. The request was denied.[113] In May 1846, a Select Committee of the NSW Legislative Council was established to examine the administration of the Tarban Creek Asylum after a series of complaints about the lack of coronial inquests into unexpected deaths, possible abuses, and faults in the design and management, in particular related to the perceived lack of medical input to guide the attendants in a consistent approach to patient care. A series of six letters by 'Iatros', widely believed to be Irish doctor, Francis Campbell who was on the Honorary Medical Staff at the Benevolent Asylum, was published in the *Sydney Morning Herald* that were highly critical of the non-medical management at Tarban Creek, citing the 1844 Lunacy Commission report in the UK and the subsequent British legislative reforms of 1845 which emphasised the medical treatment of mental diseases.[114] Although the Select Committee found little evidence of abuses, the lack of a physical restraint case register by Digby and the incomplete case documentation of Dr Thomas Lee was enough to have Digby removed and a medical superintendent installed in his place. James Dunk notes that the Select Committee's interrogation of Dr Lee, a man in his early 60s, had ageist overtones when questions were asked about his fitness to take charge of the asylum; one answer given referred to Dr Lee as being 'a very old man'. According to Dunk, 'his age quickly became shorthand for ineptitude'.[115]

Dr Francis Campbell was appointed as the first Medical Superintendent of Tarban Creek in 1848. In his first report for the year 1848, of the 39 admissions with known ages, four were aged 60 and over.[116] Insight is gained about the way some confused older people were being managed. He defended and described the persistent use of crib rooms, 'they are' he said 'intended only for the aged, infirm, diseased and mindless persons of dirty habits'. Campbell described the types of cases that might be placed in crib rooms with one being 'the mindless and the feeble, without knowing why, would leave their beds, wander around the room and annoy those inclined to rest'. He then described how the crib rooms prevented such behaviour, 'the custom has always been to confine the arm of such patients to the side of their cribs by a short chain and handcuff, leaving them the perfect power of getting out of bed should they understand and wish to maintain habits of cleanliness'. Interestingly, in the same report Campbell claimed to have completely eradicated physical restraints and by this he meant coercion chairs, strait waistcoats, muffs, leglocks, handcuffs, and collars.[117] John Bostock includes Campbell's case notes from Tarban Creek in his book *The Dawn of Australian Psychiatry* and of the four aged cases described, three had longstanding mental disorders and had been admitted before the age of 60. The fourth was a man with a psychotic illness admitted at the age of 65 after stabbing someone and after three years in the asylum remained psychotic and pugnacious.[118]

In March 1848 it was announced that the vacant Female Factory and Barracks at Parramatta, built under Macquarie's leadership and opened in 1821 to house 300 female convicts, would be used as a lunatic asylum with the proclamation occurring in December 1849.[119,120] With the overcrowding at Tarban Creek, some senile patients were transferred to Parramatta, while male convict lunatics had been transferred from Liverpool Hospital in 1848.[121] From the outset Parramatta Lunatic Asylum became an institution for incurable chronic patients many of whom had dementia and were aged and infirm.[122]

The demands on the Benevolent Asylum continued to increase spurred on by population growth through immigration and periods of economic depression such as in 1842–1843.[123,124] To curb demand, restrictions were placed on admissions with alcoholics and those of 'blatant immoral habits' excluded. By 1849 there were nearly 500 residents with 60 confined permanently to sick wards and almost half the residents were classified as sick or infirm. There were eighteen adults described as 'idiots' and whether this is due to intellectual disability or dementia is unknown.[125] Thus by around 1850 the Tarban Creek

Lunatic Asylum, Parramatta Lunatic Asylum and the Sydney Benevolent Asylum were overcrowded and included numerous older people with cognitive and mental disorders.

## Older Aboriginal People

After European settlement, Watkin Tench and David Collins frequently mentioned older Aboriginal people in their journals, particularly in the context of the smallpox outbreak of 1789 that Bennelong estimated had claimed the lives of half the people who lived in the area. The full impact of the smallpox epidemic upon the Aboriginal people in coastal Sydney is not known but the loss of many senior people with their ceremonial knowledge and primary connection with the land meant that survivors had to reconstruct their lives in new bands formed out of old and new family connections.[126]

Throughout this period the Aboriginal population around coastal Sydney struggled to adapt to European civilisation. Over the first 60 years of colonisation there was a massive decline in the number of Aboriginal people in south eastern Australia estimated as being around 95 per cent to approximately 10 to 15 thousand in 1850.[127] In the first half of the nineteenth century the Aboriginal people around coastal Sydney regrouped around acknowledged leaders Bennelong (*c*.1764–1813), Bungaree (1770s–1830), and Cora Gooseberry (1770s–1852), Bungaree's wife. As noted by Paul Irish, because they were born before the arrival of the Europeans, their knowledge of language and cultural practices was regarded as 'authentic', but the life changes brought on by needing to adapt to European civilisation were seen as 'parables about the inevitable demise of Aboriginal culture'.[128] There was a preoccupation on the effects of alcohol on their lives rather than their leadership in their community. Alcohol misuse may well have been an issue for them in their old age, Bungaree was regarded as a 'hard drinker' and Cora Gooseberry, also known as the 'Queen of Sydney and Botany', regularly frequented Edward Borton's Cricketer's Arms hotel near Sydney Markets, despite the prohibition of the sale of alcohol to Aboriginal people that was imposed by the 1838 Licensed Publicans Act.[129] There has been considerable debate about the causes of alcohol misuse in Indigenous peoples globally with the notion of 'loss of culture' leading to anomie (or normlessness) and acculturative stress, with alcohol consumption being a way of coping with psychological stress including that related to their traumatic life experiences, long being the 'accepted wisdom'. Yet modern research also notes that the cultures of Indigenous peoples do not exist in a vacuum and change in response to the broader social, political and economic environment, sharing characteristics with both traditional and colonising societies.[130] In this context in the 1820s and 1830s alcohol misuse was a major problem across all classes in Sydney and it was essentially the sight of drunken noisy and quarrelsome Aboriginal people on Sydney streets that upset the sensibilities of Sydney society and resulted in prohibition.[131]

# Chapter 3

# Population Ageing and Growth of the Asylums: 1851-1900

The second half of the nineteenth century, particularly after the 1860s, witnessed a rapid increase in the number of older people in Australia but this varied between the colonies and within the colonies. Between 1870 and 1891, due to its ageing ex-convicts, Tasmania had by far the highest proportion of people aged 60 years and over in Australia peaking at 8 per cent in 1881. Similarly, the ageing of convicts in Western Australia (WA) led to it having the second highest proportion of older people in 1881 at 5.2 per cent, but by 1901 WA had the lowest proportion of older people in the federation as the convict generation had died and the Kalgoorlie gold rush in the 1890s had attracted a young male population. Victoria had the highest proportion of older people in the 1890s due to the ageing of the gold rush immigrants from the 1850s and 60s, reaching 7.9 per cent in 1901.[1]

International comparisons show how much change occurred. In 1861, Australia had two per cent of the population aged 60 years and over and England had 7.7 per cent, but by 1901, Australia had increased to 6.2 per cent aged 60 years and over, while England had declined to 7.4 per cent.[2] Ireland had a similar increase in the proportion of older people in the population in this period as a consequence of the Great Famine of 1845–1849 with many younger people emigrating leaving behind the older generation. Those aged 60 years and over increased from 6.3 per cent in 1841 to 11 per cent in 1901.[3]

This relatively rapid population ageing, when combined with the economic depression and prolonged drought of the 1890s and early twentieth century, led to Australia's first crisis in aged care. Victoria, which by this time had the largest aged population in Australia, also experienced the worst impact of the depression, with many losing their life savings when building societies and banks crashed in 1892–93.[4] Australia was an immigrant country and this meant that ageing immigrants, many of whom had migrated to Australia during the Victorian gold rush of the 1850s and 60s, had limited family support networks. Pat Jalland commented that these economic and demographic changes 'left an ageing immigrant workforce without property or skills'.[5] Many ageing men were unmarried in part due to the sex imbalance in the colonies. Those who had labouring occupations such as mining, often had a premature end to their careers as their health was affected by the working conditions. This left many alone in early old age without adequate finances and circumstances often accentuated by alcohol misuse in the masculine pub culture.[6] Even before the 1890s, concerns were being expressed about the number of older admissions to lunatic asylums and the appropriateness of disabled older people with senile dementia being in a lunatic asylum. For example, in his 1881 Annual Report to the Victorian Parliament of the Inspector of Lunatic Asylums, Dr Edward Paley stated that those admitted to Yarra Bend with 'impairment of mind consequent of old age' would be more suitably housed in a benevolent home and that they were a burden on the lunatic asylums.[7] Yet the alternative institutions around the colonies, the benevolent asylums and invalid depots, were not particularly suitable either once the older person posed significant challenges in their ability to care for themselves or with behaviour such as wandering, self-harm and aggression.

The number of Australians in the nineteenth century who might have had dementia is unknown. Anthea Vreugdenhil made rough estimates of dementia prevalence in Tasmania, but these were not adjusted to the age profile of the era.[8] In a paper published in *Health and History*, I made more accurate estimates of dementia prevalence in each colony in the second half of the nineteenth century utilising the censuses of the Australian colonies between 1861 and 1901 that provide data on the ageing population in age bands. Dementia prevalence rates used by the Australian Institute of Health and Welfare in the 2012 edition of *Dementia in Australia* were applied to the census data.[9] These dementia prevalence rates are in five-year age bands and calculated for each sex. This allows for a more accurate estimate as dementia prevalence doubles approximately every five years over the age of 60 and dementia prevalence is higher in females than males in old age (See Figure 1, page 296).[10]

It is unclear how accurate these dementia estimates are. In many developed countries dementia incidence has declined over the last thirty years despite ageing populations, with the most likely explanation being improved health, education and lifestyle, although dementia prevalence has not changed due to longer survival with dementia.[11] Prevalence rates used for those under the age of 60 could be an underestimate based on a recent global estimate of the prevalence of young onset dementia, which in particular demonstrated that the prevalence is higher in developing countries with health, educational and life expectancy profiles more like those present in the nineteenth century Australian colonies.[12] In the nineteenth century, when the Australian population health was undoubtedly worse in old age than it is now and education was much less, these prevalence estimates have two opposing factors acting on them; poor population health and education that might increase dementia incidence but counterbalanced by shorter survival time with dementia that reduces the prevalence. Other influences include the impact of prolonged alcohol abuse. where dementia risk is increased particularly in those who have poor nourishment, and GPI would both increase dementia numbers in younger men.[13,14] These censuses also do not include Aboriginal people although their numbers had declined dramatically by mid-century and few would have been aged.[15] In 1889, Frederic Norton Manning in his examination of insanity in Aboriginal people cited the Reverend George Taphill 'it is not uncommon for the intellect of old men to give way, and for them to be insane', thus it was likely that there were some Aboriginal people with dementia.[16] Others have argued that Alzheimer's disease was relatively rare in developed countries in the nineteenth century with an estimated prevalence of around one per cent and that environmental factors might have led to the epidemic of Alzheimer cases in the twentieth century.[17] However, the overall pattern of an age-related increase in dementia prevalence and how it varied across the colonies over the second half of the nineteenth century is not likely to differ.

The estimated number of people with dementia in Australia increased from approximately eight hundred (prevalence 3.3 per cent aged 60 years and over) in 1861 to approximately nine thousand (prevalence 3.9 per cent aged 60 years and over) in 1901, an increase of around eleven-fold. The increase in dementia prevalence was due to the ageing of the 60 years and over population. In 1861, it was the 60–64 year age group that had the highest number of dementia cases in the colonies, but by 1891 the increasing numbers surviving until their seventies resulted in the highest number being in the 70–74 year age group. Tasmania with its older population profile was the exception with the highest number of dementia cases being in the 80 years and over age group by 1881. At this age dementia prevalence in males is 11.5 per cent.[18] Over two-thirds of the estimated dementia cases resided in NSW and Victoria but the impact of dementia varied across the colonies. When the estimated number of people with dementia is related to the total population in each colony, Tasmania was the most severely impacted colony due to a combination of an ageing convict population and emigration of younger people to the mainland, particularly in the period up until the 1890s after which Victoria and South Australia caught up (See Figure 2, page 297).[19] The high proportion of estimated dementia cases in Western Australia in 1881 was due to the ageing of its convicts, with the steep decline in the 1890s due to the influx of younger people for the gold rush. In each colony, the majority of dementia cases was male, a feature that did not change until the early twentieth century, which was a major factor in older asylum admissions being predominantly male.

As economic recovery occurred in the late 1890s, the number of aged poor grew, in part due to the new jobs being more likely to be offered to younger more active men. Many became homeless leading to a more than doubling of older people being admitted to government homes and benevolent asylums across the country in the 1890s.[20] There had been a series of scandals about the ill-treatment of the aged and infirm in government and benevolent asylums in the 1880s and so this was not regarded as a good solution for that reason alone. It was in this broad context that inquiries into old age pensions were held in NSW, Victoria and South Australia in the late 1890s. It was the 1896 Select Committee of the NSW Legislative Assembly that had the greatest long-term impact as its report, along with the New Zealand *1898 Old Age Pensions Act*, influenced the Commonwealth inquiries of the next decade and the ultimate establishment of the Commonwealth old age pensions in 1908 which replaced state pensions. The NSW Select Committee report recommended that pensions for those who had lived in NSW for at least 15 years (which became 25 years in the eventual Act) should be given as a free gift without distinction between the deserving or the less deserving. It became the basis of the NSW *Old Age Pensions Act, 1900* that came into force in 1901. It was means tested, excluded Australian Aborigines, aliens and 'Asiatics', and although it had an exclusion of 'unsatisfactory moral character' requiring evidence of 'sober and respectable life' for at least five years, it was more progressive than the Act in Victoria.[21,22]

This NSW approach was in contrast to the reports from the Victorian and South Australian Royal Commissions in 1898. The Victorian Royal Commission distinguished entitlements based on whether the person was 'deserving' or not, while the South Australian Royal Commission focused on a very limited scheme in part due to the lack of resources in that colony. The more restrictive Victorian pension scheme was enacted in 1899 and until replaced by Commonwealth pensions, there was a marked difference in old age pension eligibility between NSW (39 per cent) and Victoria (16 per cent).[23]

During the second half of the nineteenth century each colony developed lunatic asylums and benevolent asylums or invalid depots for the 'destitute', which in the last two decades of the century increasingly meant for the aged and infirm. The growth of lunatic asylums in this period is quite startling. In 1850 there were four lunatic asylums in the Australian colonies with around 460 patients; by 1900 there were 19 lunatic asylums with over 12,000 patients and yet still most colonies reported overcrowding in their asylums.[24] At a time when the overall Australian population had increased by around fourfold, the population in lunatic asylums increased by around 25-fold. While there were numerous factors that undoubtedly contributed to this increase, one of them was the rapidly ageing population and limited social supports available for ageing 'mentally feeble' older people. Yet, despite this population ageing, no colony organised their lunatic asylums on the basis of age. Classification was largely based on degree of behavioural disturbance, state of physical health, and by whether it was believed that a cure could be achieved, with the majority of older patients being regarded as unlikely to improve and often classified as quiet chronic cases.

Growth of asylums was an international phenomenon and in this context there were concerns in the British Colonial Office that were triggered by an inspection of the lunatic asylum in Kingston, Jamaica in 1859 which found evidence of abuses and poor conditions. In 1863, the Duke of Newcastle,

Secretary of State for the Colonies, requested information from the 43 colonies administered by the Colonial Office about their public hospitals and asylums. The issues covered included whether there were asylum provision, regulatory framework, monitoring and inspection, medical influence, staffing level, and use of restraints. Around two-thirds of colonies in the British Empire responded and the findings were distributed confidentially to the colonies in 1864.[25] The extent to which this interrogation led to changes in the administration of lunatic asylums in the Australian colonies is unclear but only three Australian colonies responded (Tasmania, Victoria and Western Australia).[26]

Beyond providing institutional care for people with mental disorders, there were few treatments available in the nineteenth-century lunatic asylums that altered the course of mental disorder. The treatments used in Australian lunatic asylums were generally the same used to treat the insane in asylums in other parts of the western world but were largely derivative from those used in Britain.[27] Moral treatment principles guided the approach to care in the asylums, but often the overcrowded, and in some of the colonies substandard accommodation, prevented their application. While physical restraints were not regarded as desirable or therapeutic, as the asylums grew restraints were used more frequently. Mechanical restraints included camisoles, straitjackets, muffs, gloves, ankle straps, the restraining chair where the patient was tied to the chair with bedsheets, and 'utica-cribs' where the bed was in the form of a closed in cage. Chemical restraints essentially used the sedative properties of drugs such as opiates, chloral hydrate, mercury, digitalis, bromides and hyoscyamine, to temporarily allay excitement in excited and restless patients. Continuous use was regarded as harmful.[28,29] David Roth examined the use of chemical restraints at Callan Park Hospital between 1877 and 1923, noting that for the period 1877–1900 medications were routinely recorded in the medical casebooks but thereafter the records became much less reliable. Opiates were used in around 30 per cent of the patients in his study and overall 50 per cent of patients were chemically restrained at some point during their admission.[30] This mirrors the twenty-first-century situation where modern tranquillisers such as the antipsychotic drugs have a role in short-term treatment of agitation, aggression or psychosis in people with dementia, but continuous use has little benefit and might cause harm.[31] Seclusion rooms were also frequently used but how often they were used without mechanical restraints and locked doors, which was felt to be the optimal type of use, is not clear. Cold baths and showers were used to quell restless and disturbed patients.[32] A rudimentary form of electrical treatment was used at New Norfolk Asylum from the 1850s to the 1870s, not to produce a convulsion as in modern day electroconvulsive therapy (ECT), but to shock the patient. It is not clear as to the extent to which it was regarded as a punishment rather than a treatment.[33] Some longstanding treatments such as purgatives, emetics, laxatives and bloodletting were used to evacuate noxious 'humours' from the body were still commonly in practice despite lack of evidence for benefit.[34] None of these treatments had efficacy in reducing symptoms of psychosis, mood or cognitive disorder, they merely exerted some level of behavioural control. There did not appear to be any age-related selectivity in their use.

Ageism remained an issue in this period as these examples of journalism testify. Concerns about the eccentric behaviour on and off the bench of 77-year-old District Court Judge Forbes led to the *Queanbeyan Observer* in July 1896 describing him as 'poor, silly, worn out and senile' for denouncing the public schools of the colony as 'breeding grounds of idleness, crime and immorality'.[35] And then in 1898 the *Clarence and Richmond Examiner* in its obituary for the politician the Honourable George Alfred Lloyd, who died at the age of 82, described him as having 'outlived his usefulness by considerably more than a decade. How many people like him in this respect there have been!'[36] At the turn of the century the prevailing medical and literary views in Australia emphasised the physical decline associated with ageing and it is unclear how this shaped public opinion.[37]

Older Aboriginal people are not specifically mentioned in reports from the lunatic asylums in the late nineteenth century but in 1889 Frederic Norton Manning, the Inspector General of Asylums in NSW, presented a paper at the Intercolonial Medical Congress of Australasia about 32 cases of insanity in Aboriginal people encountered in the asylums in NSW and Queensland, the first report on the mental health of Aboriginal people in the medical literature.[38] In his introduction Manning cites the work of Edward Curr and states that 'from the accounts published by explorers and early colonists, insanity was a very rare affliction among the Australian Aborigines whilst in their primitive and uncivilised condition'. He describes the ways that he understood Aboriginal people had dealt with various types of mental maladies including 'if demented and helpless he was left to die'.[39] Manning then goes on to say that as European contact increased and the Aboriginal people 'became acquainted with the vices and the cares of civilisation, we find more frequent notices of mental disease'.[40] James Dawson's *Australian Aborigines* published in 1881 about the language and customs of several tribes of Aboriginal people in the Western District of Victoria is cited with reference to suicide being uncommon but that it had increased since alcohol had been used and since the laws of consanguinity in marriage had been disregarded. Manning claimed that the rates of insanity amongst Aboriginal people was increasing and in NSW had passed from a level at which it was almost unknown to being in 1889 almost double that of the European population.[41]

Manning then described the 32 cases (18 from NSW, 14 from Queensland) but no ages are given. Probably his most important observation was about the perceived causation, 'the chief share was due to civilisation and its accompanying vices'. Alcohol was regarded as the main culprit resulting in presentations to the asylums with features of mania that passed very quickly into dementia with poor self-care and incontinence – 'indescribably dirty habits'.[42]

Two prominent Aboriginal persons lived to old age in the second half of the nineteenth century and each demonstrated the impact of European influence on their lives. The first, William Warrell (also known as Warrah Warrah) was a cousin of Cora Gooseberry, the widow of Bungaree who was one of the key Aboriginal leaders in Macquarie's time through until his death in 1830. Warrell was born in the 1790s started to frequent Sydney in the 1840s. In the 1840s and 1850s, despite prohibition of alcohol sales to Aboriginal people, Warrell would regularly attend Edward Borton's Cricketer's Arms hotel with Cora and his drinking habits became well known. His image was used by famed local silversmith Julius Hogarth in the 1850s as the model for a series of statuettes and he was regarded as the last of the tribal celebrities. As he aged he developed a condition that affected his legs and caused severe lameness. He was a cripple and was mockingly given the nickname 'Ricketty Dick'.[43] According to Grace Karskens, as his immobility increased, his once good nature became 'irritable' and a 'terror to children'. Eventually when he could no longer walk he set up camp on South Head Road at Rose Bay where passers-by threw sixpences into his gunyah. William Charles Wentworth paid for food to be provided for him.[44]

When his condition deteriorated, Warrell was offered accommodation at the Benevolent Asylum, but having stayed there briefly in the 1840s, he declined. Warrell died in 1863 aged in his mid to late 60s.[45]

The second is Truganini who was born on Bruny Island in Tasmania and raised in her own clan. The decimation of the Tasmanian Aboriginal clans in the 1820s and 1830s, during wars precipitated by European colonisation, resulted in an attempt to resettle the few remaining Tasmanian Aborigines on Flinders Island in the 1840s. Wooredy, Truganini's husband, died in his mid-fifties en route to Flinders Island in 1842 and it was noted in contemporary reports that he had rapidly become 'imbecile' in his last year of life. Cassandra Pybus speculates that this might have represented the last stage of neurosyphilis (GPI), syphilis being prevalent in the Aboriginal population at the time. This settlement on Flinders Island failed with many of those resettled dying. In 1847 the forty-six remaining Aboriginal people were transferred from Wybalenna on Flinders island to an old convict station at Oyster Cove located on the Tasmanian east coast south of Hobart and across the D'Entrecasteaux Channel from North Bruny Island.

At Oyster Cove through the 1850s to the early 1870s this last remnant of the Tasmanian clans in Tasmania dwindled and ended with the death of Truganini in 1876 at the age of about 64. It was a microcosm of the ill-effects that repeated trauma, dispossession and destruction of traditional lifestyles has had on Aboriginal people across the country. From an early stage disreputable men built huts on the nearby Crown land and traded alcohol for sex. In 1855 the colonial surveyor James Calder examined the Oyster Cove station and was given distressing accounts by local publicans about the states of intoxication of the women and scenes of immorality with white men in the open.

Truganini had endured a lifetime of repeated traumas including parental death, sexual abuse, violence, partner deaths, loss of her land and lifestyle from childhood, disappointments from repeated broken promises by the Aboriginal Protector George Augustus Robinson, and witnessing the near extermination of her people. Her resilience was remarkable. Truganini's closest friend, Dray, a woman in her mid-70s and from Truganini's clan, died in 1861 and this was a loss that she found hard to endure. In 1863, Truganini who was aged in her early 50s, was one of seven people kept in a police lockup overnight for being senseless drunk. And then towards the end of life she realised that when she died various learned Societies such as the Royal Society of Tasmania would try to claim her body 'for science' as had been happening after the deaths of her last few compatriots. She made her views clear that this was not to happen to her and indicated to Reverend Atkinson while on a boat in the D'Entrecasteaux Channel that this was where she wanted to be buried. The thought of this one last insult was very upsetting to her. Efforts were made to respect her wishes and she was buried 'in secret' but after two years the Royal Society requested disinterment. For years her skeleton was on public display in the Tasmanian Museum until 1947 even though this ignored the explicit conditions of disinterment. Eventually her remains were cremated in 1976 after a lengthy legal battle by the Tasmanian Aboriginal Centre and her ashes scattered in the D'Entrecasteaux Channel which fulfilled the promise made to her by Reverend Atkinson.[46]

# Chapter 4

# New South Wales 1851–1900

Francis Campbell continued as Superintendent at Tarban Creek Asylum until 1867, while Dr Patrick Hill, the former medical officer for Liverpool Lunatic Asylum, was Superintendent of Parramatta Lunatic Asylum until his death in 1852.[1] Hill's replacement, Dr Richard Greenup had a reputation of being kind and concerned about patient welfare, yet was in favour of using a variety of mechanical restraints for violent or self-injurious behaviour. He held the post until his death at the hands of one of the patients in the asylum in 1866.[2]

Overcrowding and staff shortages plagued the asylums through most of the 1850s and 60s as would-be prospectors headed for the goldfields and abandoned jobs in the city. This was accentuated by the low wages and poor conditions of employment of the attendants. At Parramatta Lunatic Asylum convicts and recovering patients were being employed as attendants and lacked the qualities necessary for the job. Although wages improved, complaints of poor pay persisted.[3] During the 1850s the Parramatta Lunatic Asylum operated as a mix of benevolent asylum and lunatic asylum as it would accept the admission of destitute patients suffering other forms of chronic disease. It assisted with overcrowding at Tarban Creek, particularly female patients, but would also accept admissions from Sydney and Liverpool Benevolent Asylums. It became a repository for the harmless patients with dementia which in this era included younger patients with secondary dementia due to chronic psychoses as well as older people with senile dementia. By 1855 there were 279 patients in the Parramatta asylum.[4]

With the continued overcrowding at Tarban Creek, work began to enlarge the asylum but progress was slow. While Campbell was on leave of absence in

1854, his replacement Dr George Walker wrote to Henry Parkes in the Legislative Council with concerns about delays in transferring patients from gaol to asylum and, while incarcerated in gaol, being subject to cruelty and abuse with injuries apparent on arrival at the asylum. A Select Committee Commission of Inquiry was held in 1855 with similar terms of reference to the 1846 inquiry. The report was very critical of the facilities at Tarban Creek but not the care.[5] Another Select Committee of Inquiry was held in 1863–64 after the social reforming Catholic Bishop Robert Willson from Hobart visited Tarban Creek and Parramatta asylums and wrote to the Colonial Secretary with scathing criticism of the conditions in both asylums. The Inquiry largely came up with similar findings to the previous inquiries, notably that overcrowding, poor facility design and location each contributed to the lack of proper patient classification though the care and treatment of patients was regarded as adequate. The Inquiry heard that difficulties in staff recruitment meant that there was only one attendant for every twenty patients which contrasted to the ratio of one to ten adopted in England.[6]

In this period an explorer from the early part of the century, Gregory Blaxland, died by suicide in 1852 at the age of 74. A free settler who arrived with his family in 1805, Blaxland had concerns that his coastal landholdings were inadequate to sustain his livestock, and in May 1813 set out with William Charles Wentworth and William Lawson to cross the Blue Mountains. They achieved success by following the mountain ridges instead of the valleys to Mount York and then subsequently past Cox's River to a hill they named Mount Blaxland from which they could see the pastures that they were seeking. He retired from public life in the late 1820s after being found by Governor Darling to have acquired land by deception.[7] He endured a series of losses with the death of his wife in 1826, two sons and others close to him and was reported to be heavy at heart.[8] In the last six months of his life he suffered pains in the head and general debility for which he was being treated by his physician. For the three days before his death he had requested that a neighbour sleep in the adjoining room as he was feeling light-headed. He felt most afflicted in the hot weather at which times he became a little 'delirious'. On New Year's Eve 1852 it was a particularly hot day and he had commented at breakfast that he felt not so well because it was hot. At eleven in the morning he was found hanging.[9] Chronic pain is a well-established precipitant for suicide but in addition to that Blaxland seemed to be having difficulties in coping with his overall life situation.

Francis Campbell retired at the age of 70 in 1867 and Frederic Norton Manning was appointed as Campbell's successor in 1868. He was selected by NSW Premier Henry Parkes with whom he developed a close friendship. He was immediately sent abroad to examine asylums, their management and staffing to inform the government about what was required to reorganise asylums in NSW.[10] His comprehensive report included recommendations to abandon the Parramatta asylum; that Tarban Creek should either be altered to bring it into harmony with institutions in England or abandoned; that new small asylums be built in three country towns; that a new large 500-bed asylum be built in Sydney; and that an Inspector for the Insane with legal and executive powers over asylums be appointed.[11] A key theme was that the asylums should be regarded as hospitals where treatments were applied with care and skill rather than as prisons. He recommended that the Tarban Creek Asylum be renamed as 'The Hospital for the Insane, Gladesville' in order to impress on patients that they were there for treatment and cure.[12]

The Lunatic Reception House was opened at Darlinghurst in July 1868. This served a number of purposes with one of the most important being that it was where dangerous patients could be sent by justices as an alternative to gaol while awaiting transfer to a lunatic asylum. This of course addressed the concerns that George Walker had in 1854.[13] In modern parlance, the reception house served as a psychiatric emergency centre allowing some patients who did not require admission to a lunatic asylum to be discharged after observation. By the 1880s, around two-thirds of reception house admissions were discharged as recovered within a few days, largely because many had alcohol-related presentations including delirium tremens.[14]

When Manning took over the superintendency of Gladesville Hospital in October 1868 he found the conditions to be appalling and in need of reform. Accommodation was provided for 300 patients yet 650 were being treated; some were sleeping in corridors, others in dining rooms. There was a lack of space for recreational activities. Ventilation was poor, the windows were set so high in the walls that patients could not look out at the views, and the artificial lighting was very primitive. Washing facilities were old fashioned and needed repair, while every patient was bathed weekly with three patients using the same water. Shower baths were used as punishments. Toilets stank as did the rat infested dirty store rooms. The kitchens were poorly equipped, the unpalatable food being served on circular tins. Clearly the staffs' lack of awareness of basic principles of hygiene was an issue in these squalid conditions.[15]

Manning held the position of medical superintendent of Gladesville Hospital until his promotion to Inspector-General of the Insane in September 1879. Over the decade Manning submitted annual reports to government with the common theme being the overcrowding of the facility. He also documented the improved recreational activities and conditions that he championed for the patients. His report for 1877, published in the *Sydney Morning Herald*, was the first to mention older admissions where he simply comments that twenty-four were aged 60 years and over.[16]

New wards were built and various facilities were used as temporary asylums but always as a reaction to these reports rather than in anticipation of future needs. One such facility was Tucker's private 'Licensed House for Lunatics' at Cook's River, Tempe, which had few private patients and was largely operating as a government-funded annex of Gladesville Hospital.[17] According to Manning's Annual Report for 1876 there were 125 quieter female patients with chronic disorders residing there.[18] The new city asylum recommended by Manning in his 1868 report had its beginnings with the purchase of the Callan Park Estate in 1873. The mansion was fitted and furnished in 1876 for quiet convalescent patients and managed as a ward of Gladesville Hospital.[19] Although Callan Park Hospital for the Insane opened as a separate hospital in 1878 with the transfer of 44 patients, of whom eleven were aged 60 years and over, it was not completed until 1887.[20,21]

Meanwhile, Parramatta Asylum continued with little change, the main building still being the old Female Factory from the Macquarie era. An 1877 report by 'A Pilgrim' in the *Freeman's Journal* described it as 'an odd remnant of Dante's Inferno'. The sick room was described as a 'happy compromise between a stable and a dog kennel, and possesses the odours of the two combined'. The conditions under which these patients with chronic mental disorders including older people with dementia were living did not provide much encouragement for improvement.[22] In 1879 Manning was asked by the Colonial Secretary to inspect the asylum and he was saddened by what he found and felt that those who were expected to live in such accommodation should be 'profoundly pitied'. For Manning, the rebuilding of Parramatta Asylum was a priority and in June 1885 a new building was completed,[23] but Manning was concerned that the 'sick ward', the last remaining section of the old Female Factory, was in poor condition and needed to be pulled down. The Official Visitors had commented that 'the sick appear to be the last to have proper accommodation made for them'.[24]

The *Lunacy Act of 1878*, into which Manning had much input, established a more centralised administration of mental health services in NSW with the creation of the office of the Inspector General of the Insane that had oversight over all public and private mental health facilities, uniformity in their procedures including admission and discharge processes, use of restraints and other patient safeguards including Official Visitors.[25] The Act also combined the notion that the lunatic not only needed to be prevented from being a danger to others, but also needed protection from being a danger to themselves.[26] After the introduction of the 1878 Act, transfers from the Benevolent Asylums noticeably decreased.

Annual reports became a statutory obligation for the Inspector General of the Insane to cover the state of mental health services in NSW and were continued in an evolving format until 1971, with the reports from 1881 onwards retained in the State Library of NSW. Data on admissions, discharges, and deaths were provided by age group and allow for analyses of the older cohort. In Manning's first report in 1879, as partially published in the *Sydney Morning Herald*, he provided information about the 1878 calendar year and he notes that there had been 33 (6.1%) admissions, readmissions and transfers of patients aged 60 years and over and comments that the number of aged patients was increasing, a situation that was also occurring in Victoria. Patients aged 60 years and over under care during the year numbered 281. Manning recommended that 'demented and epileptic' patients be housed at Newcastle Hospital with the 'idiot children' being relocated, but this did not occur.[27]

In his 1882 report, Manning demonstrated that he understood the importance of relating the number of mental health admissions to the size of the general population by age group. Presumably drawing on the 1881 NSW Census, he calculated the proportion of insane admissions per one thousand people in the population. For males the rates peaked at 10.96 per thousand in those aged 70 to 80 years. For women, the rates peaked at 11.64 per thousand in those aged 60 to 70 years.[28] Here there was clear evidence that older people had higher rates of admission than other age groups.

Over the last 20 years of the nineteenth century, the proportion of admissions age 60 years and over steadily increased from 8.2 per cent to 9.9 per cent. Old age and chronic physical health issues were increasingly seen as the 'apparent or assigned' causes of insanity. The number of cases with a diagnosis of senile mania, senile melancholia or senile dementia steadily increased. With dementia diagnoses, the most notable changes were the increase in senile dementia cases and reduction of primary dementia cases, a diagnosis previously used more frequently in younger people with chronic psychoses. There was also an increase in GPI (dementia paralytica) but few cases occurred in those over the age of 60.

Throughout the 1880s Manning repeatedly drew attention to aged admissions with dementia and physical disabilities, being of the view that they would be more appropriately housed in a different type of institution. In 1883 he again recommended that Newcastle Hospital might be set aside for 'aged, demented and quiet epileptic patients' as there were now 400 such patients. He commented that:

> 'they are harmless, require comparatively little care and attention, and as far as their mental condition is concerned are absolutely beyond cure or alleviation. In Great Britain cases of this kind are maintained in Poor-houses or in separate Institutions in which the attendants are fewer in number, the medical supervision less constant, and the dietary less liberal than in Institutions for acute cases of insanity … with the result that there is a very considerable saving in the expense of maintenance.'[29]

He also mentioned that the new Sunbury Hospital in Melbourne was an asylum of this type and the maintenance rate was two-thirds of the Kew and Yarra Bend asylums. By 1892 Manning had softened his comments somewhat and recognised that brief admissions had a role even if long-term care was not appropriate:

> 'In no case was it possible to say that the patient was not insane and a fit subject for hospital treatment; but in a few, after a short period

of rest, treatment, and careful feeding, it was possible to send on the patients to one of the Asylums for the Infirm and Destitute, the mental condition being that of dementia from old age or other cause temporarily aggravated by penury or exposure.'[30]

While Manning's comments might seem discriminatory and failing to recognise the challenges of geriatric nursing, many of these patients were in mid-life and able bodied. There were many incontinent patients, for example in 1887 out of 715 patients at Gladesville Hospital 43 patients had urinary incontinence and 21 faecal incontinence at night, and yet the comment was that 'the number of old & helpless cases has diminished, number of wet and dirty cases decreased'.[31] These were not just age or dementia-related. In 1893 at Rydalmere it was estimated that about half of the cases of urinary incontinence were due to epilepsy.[32]

Manning's reference to having an institution more like a poorhouse than a hospital is the nineteenth-century equivalent of recognising that, in general, people with dementia do not require daily medical care in a hospital and that a poorhouse is a less medicalised option. It took another eighty years before the nursing homes in the 1960s became the main locus of long-term residential dementia care in Australia. Manning understood the social context of many of the admissions. In 1884 he noted that pastoral and commercial depression in the colony was the precipitant for many admissions and that 'in more prosperous times people are able and willing to keep their imbecile and demented relatives at home'. He also commented on how it was easier for people with mental disabilities to gain employment in more prosperous times, and thus presumably be able to fend for themselves.[33]

Those with dementia who had the resources could remain at home. Hamilton Hume was an explorer best known for his return journey to Port Phillip with Captain William Hovell in 1824–25. Their party passed many important locations in southern NSW and Victoria not previously seen by Europeans including the Murray River and its tributaries and agricultural and grazing lands between Gunning and Corio Bay. The Hume Highway, Hume Dam and Lake Hume are named after him. In 1853, in his mid-50s Hume quarrelled with Hovell when he felt that Hovell, at a function in Geelong, had downplayed his role in the expedition. Printed pamphlets were exchanged and their friendship ended. In his 60s Hume's health started to decline and in 1865, when aged 68, he then quarrelled with his nephew with whom he had been close, and they parted their ways. His health deteriorated rapidly, he was almost totally deaf, his memory was failing and he became totally obsessed with the idea that his role in the 1824 expedition had not been restored with the general public. He died in 1873 at the age of 76. Hume's increasing obsession with his legacy as an explorer, which was built on a grudge, was likely fuelled by his cognitive decline in late life.[34]

The medical casebooks of patients admitted to NSW Hospitals for the Insane in the nineteenth and early twentieth centuries are retained at the NSW State Archives. In order to better understand the types of disorders, behaviours, and symptoms that were present in older admissions in this period, I examined the medical casebooks of 226 patients admitted to Gladesville or Callan Park Hospitals aged 60 years and over between late 1849 and 1905 and published it in the *History of Psychiatry*. The quality of the admission notes from Gladesville Asylum was poor in the 1850s and 1860s. There was a tendency to state a conclusion about the mental condition of the patient with little description of the history, symptoms or behaviour to justify it, while in 22 per cent of cases no diagnosis was provided. The quality of the medical casebook notes improved in the 1870s and this was maintained. Mania in one of its forms (including mania, delusional mania, or senile mania) was the most common diagnosis (36.7%), followed by dementia (including senile and organic) (31.9%) and melancholia (including senile, delusional, a potu) (17.7%). Other diagnoses were made in five per cent, three cases were judged to be 'not insane' (1.3%), while no diagnosis was made in 17 cases (7.5%). Alcohol misuse was identified as being an issue in 18.5 per cent of male admissions. Over 35 per cent of admissions displayed verbal and/or physically aggressive behaviour, while suicidal behaviour was present in 24 per cent, and 20 per cent feared that they might be harmed, usually due to delusional beliefs. GPI was identified as a possible issue in three cases. It is possible that some older cases of GPI were being misdiagnosed as a form of dementia but it seems unlikely to have been in large numbers.[35]

One aim of the study was to determine the relationship between these nineteenth and early twentieth-century diagnoses with modern psychiatric diagnoses. Melancholia diagnoses had the highest concordance with 82.5 per cent of melancholia cases being assigned the possible or probable modern diagnosis of major depression. In particular, a diagnosis of delusional melancholia was closely related to the current diagnosis of major depression with psychosis. Dementia diagnoses were next with 65.2 per cent assigned the possible or probable modern diagnosis of dementia. Symptoms of psychosis were present in over 40 per cent of dementia cases. The least robust were mania diagnoses which were concordant with different modern diagnoses depending on the subtype. Those diagnosed with acute, chronic or recurrent mania had 54.2 per cent concordance the possible or probable modern diagnosis of mania, while senile mania had 39.4 per cent concordance the possible or probable modern diagnosis of dementia, and delusional mania had 42.3 per cent concordance the possible or probable modern diagnosis of schizophrenia. Many other diagnoses were represented in small numbers.[36]

Over the study period, no case was diagnosed with delirium even though this was a well-established diagnosis of the time. The importance of identifying delirium is that it represents the mental manifestation of an underlying physical disorder requiring treatment, which would usually be best in a general hospital rather than a hospital for the insane. From a twenty-first-century perspective, there were at least thirteen possible delirium diagnoses, some in association with dementia, some dying within a week or two of admission with autopsies revealing lung infections, severe cardiac disorders, and strokes. One example involved a man in his early 60s who was incoherent, agitated, complaining of pain in the lower ribs which persisted and radiated to his scapula over the next week as symptoms of a lung infection became apparent with laboured respiration before he died. The post-mortem showed both lungs to be severely inflamed and congested. There was no mention in the recorded history of how long he had been unwell.[37] One of the key factors that alerts twenty-first-century clinicians that confusion and other cognitive changes in an older person might be due to delirium rather than dementia is the short course of illness of days to weeks found in delirium as compared with dementia which has a course of months to years. In no case was the symptom course identified as being an issue of importance by the admitting doctor. Senile dementia was diagnosed even when the history of mental state change was only a matter of weeks. What is unclear from these cases is whether the treatments available in a nineteenth-century general hospital would have made any difference to the outcomes.

The medical casebooks provide indications of the challenges that these older people and their families were facing. Severe behavioural change in which the older person endangered the lives of others or themselves was a common issue precipitating admission. In many cases the behaviour change had been present for months, for example, one man in his mid-70s had:

> 'been getting childish for seven years; for the last four months has had attacks of excitement and violence. He fancies that larrikins were constantly annoying him, threatened to commit suicide and broke the furniture.' [38]

Wandering away from home in a confused manner was a frequently mentioned behaviour with justifiable concerns that their wellbeing was at risk. One man in his 70s who had a long history of being impaired was found wandering in the bush in a confused delusional state and when admitted was feeble, debilitated from diarrhoea and died a week after admission.[39] A woman in her early 60s diagnosed with dementia:

> 'lately has become so addicted to wandering into the bush where on several occasions she has been nearly starved that her husband has become fearful of some fatal accident and thought it best to place her in an asylum.'[40]

In most cases wandering away from home was associated with other challenging behaviours and mental symptoms such as delusions.

Inability to self-care was the second common issue associated with admissions. Refusal to eat, often due to delusions that food was poisoned, was not uncommon and in an era devoid of antipsychotic drugs, the stomach pump was the only treatment available to keep the patient alive long enough in the hope that the delusions would resolve and allow the patient to feed themselves. A widow in her 70s had been unwell for four weeks being restless and excited with incoherent speech, moaning inarticulately and unable to sleep. She was tearing her clothes off, miserable and melancholic in appearance, refusing food due to delusions it was poisoned, and had a pale, dry, furred tongue suggestive of dehydration. Despite use of the stomach pump to feed her, she deteriorated and died after 3 weeks.[41]

Having 'dirty habits', in other words being incontinent of urine and/or faeces, was a frequent issue found in admissions in people with more advanced dementia. As in contemporary society, this appeared to be a factor leading to admission. Problems with self-care were often related to physical debility. One single blind man in his early 60s was admitted from gaol with the following medical note:

> 'the whole of his buttocks, sacrum, upper part of his thighs are one mass of inflamed sores and excoriations; he is feeble as to be nearly incapable of walking and is ill-tempered as a porcupine.' The malady was put down to 'senile imbecility' and he was regarded as an eccentric blind man, 'helpless but not a dangerous lunatic'. [42]

It is also clear from these medical notes that the admitting doctors in the 1850s and 60s often assumed that the cause of the mental disorder was age and that this meant that the outlook was poor, with comments such as 'his psychopathy is probably that of the aged',[43] 'it is enough to know that he is imbecile from old age',[44] and 'his great age and infirmity make history less necessary as he is beyond cure'.[45] This last comment is actually the exact opposite of what is now regarded as best clinical practice whereby collateral history from an informant who is aware of what has been happening is essential. Ageing ex-convicts were not uncommon and accounted for nearly ten per cent of older admissions between 1850 and 1870.

An additional twenty-seven cases were examined that represented transfers of long-stay patients included eleven males transferred from Gladesville to Callan Park when it opened in 1878 and sixteen females transferred from Cook's River Licensed House to Callan Park in 1886. They provide some understanding of the mental state of long-stay patients that is not otherwise apparent from the skimpy progress notes. It is clear from these admission notes that considerable psychopathology was still present although in many cases the florid psychotic symptoms had subsided leaving a range of less severe chronic delusions, cognitive impairment, behavioural disturbances and depression, with evidence of impaired self-care and function. The extent to which institutionalisation contributed to these residual symptoms is not clear.

Some examples include a man in his mid-60s who had been in hospital for seven years with a diagnosis of melancholia who was described after transfer to Callan Park as:

'morbid and melancholic and although he never makes any reference to his delusions they no doubt exist though they are not so vivid as to occasion the acute mental distress from which he before suffered. He wanders aimlessly about, is unable to occupy himself & appears to take very little interest in what is happening about him'[46]

Another man in his mid-60s, who had been in hospital five years with a diagnosis of delusional mania, was described on transfer as:

'extremely eccentric, is very loquacious, given to singing and hilarity and has a great opinion of his own powers & capabilities. He draws elaborate sketches of bridges, houses etc. which he is ready to present to any visitors and to which he attributes an absurd value. He is cleanly in habits & quiet at night.'[47]

A third example is a woman in her early 60s who had been hospitalised for eleven years with a diagnosis of delusional melancholia with symptoms of auditory hallucinations, persecutory delusions and irritability. When transferred to Callan Park she was described as suffering from secondary dementia, showing 'much mental enfeeblement, but is quiet, tidy, inclined to be useful, very deaf'.[48]

Perhaps the ageing long-stay patient who became best known during the mid-1890s was William Cresswell, who was put forward by Sydney lawyer Edward Priestman as a claimant to being Sir Roger Tichborne, the heir to the Tichborne baronetcy who had been presumably lost at sea in 1854.[49] This was not the first time that a person in Australia had made such a claim. In 1865 Thomas Castro, a bankrupt butcher from Wagga Wagga, put forward a claim which eventually led to a series of sensational long running civil and criminal trials in England the outcome of which saw Castro, under his real name Arthur Orton, convicted of perjury and sentenced to 14 years imprisonment. Creswell knew Arthur Orton while working in the Gippsland and Queanbeyan districts in the late 1850s and early 1860s.[50] Both bore some resemblance to the missing heir. Creswell was admitted to Gladesville Lunatic Asylum in 1869 at the age of 40 but was now residing in Parramatta Asylum. There had been public mention of Cresswell in relation to the Tichborne case in 1871 when one of Orton's junior counsels visited Wagga Wagga to gather evidence,[51] and again in 1884 when a representative of the 'Tichborne Release Association' in London attempted to obtain Cresswell's release from Parramatta Asylum to take him to England to promote his claims as Tichborne, Orton at this point being imprisoned. A Sydney court declined to release Cresswell.[52] In 1894, Edward Priestman, representing Reverend Edward Williams a Catholic priest from Devonshire, again attempted to push the claim that Cresswell was Roger Tichborne. There was considerable interest in the Sydney press. Eventually a Royal Commission was held in 1898 that determined Cresswell was not the missing heir but also recommended his release from the Parramatta Hospital. By this time Cresswell was a somewhat eccentric passive man often talking incoherently to himself but without evidence of florid psychosis.[53] Despite efforts to obtain his release Creswell died in the Parramatta Hospital in December 1904 of 'senile decay' at the age of 75.[54] Cresswell had never been the instigator of the claim and indeed during the Royal Commission denied that he was Tichborne.

By 1888 Manning was aware that the growing number of older people in the asylums was not just due to the increase in older admissions but was also due to the ageing of chronic cases in the hospitals. Many older long-stay chronic patients were transferred to Parramatta Hospital or Rydalmere Hospital, the latter opening in 1888 in the nearby old Protestant Orphan School that had closed in 1886. Rydalmere was initially a branch of Parramatta Hospital and by 1890 there were 120 male patients there. It became an independent hospital in 1891.[55]

From 1883, the NSW Inspector-General Annual Reports used the 1882 Medico-Psychological Association 'Form of Insanity' Classification in reporting the admitted, recovered, deaths, and 'remaining in hospital' for each diagnosis.[56] The 'senile' categories give a suggestion of the outcomes of older admissions by diagnosis although as noted at Hanwell Asylum in England during the same period, at least 50 per cent of those aged 60 years and over were not given a 'senile' diagnosis.[57] The number of patients aged 60 years and over who were 'under care' in any given year steadily increased, almost doubling between 1880 and 1900, although as a proportion of all cases under care the change was less dramatic as in all age groups there was an increase. The outcomes for older patients were not as good as for younger adults, which is not surprising as many had dementia. The proportion of older admissions that recovered was consistently lower than the overall rates of recovery, although this fluctuated between 1880 and 1900, and was particularly low for those with a 'senile' diagnosis. The number and proportion of deaths in those aged 60 years and over steadily increased with many of these being in the long-stay chronic patients admitted at a younger age, while those with a 'senile' diagnosis nearly doubled over the period. Older people were particularly vulnerable to contracting infectious diseases. In the 1880s, when there were concerns about water quality at Gladesville, deaths from typhoid, dysentery and diarrhoea were more common, while the influenza outbreak of 1891 caused 24 deaths mainly in older patients.[58] But overall cerebral disease was consistently the most prominent identified cause of mortality.

By the turn of the century around ten per cent of lunatic asylum admissions were aged 60 years and over which was nearly double the proportion of this age group in the NSW population (5.6 per cent). A high proportion of the older admissions died in hospital as witnessed by the number of deaths with a 'senile' diagnosis that increased from 29 per cent of deaths aged 60 years and over in 1881–1885 to 43 per cent by 1896–1900. The ageing of the chronic long-stay population had resulted in a near doubling of the number of older people in care in the asylums between 1880 and 1900. Yet it is important to note that the proportion of older patients under care had increased by less than one per cent over this period as overall there was a near doubling of patients under care; the drivers of increasing numbers of patients in the lunatic asylums occurred across the age range.

## Benevolent Asylums and Hospitals for the Aged and Destitute

The perennial overcrowding at the Sydney Benevolent Asylum in Pitt Street was temporarily relieved in 1851 when the Benevolent Society was given the use of the vacant Liverpool Hospital, formerly a convict hospital. Male inmates were transferred there leaving the Sydney Asylum for females thus establishing a principle of separate institutions for males and females that continued for over a century. For the first time in NSW, a medically qualified manager, J.C. Russell, was appointed to manage the Liverpool Asylum.[59] The relief was short lived. In 1856, when the railway extended to Liverpool, the combined number of inmates at Sydney and Liverpool was 550 and by 1859 it was 691 with Liverpool grossly overcrowded.[60]

Shortly before NSW attained self-government in 1855, the Government constituted a board to enquire into the operation and general management of the Benevolent Society. There had been mounting concerns that despite increasing Government support of the Society,[61] it had little say in its policy and management.[62] The Mayne-Mereweather Report, was presented just before self-government but it was not until 1862 that firm action occurred. Charles Cowper, the NSW Premier who was also a member of the Society's General Committee, suddenly announced that the Government would take over the care of the aged and destitute requiring residential facilities, while the Society would remain in control of outdoor relief, supported by a pound for pound subsidy, as well as destitute children and maternity cases.[63] The Liverpool Asylum was placed under a new board of Government Asylums for the Infirm and Destitute, the women in Sydney Asylum were transferred to the Immigration Barracks at Hyde Park, while a third asylum was established at Parramatta in the buildings of the old military hospital which took the overflow from Liverpool and functioned as a receiving house for aged and infirm men. The Board was largely inactive, supervision and inspections were irregular and of limited scope. Conditions within the asylums were variable with the Hyde Park Barracks regarded as being reasonable, while Liverpool had callous and harsh discipline and so the men preferred Parramatta despite its reputation for poor living conditions. The 1873 Royal Commission on Public Charities took evidence about the harsh discipline of James Denis, the Master at Liverpool, along with the poor conditions at Parramatta. It was unimpressed with the Board and its management recommending that the board be abolished.[64]

Between the 1850s and the 1870s transfers from the Benevolent Asylums to the lunatic asylums were a concern. Many were old and infirm and a drain upon charitable resources with no prospect of recovery with the lunatic asylums being used as charitable institutions of last resort.[65] In December 1863, George Walker the surgeon of the Hyde Park Asylum, attempted to draw to the attention of its management the challenges in getting the required two medical certificates to transfer aged lunatic inmates to a lunatic asylum. He noted that inmates of advanced age were prone to attacks of senile mania and dementia. He pointed out that the medical certificates were worded that the patient 'would be benefited by treatment in such asylum' and that the difficulty arose that doctors brought in to furnish the necessary documentation were reluctant to do so as they doubted that any benefit could accrue from such transfer. He noted that one such inmate had died from 'exhaustion produced by violent paroxysms of acute mania' and that the limited accommodation at Hyde Park meant that noisy insane inmates had to be housed with other sick patients which was prejudicial to their recovery. He advocated that such patients would be more appropriately managed in a lunatic asylum and that it might be best to reword the medical certificates to facilitate such transfers and thought this should be drawn to the attention of the Colonial Secretary. In a reply that he ordered to be published, the Colonial Secretary stated that he could not see the force of Dr Walker's objection about the wording of the certificates as he noted that Dr Walker had acknowledged the benefit of lunatic asylum admission and that there was nothing in the certificate that precluded lunacy arising from old age. Of course the Colonial Secretary by intent, or otherwise, ignored the thrust of Dr Walker's concerns which related to how other doctors interpreted the wording of the certificates.[66]

The medical officers in the lunatic asylums had a different perspective to Dr Walker. In the medical casebooks of Gladesville Hospital, the admitting doctors frequently commented about the lack of information accompanying the patients on transfer and the inappropriateness of the admissions. For example, one man in his 60s who had been living in a benevolent asylum for some years, was transferred to Gladesville after failed cataract surgery. The admitting doctor commented 'the only reason of his transfer so far as I can judge was to rid the benevolent asylum of a burden',[67] and a woman in her 70s was described as 'in articulo mortis; she is pale emaciated; haggard and weak, so much so that the escort had much difficulty getting her from the punt to the asylum.'[68] There were also concerns about the quality of care that had been provided in the benevolent asylum. A man in his 70s, described by the admitting doctor as 'an aged wreck of humanity', was:

> 'covered wherever there is a hair on his body with the pediculosis pubis in countless numbers. This sufficient is enough to drive a man crazy. His legs are covered with sores, the left leg in particular is on the lower half a uniform ulcer.'[69]

He died within a month of admission. Another man in his mid-70s with sunken eyes, a wasted face, quiet and inoffensive in a state of senile dementia was transferred:

> 'in almost an unparalleled condition of disgraceful neglect, literally swarming with vermin with which his clothing was alive and his body so thickly populated as to be swept off it by handfuls ... it seems hard therefore to conceive on what grounds he would have been certified as a fit and proper person to be removed here' [70]

Over the last quarter of the nineteenth century the NSW State Hospitals and Asylums for the Destitute and Aged kept growing in number and size. In addition to the Liverpool and Parramatta George Street Asylums, in 1880 the Parramatta Macquarie Street Asylum for blind men and aged men with defective sight and senility was opened. In 1886 the 306 women housed at Hyde Park were transferred to the Newington Asylum for Women located at the Blaxland property at Silverwater on the Parramatta River about 16 kilometres from Sydney, while in 1893 the new Rookwood Asylum (the future Lidcombe Hospital) was established for aged and infirm destitute men to relieve overcrowding at Parramatta Asylum. In 1896 it became the main State asylum for men and at that time there were 581 inmates, with accommodation increasing to 800 in 1899.[71]

Brian Dickey notes that the Asylums for the Aged & Destitute accumulated a growing proportion of hospital cases. 'In the 1880s, as many once able-bodied destitutes lapsed into senility, 25 per cent of the inmates were hospital cases.'[72] Cyril Cummins commented that these asylums were operating as 'auxiliary hospitals – part poorhouse and part chronic diseases hospitals. Their facilities were limited, their policies restrictive, penny-pinching and open to frequent criticism'.[73] They were the nursing homes of the late nineteenth century for those with chronic incurable illnesses, particularly in people with no family support. A study by Anne O'Brien on NSW benevolent asylums between 1880 and 1896 reported that of three hundred inmates 92 per cent were immigrants and 64 per cent had no living relatives.[74]

Due to the frequent complaints about the Liverpool, Newington and Parramatta Asylums, a Government Asylums Inquiry Board was established in 1886 and reported in May 1887. It noted that the asylums were full, about 70 per cent were over the age of 50, 84 per cent of whom were men.[75] The Board was particularly critical of the conditions and staff at Newington and Parramatta. The adverse findings were numerous; lack of recreational space, poor food quality, brutal treatment by wardsmen, untrained illiterate unkind inattentive wardswomen dispensing medication in hospital wards, and the carelessness and neglect of the medical officer.'[76] The criticism of the Macquarie Street, Parramatta Asylum included that 'the evidence is incontrovertible of the gross brutalities practised upon helpless inmates by the wardsmen who were appointed by the matron.'[77] Many of the victims were identified as having senile dementia or other forms of limited mental capacity.[78] The Board went on to make it clear that they could not believe that the matrons were unaware of the atrocities, and that even if they were unaware, the assumption would be 'that they systematically neglected the work for which they had been paid.' [79] The medical superintendent of the three asylums, Dr Charles Rowling, was strongly condemned for negligence and brutality.

As Pat Jalland remarked:

> 'it was highly unusual for an Inquiry Board to take a stand so strongly opposed to the senior staff of the asylums in favour of the numerous brave inmates who had made allegations to the Governor, the Board, and the press. Such charges were usually dismissed for lack of evidence, as the product of inmates' minds confused by disease, dementia, and alcohol.'[80]

One of the main recommendations of the Inquiry Board was the need to establish a 700 bed Central Sick Asylum for those who had chronic illnesses constructed as a hospital with a Resident Medical Officer and a small staff of trained nurses. It still foresaw that less infirm inmates of the benevolent asylums would do part of the work but 'these should never be engaged in cooking, nursing, or the like'.[81] Although trained nurses were employed following the inquiry, the proposed Central Sick Asylum was not established. By the turn of the century, NSW governments had not undertaken asylum reform in part because they believed that the establishment of old age pensions would resolve the problems by reducing numbers.[82] Throughout the second half of the nineteenth century the Benevolent Society remained responsible for outdoor relief in NSW. But during the depression in the 1890s when employment was hard to come by for people over the age of 60, the number of people receiving outdoor relief from the Benevolent Society nearly trebled between 1891 and 1897.[83]

In an era in which the press reported the details of attempted suicides before and after the criminal proceedings,[84] it is noteworthy that being a resident of one of the Asylums for the Aged and Destitute was no protection from self-harm. Some became depressed, such as a 60-year-old woman who attempted to hang herself at Newington Asylum eight months after returning from being with her daughter and becoming 'very disconsolate several times saying that she would end the life that had become unbearable to her, but as all these threats were put down to the grumblings of senility not much notice was taken of them.'[85] Others had difficulties with institutional living, an example being an 80-year-old man from the George Street, Parramatta Asylum who had 'been offended at being put out of his seat at the mess table' and subsequently impulsively cut his throat.[86] The outcomes of the court hearings for attempted suicide were quite variable, including imprisonment for periods ranging from the rising of the court to many months, discharge on their own recognisance, and occasionally committal to the Reception House for further assessment. Many of those imprisoned were specifically ordered to the gaol hospital for medical supervision. For those older people noted to have difficulties with self-care and finances, it was common for the court to recommend admission to an Asylum for the Aged and Destitute. An example was a 'decrepit' 64-year-old man who had cut his throat and was imprisoned for three days to facilitate transfer to a benevolent asylum.[87] But some were not keen to go to an asylum, such as a 78-year-old miner who cut his throat when drunk and was initially sentenced to the rising of the court and subsequently to be sent to the benevolent asylum. He refused stating 'I can get my living by working, and I don't want charity'. The magistrate changed his sentence to gaol for 14 days.[88]

By the end of the century, although asylums were overcrowded, in the absence of adequate community support, many older people had few alternatives especially if they mental or physical disabilities.

# Chapter 5

# Tasmania: An Ageing Nineteenth Century Convict Colony

Nineteenth-century Tasmania was the first Australian jurisdiction to grapple with the effects of population ageing and its impact on mental function. As discussed in chapter 3, the estimated dementia prevalence in Tasmania was higher than in the other colonies throughout most of the second half of the century and this was reflected in the challenges experienced by its institutions.

Governor King authorised the colonisation of Van Diemen's Land (the future Tasmania) in 1803 with the intent of relieving the settlement in Sydney of its most dangerous convicts.[1] The first hospitals were improvised small wooden huts that were opened at Hobart in 1804 and Launceston in 1808.[2] No provision was made for the mentally ill and those who could not be managed in their home had to be sent to the Castle Hill Lunatic Asylum in Sydney.

Few in the population were in a position to support the aged and infirm as they were often struggling themselves. For example, in 1814 when there were approximately 1900 people in the colony, only 40 per cent were 'off the store', that is, living independently of Government supplies.[3] In 1819, a room was rented for the aged and chronic sick to relieve pressure on hospital beds. Lack of a Benevolent Society was keenly felt but it was not until 1829 that Lieutenant-Governor Arthur funded the Benevolent and Stranger's Friend Society. Other Benevolent Societies in Hobart and Launceston in the 1830s did not survive due to financial difficulties, in part because of the lack of government support.[4] An example of the problems that were emerging was reported in the *Launceston Advertiser* in 1832 where an elderly beggar, suffering from severe palsy and formerly on an invalid ticket but now a free man, was witnessed. It was suggested that 'as this poor fellow cannot work, we think his rations ought to be continued to him for the remainder of his wretched existence, and be prohibited from begging'.[5]

In 1827, the first asylum in Van Diemen's Land was established at the town of New Norfolk situated about 35 kilometres up the Derwent River from Hobart. Barracks for incurable convicts were converted to house the colony's invalids and the first admission of a designated insane patient occurred in 1829. Permanent buildings for the insane at the New Norfolk Invalid Hospital and Lunatic Asylum were not completed until 1833 with buildings arranged around a courtyard and able to accommodate 40 patients of each sex.[6,7] Most mentally ill patients were still being managed in the Colonial Hospital in Hobart Town and it was a number of years before this changed. For example, of 109 patients in 1833, only 20 were designated as lunatics but by 1842 the number of insane increased to 55.[8,9] The majority of the patients were physical invalids or aged infirm and it was soon overcrowded. Built for 150, by 1838 there were 279 inmates of whom 100 were capable of some work but not sufficient to live independently.[10] In Anthea Vreugdenhil's study of older admissions to the New Norfolk Lunatic Asylum only eleven people aged 60 years and over were admitted between 1830 and 1850, all were paupers, most were convicts. In the 1840s, this represented twelve per cent of lunatic admissions.[11]

Most of the older people in this era were admitted to New Norfolk as invalids; how many of these had dementia is not known. There were few activities available and as noted by Joan Brown, 'in general the invalids loafed the day away and in the process probably brought on an earlier onset of senility'. Some men hired themselves out in the town, got drunk on the proceeds and brought attention to themselves. Conditions at New Norfolk were frequently criticised, sometimes for ill-treatment and sometimes for leniency. The doctors were at times accused of neglect.[12]

Ageing and infirm ex-convict pauper patients in the hospitals had from 1839 been recognised as the main reason for increasing costs; thus only indoor relief was provided for the aged and infirm, a policy designed to control expenditure but one likely to have encouraged institutionalisation. In 1848 Lieutenant-Governor Denison tried to induce the British government to accept ex-convicts as being chargeable to them if they became dependent on government aid for up to 10 years after expiry of their sentence. The British government did accept responsibility for those aged 60 and over at the time of arrival in the colony and for those who through age or infirmity (including mental infirmity) were unable to support themselves at the expiration of their sentence. With this response the colonial government with inadequate revenue ceased outdoor relief and only admitted the aged and disabled to institutions if they were totally destitute.[13]

It was not until 1846 that Tasmania had its first mental health legislation, the *Treatment of Insane Persons Act*, which specified the admission process for lunatic asylums requiring an Order by two Justices of the Peace and documentation of insanity by a medical practitioner.[14] Before that the legality of detention of non-convicts at New Norfolk had been repeatedly queried. In 1846 female invalids were transferred to the Colonial Hospital Hobart. New Norfolk became entirely a lunatic asylum in 1848 with the invalid male patients being transferred to the Impression Bay (now known as Premaydena) depot at Port Arthur, a former convict station. While the majority of the invalids cooperated, 26 older men refused to go as they said that they did not want to go to a penal settlement, thirteen changed their mind while the rest were evicted. In May 1848, there were 450 invalids at Impression Bay depot and mostly described to be in very poor physical condition due to age, accident or disease.[15]

Van Diemen's Land became self-governing in 1856 and was renamed Tasmania, in part at least to disconnect the colony from its convict past. Even when English novelist Anthony Trollope visited Tasmania in 1872 he reported that the name Van Diemen's Land was 'odious to the ears of Tasmanians, as being still tainted with the sound of the gaol and harsh with the crack of the gaoler's whip'.[16] As noted in Chapter 3, Tasmania had an ageing population in the second half of the nineteenth century due to the exodus of younger people to the mainland from the 1840s onwards, a depressed economy, and the ageing of the emancipist population which put pressures on the Tasmanian asylums in part due to the prevalence of dementia.[17]

The main dynamic for the rise of the asylum in Tasmania was the decline of the penal system that had housed, fed, and worked where possible, convicts who were insane or infirm. The provision of mental health care and other services was viewed by Tasmanians as a responsibility of government as it had been responsible for transportation and the creation of social dependents.[18] By the 1850s around

75 per cent of those admitted to New Norfolk Lunatic Asylum were convict paupers.[19] Throughout the nineteenth century many patients at New Norfolk had previously been cared for in some other institution for social dependents such as the New Town Charitable Institution or Launceston Invalid Depot and their successors.[20] Indeed, since establishment, the New Norfolk asylum had been administered by the Convict Medical Service, the focus being on security and control which was accentuated by its isolation from the rest of the colony allowing for lax standards of care and a perceived lack of focus on treatment. Repeated complaints about the mistreatment of the insane, which were strongly denied, along with the end of transportation in 1853, led eventually in October 1855 to the colonial government taking over the administration of New Norfolk Asylum with a Board of Commissioners and a new medical officer tasked to turn it into a civil hospital.[21]

The Board of Commissioners identified many problems with the accommodation at New Norfolk with one key issue being the lack of separate accommodation and eating arrangements for the 'better classes' from the pauper convicts.[22] In the mid-nineteenth-century Tasmania, pejorative attitudes towards emancipist and convict aged and infirm invalids were prominent, particularly those who were unable to work and support themselves. Social historian Andrew Piper commented 'invalids felt the full brunt of the "hated stain" and were seen as carriers of a moral contagion which had its greatest impact on women who were seen as disseminators of immorality'.[23] This contributed to an 'out of sight, out of mind' attitude whereby institutions were preferred as the solution rather than support for aged invalids to live in the community.[24] It also contributed to the decision to focus early efforts to modify the asylum by building better accommodation for the 'superior patients' with a Gentlemen's Cottage completed in December 1859.[25]

*The 1858 Insane Persons Hospital Act* was the first comprehensive mental health legislation in Tasmania that provided the legal framework for the detention and care of the insane at New Norfolk.[26] The Board of Commissioners were replaced by Official Visitors and recording requirements were specified for admissions. In 1859, a Joint Committee of Parliament was appointed to inquire into the accommodation at New Norfolk.[27] Although Principal Medical Officer Dr Robert Officer had previously drawn up the plans for the buildings housing the insane at New Norfolk, now that the whole institution was a hospital for the insane he asserted that the buildings were not designed for their care and the institution was not fit for the purpose.[28] The amenities were regarded by the Joint Committee to be unsatisfactory and were felt to be contributing to the low rate of recovery compared with asylums overseas. While consideration was given for the construction of a purpose-built lunatic asylum along the lines of the contemporary English asylums, the colonial authorities decided to remodel New Norfolk to bring it closer to an environment that could facilitate moral treatments.[29] In the mid-1860s New Norfolk still lacked the apparatus for hot and cold water and shower baths.[30] For the rest of the nineteenth century lack of funds meant work undertaken was piecemeal, repairs and modifications were repeatedly delayed.[31]

In 1879 the Government proposed to move the 'imbeciles' to an invalid depot but the Commissioners were opposed to it stating that only six patients could be moved without danger to themselves or others and that their age and debility meant that it was absolutely necessary that great attention should be given to them.[32] In late 1879 Martha Laland, formerly of the Melbourne Benevolent Asylum, was appointed as matron after her predecessor had been dismissed. She was shocked by the primitive conditions that confronted her. The sick ward, under the charge of an untrained nurse, was situated in a gloomy, unventilated, damp location and next to a foul drain. The epileptic patients, instead of being managed together, were scattered around the asylum, and due to their incontinence spread filth around the institution. There were no night nurses with the day nurses having to sleep in the wards with the patients.[33]

A Royal Commission in 1883 criticised the Government for neglect and poor funding but its recommendations were ignored.[34] A Select Committee in 1884 enquired into the staffing and noted that half of the nurses and attendants had less than a year of experience. Breaches of discipline were being overlooked, charges of cruelty and ill-treatment of patients were not being investigated by the doctors. Low pay, the ongoing sleeping arrangements with the patients, and lack of leave to be with their families were seen as factors contributing to the problem.[35] In the second half of the nineteenth century, there were seven Government inquiries into the New Norfolk asylum that had similar recommendations with similar outcomes. Authorities believed that as most of the patients were ex-convicts, when they died the need for accommodation would diminish, which impacted on decisions about the asylum. This meant that the environment for the treatment of the mentally ill at New Norfolk remained substandard, even by standards of the day, for the rest of the nineteenth century and overcrowding worsened through the 1890s.[36,37]

Anthea Vreugdenhil analysed the mental health admissions to New Norfolk aged 60 years and over for the period 1830 to 1899. In the nineteenth century there was no separation of the older from the younger patients; males and females were separated, as were for the most part, acute and chronic refractory patients. There was also a sick ward for those with severe physical ailments. Of the 2258 admissions, 328 (14.5%) were aged 60 years and over, with even higher proportions in the 1870s (17%), 1880s (16%), and the 1890s (16%). Only 30 per cent of older admissions were married in the 1830s–1859 but by the 1890s this increased to 54 per cent. While all of the older admissions from 1830–1859 were paupers, this declined over subsequent decades to 17 per cent in the 1870s and six per cent in the 1890s, with an associated increase in those described as labourers or domestics to around a half of the admissions. Clearly many of the admissions had limited financial resources. The two main 'causes' of insanity identified by the medical officers were 'old age/senile decay' (35%) and alcohol (22%). Throughout, the proportion of admissions aged 60 years and over was higher than in the general population. This was particularly the case for males who comprised around three quarters of the older admissions peaking at 81 per cent in the 1890s. Vreugdenhil suggests that this might relate to males being in worse physical health and having more severe mental disorders than females with accompanying higher mortality and females more likely to become long-stay patients.[38] But it is likely to be more nuanced than that.

To obtain a better understanding of the older admissions, I examined the medical casebooks from the period 1848–1873 which are available online through the Archives Agency, Libraries Tasmania.[39] In this period there were 84 completed admissions aged 60 years and over. The average length of stay of females (61.8 months) was more than double that of males (28.2 months). This was not just due to mortality as more males (31%) were discharged than females (19%) with 75 per cent of discharges occurring within a year of admission. However, more males died within 12 months of admission (25%) than females

(19%). In discharges and deaths that occurred within a year, most occurred within three months of admission.

Although the medical casebooks of this era have sparse information about the admissions compared with case notes today, there is usually enough to gain a reasonable sense of the broad issues involved. As previously noted, the diagnoses used by the medical officers are not particularly helpful, most were diagnosed with either 'amentia', 'mania' or 'dementia'. Four admissions related to suicidal behaviour. Only five of the patients in the period from 1848 to 1873 had insufficient information to establish a possible contemporary diagnosis. Thirty of the remaining 79 admissions (38%) had a possible twenty-first-century dementia diagnosis.

Around a quarter of the patients had admissions of up to three months duration before death or discharge. Examination of the casebook histories of the fourteen cases that died within three months of admission revealed a range of issues that can be broken down into two broad groups. The first group were terminally ill patients; some were palliative hospice type cases ailing from chronic physical infirmity attributed to senility and sent to New Norfolk to die. For example, a poor man in his 90s who had been living on charity for years, was admitted as an 'object of charity' and was becoming an 'imbecile with age'. He was extremely helpless, living in dirt and filth. He was troubled with rheumatism and suffered from bronchitis.[40]

Others were delirious from disorders such as tuberculosis, dysentery, and gangrene that in modern hospital practice would have been potentially remediable and treated in a general hospital. In this era the absence of fever meant that a person who had other features of delirium was usually treated in a lunatic asylum as insane. For example, a single man in his 60s was incoherent and rambled in his conversation verging into idiocy, refused food, and was restless at night, defecating in his bed with watery stools. He looked very ill with a cadaverous countenance, blue lips, and was scarcely able to walk. He died two days after admission the post-mortem revealing ulcerated intestines and tuberculous lungs.[41]

The second group of admissions died from hospital-acquired complications, some from unpredictable disorders in that era such as strokes and status epilepticus, others from complications of falls in the hospital. An example was a woman in her 70s with a likely history of alcohol abuse, who was confused and incoherent for two weeks after admission then fell out of bed sustaining a head injury. Gradually she declined and died. The post-mortem noted that there was blood in the brain sinuses presumably from the head injury.[42]

Examination of the eight patients who were discharged within three months indicate that severe mood disorders, acute transient psychoses, and alcohol-related disorders were the main problems. Here are two exemplars. The first was a single man in his 60s with recurrent mania. He had two brief admissions characterised by physical overactivity, incoherence, agitation, delusions of grandeur and violence requiring restraints. They settled within weeks of admission. On his third admission, he was discharged after five months to work as a wardsman so they could monitor his progress but he relapsed six months later and remained in the asylum for 15 years with periodic relapses until his death.[43] The second was an ex-convict in his 60s with symptoms consistent with severe major depression on the background of having committed incest. He had a ten-month history of remorsefulness and ejaculations that he was 'damned to all eternity', with periods of incoherence in speech and being unable to comprehend questions. In the three weeks before admission he had been indolent and helpless in manner. In hospital, he gradually improved.[44]

The absence of clear evidence of insanity was another reason for discharge, even if there was evidence of cognitive impairment that was likely consistent with mild dementia. Around a third of those who remained in hospital for over three months had presentations consistent with dementia, often associated with behavioural change or psychosis. Many were dangerous and threatening violence to family members or others in the community. Even with current interventions and support services to address these issues in the community, many such patients still require long-term residential care. Thus, it is understandable that in the nineteenth century admission to New Norfolk was the best option available. For example, a married labourer in his early 60s had a six-year history of cognitive decline. He was unable to give his age, where he lived, or details of family members. He was wild, abstracted, and unable to concentrate. His wife stated that he was sometimes dangerous, threatening to strike people with an axe or other weapon he may have in his hand. He died 12 months after admission.[45]

It is not clear what specific treatments these patients with dementia would have received apart from basic nursing care. Admission notes documenting the disturbed behaviour that precipitated admission were rarely accompanied by any progress notes. The extent to which there would have been any activities appropriate for people with dementia is questionable. Given the very poor quality accommodation, bathrooms and lavatories, conditions for nursing often incontinent patients were dreadful. Most of the patients are repeatedly described as 'unchanged', or with 'increasing imbecility', or becoming more feeble and debilitated. Anthea Vreugdenhil reported that many became debilitated towards the end of life and would have most likely been bedbound and nursed in the sick ward.[46]

Chronic psychoses of various types including paranoid psychoses, alcohol-related psychoses, severe depression and chronic mania accounted for most of the other cases. Some were clinically diagnosed with GPI but this was before diagnostic tests were available and so accuracy is questionable in older people. Other cases were complicated by epilepsy and physical ailments including paralysis, chronic pain, arthritis, and sensory impairments. For most patients the clinical notes do not provide a good indication of the duration of the psychoses; only those whose behaviour caused disruption were likely to get an entry to that effect. Social circumstances likely contributed to the prolonged admissions, in particular most of the men were either single or widowed and had no informal carer. In contrast the majority of the women were married and while it is speculative, one wonders how many of the husbands were willing or able to take on the caregiving role. Indeed, in one case the husband had moved to Melbourne and proved uncontactable. Some of these cases had entries suggesting that there was no reason related to insanity for the patient to be in an asylum; in one case the doctors thought the patient was malingering. In the cases I examined, around twenty per cent of admissions aged 60 years and over remained at New Norfolk for five or more years, while ten per cent were there ten or more years. The extent to which this represents ongoing insanity, institutionalisation, or chronic physical infirmity (or a combination of these) is unclear from the records.

## Other Tasmanian Hospitals for the Insane

Although the New Norfolk Hospital for the Insane was the principal institution that admitted insane patients during the nineteenth century there were others too. To relieve overcrowding at New Norfolk, patients were sent to Impression Bay in the 1850s. Convicts were initially treated on the Tasman Peninsula at Saltwater River from around 1850 and then later transferred to Port Arthur Asylum in the late 1850s.[47] A purpose built lunatic asylum for 100 patients was completed at Port Arthur in 1868 and located next to the invalid depot. The asylum was a model structure with every care being taken to provide comfortable accommodation, a contrast to New Norfolk.[48] When Anthony Trollope visited Port Arthur in 1872 he noted that 'the lunatic asylum and that for paupers have no appearance of prisons'.[49] It quickly became overcrowded but there were no efforts to extend it.

When the Female Factory at the Cascades closed in 1877, the patients from Port Arthur, a mix of invalids and lunatics, were transferred to the vacated hospital at the Cascades. There were 100 male patients classified as lunatics and of these, 84 were regarded as 'Imperial Lunatics' which meant that the convict had been declared insane during his period of servitude and the costs of care would be covered by the Imperial (British) Government.[50] The rest were transfers from New Norfolk or Cascades Asylums of 'colonial' patients either due to overcrowding or being too violent. As transportation had ended 24 years earlier, this was an older cohort of patients. The casebooks reveal that there were 41 men aged 60 years or older at the time of transfer, and overall the mean age of those transferred was 57.3 years.[51] Having over 40 per cent of patients aged 60 years and over in a lunatic asylum was not seen elsewhere in Australia until the second half of the twentieth century. The Cascades lunatic asylum, which was totally unsuited for the purpose, closed in 1890 with patients being transferred to New Norfolk which was the only lunatic asylum in Tasmania at the turn of the century.[52]

### Invalid Depots

Tasmania had a poor reputation regarding the quality of its institutions for the aged and infirm where treatment could be inhumane and inappropriate.[53] The Government-run invalid depot at Impression Bay was predominantly for convicts or ex-convicts and after transportation ended in 1853, the number of invalids dropped to 238 in 1857 when it closed. In the second half of the century a number of charitable invalid depots opened with their main focus on aged care. Andrew Piper reported that in 1875, 59 per cent of all charitable institutional inmates were aged 65 years and over, increasing to 72 per cent in 1901, while during the same period more than 80 per cent were aged 55 years and over.[54] These were the nursing homes of the day although most of the inmates were paupers and the style of care was punitive with authoritarian control.

The charitable invalid depots were seriously underfunded, understaffed, and overcrowded, the latter easing in the 1890s. Historian John Hargrave reported that the total number of invalids in gaols and depots grew from 400 in the 1860s to 600 in 1880, dropping to 580 in 1890 before dropping to 300 by 1900 as the ex-convicts, who comprised more than 90 per cent of inmates, died.[55] Launceston Invalid Depot was particularly overcrowded and by 1882 it averaged 140 male inmates with a mean age of 67 years, with a further 42 females housed in the gaol.[56] Until the late nineteenth century there were no outside nursing staff with the practice being to select the more able of the invalid inmates and pay them a modest wage to assist their fellow inmates. In the 1880s the Invalid Depot Superintendents repeatedly expressed concern about the capacity of the ageing and infirm nurses to provide care to their fellow inmates. John Witherington, who was in charge of Brickfields and later the New Town Charitable Institution, did not keep apace of the ageing population under his care, resisted classifying the inmates and opposed the idea of employing trained nurses.[57]

There was repeated criticism by the public and the press, with one report in 1884 in the *Hobart Mercury*, providing an analogy of the invalids to an ancient mill near the property boundary of the New Town Invalid Depot as 'both are decayed past resuscitation'.[58] As reported by Joan Brown, 'in the 33 years, 1857–1890, no less than seven Royal Commissions, four Special Commissions and twelve Select and Joint Committees probed into various aspects of the Charitable Institutions'.[59] But there was little action to rectify the situation with continued inadequate funding and lack of recognition that the staff were doing their best in very difficult circumstances. As with New Norfolk, the lack of planning seemed predicated on the view that once the ex-convicts died the problems would be resolved.[60]

How many of these aged invalid depot inmates had mental disorders, particularly dementia, is unknown, though undoubtedly many did. It is likely that if an inmate's behaviour became an issue such as with violence, self-harm, or by disrupting the other inmates, transfer to New Norfolk Lunatic Asylum would occur. Yet it did not happen too often. Using the New Norfolk Invalid Asylum case books, in the four years from mid-1885 to mid-1889 there were only five male admissions aged 60 years and over transferred from an invalid depot and similarly in the three years from October 1881 to September 1884, only three women aged 60 years and over were transferred from an invalid depot.[61]

Here are two examples that demonstrate the types of behavioural disturbances that warranted transfer. A pauper labourer widower in his 80s with severe memory impairment and incoherent conversation was transferred from Launceston Invalid Depot because, for the previous month, he had been noisy at night and calling out when alone. He was irritable, refusing food and medicine, as he thought they were poison.[62] A single labourer in his 70s with a 6-month history of incoherence and disorientation was sent from the Launceston Invalid Depot because he kept trying to abscond to Deloraine. He was repeatedly tearing off his clothes and wandering around naked.[63]

## Older people with dementia and mental disorders residing in the community

Casebook admission records often note that the patient had for a long time been recognised in his local community as having some form of mental disorder and usually it was some serious behavioural change that led to admission. Support available in the community was limited. Outdoor relief was initially by grants which were originally intended to support the aged paupers until there was a place available in an invalid depot.[64] By the early 1880s it was cheaper for charitable organisations to subsidise the pauper aged and infirm through outdoor relief rather than in an institution. As there was a policy of forced separation of married couples in institutions, it was an effective means to aid couples and was particularly popular for rural elderly.[65] In the last few decades of the nineteenth century the ratio of older males to older females got closer to parity in Tasmania. Between 1850 and 1870 there were around 2.5 times the number of males aged 60 years and over in Tasmania than females aged 60 years and over, but by 1901 it was only 1.1 times.[66] More older people were married or had partners, which in itself provided some comfort, and fewer were ex-convicts.

Suicide provides one measure of community mental well-being. Age-standardised suicide rates in the period 1860–1899 in Tasmania were generally lower than those reported in other colonies. Males aged 65 years and over had suicide rates of 30.6 per 100,000, slightly lower than the peak in the 50–64 year age group with 31.4 deaths per 100,000 population. Females aged 65 years and over had very low suicide rates of 2.9 per 100,000, much lower than the peak in the 50–64 year age group with 9.7 deaths per 100,000 population. The 1890s, when there was economic depression, saw male suicide rates peak particularly between 1890 and 1894.[67] However, it is well accepted that suicide rates from nineteenth-century Tasmania are an underestimate with a range of reasons including concealment (suicide was a crime at the time), benefit of the doubt and mistakes contributing to it. Even during the nineteenth century the relatively low suicide rates in Tasmania compared with other colonies prompted comment by Hayter, Victoria's Registrar General.[68]

In the nineteenth century attempted suicide was a criminal act and was reported in the press. In May 1890, an 89-year-old married woman from Launceston, very feeble and nearly blind, used an old table knife to deeply gash her forearm (although a briefer report indicated that she cut her throat) while her husband was at work. After being treated at the general hospital, in the police interrogation she gave no reason for her act and while she initially said that she would 'again endeavour to do away with her existence' she later recanted. She was remanded by the City Police Court for a week on a charge of self-murder.[69,70]

The economy picked up in Tasmania in the mid to late 1890s with the silver and copper mining boom on the west coast and increased migration.[71] Outdoor relief to older people, particularly married couples increased through this decade.[72] Thus by the turn of the century and the pending federation the circumstances for older people in Tasmania appeared to be improving.

# Chapter 6

# The Ageing Effects of a Gold Rush: Victoria in the Nineteenth Century

With the gold rush of the 1850s, Victoria's population exploded growing from around 76 thousand to over half a million by 1861. This was accompanied by marked economic expansion. With the younger prospectors, merchants and their families migrating to Victoria, in the 1860s and 1870s there were relatively few older people in Victoria. By the 1880s this was changing and by 1901, with 94,745 (7.9%) aged 60 years and over, Victoria had the highest proportion and number of older people in the Federation.[1] Towards the end of the century, some of the smaller goldfield towns where the mines had closed and children moved on had around 10 per cent older people in their communities.[2]

### Lunatic Asylums

By the 1840s there was a need for accommodation for the insane and extra cells were built at Collins Street West Gaol, with the more disturbed patients being transferred to Tarban Creek Asylum.[3, 4] Yarra Bend Asylum was opened in 1848 as a single storey bluestone rectangular structure with high walls and an architectural style reminiscent of contemporary penal establishments. It had extensive grounds and was isolated from the town of Melbourne.[5] Initially it was a ward of Tarban Creek Asylum until the separation of Victoria from NSW in 1851 at which point it adopted the name Yarra Bend Asylum.[6]

Over the next twenty years overcrowding was a perennial problem. In 1856 the Asylum Board had recommended that Kew Asylum be built as the second Melbourne lunatic asylum even though it was only 300 yards from Yarra Bend but its construction was a stop start affair being abandoned in 1858.[7] Construction recommenced in the mid-1860s along with the building of regional asylums at Beechworth and Ararat, both opening in 1867 along with Cremorne Private Asylum, for 'women of harmless & peaceable demeanour', that was licenced in the same year.[8,9] From the outset, Beechworth Asylum was primarily a long-term care institution and the admissions were usually middle-aged or older patients with chronic unremitting mental disorders transferred from Yarra Bend Asylum. One of the transfers in 1867 was 67-year-old Robert Coates, a professional landscape gardener in good physical health, who remained at Beechworth for five years and was instrumental in planning the gardens of the asylum.[10] Kew Asylum eventually opened as a ward of Yarra Bend in December 1871 but was not completed and gazetted as an independent asylum until October 1872.[11]

Dr Edward Paley was recruited from England in 1863, appointed medical superintendent at Yarra Bend and became the Inspector of Lunatic Asylums.[12] The *1867 Lunacy Act* specified that a register of patients admitted to a lunatic asylum be kept including the demographic details of the patients, diagnosis, cause of insanity, state of health and outcome.[13] The first information about the number of older patients in Victorian lunatic asylums is covered in Paley's 1868 annual report to the Victorian Parliament that was based on the case register. There were 27 patients aged 60 years and over (3.1 per cent of admissions) admitted to Victorian lunatic asylums in 1868, with one recovery and three 'relieved' at discharge. Five patients aged 60 years and over died.[14] The type of circumstances that resulted in these older admissions is exemplified in this 1865 report from *The Argus* about the commitment of a 66-year-old man on a charge of lunacy:

> 'The overt acts of insanity deposed to by the witnesses amounted to nothing more than an enumeration of acts of puerility too often accompanying failing powers. The old man was weak and harmless; was in the habit of pulling the fire about, and sometimes scattered the ashes; was restless in bed, and pulled the clothes about; talked about ropes, and one day half strangled the cat. He was remanded for medical examination.'[15]

Although in the 1868 report Edward Paley did not specifically identify older admissions as a concern, he did note under the heading 'incurable imbecile patients' that many patients 'unoffending in their habits, weak in mind, and feeble in body' had been admitted from hospitals, benevolent asylums, and gaols, who required care but not in an asylum. Paley drew attention to the practice in England where such patients were looked after in workhouses.[16]

In 1870 Yarra Bend housed 1043 patients making it one of the largest asylums in the world. In his 1870 annual report, Paley reviewed the data on over five and a half thousand admissions from 1848 to 1870. There were 1200 chronic permanent cases who remained in the asylums and it was the growth of this category that was pushing the need for more beds. Here for the first time he identified 'old men and women in their dotage' as one category (others included the paralysed and infirm, non-violent epileptics, the intellectually disabled, and vagrants) within a group of 'weak-minded persons' in the 'imbecile class of insane' who were 'incurable' and 'with some degree of care usually harmless' who did not require care in a lunatic asylum and asserted that such cases were not treated in lunatic asylums in England.[17]

By 1872 Paley was very clear that having such 'imbecile' patients in the lunatic asylums was detrimental and gave four broad reasons: it impacted upon the chances of the curable recovering; the 'imbecile' patients had their liberties restricted in the same way as others and that was an injustice; it cost nearly double to care for 'imbecile' patients in lunatic asylums compared with benevolent asylums; and beds taken by 'imbeciles' means more beds would be needed for 'lunatics'.[18] In the same report Paley noted that it would be impractical to send 'imbeciles' back to the benevolent asylums as they were already overcrowded. He speculated whether the building of a less restrictive facility in the grounds of Yarra Bend or Kew might be the answer, such as Leavesden and Caterham in England, or alternatively, a 'boarding out' system with family could be trialled.[19] While none of these reasons and suggestions were specifically about older people with dementia, they were included within the broad group of patients that Paley was concerned about.

By 1876 disillusionment had set in about the design of Kew Asylum as was revealed during the Kew Inquiry of that year after a sudden and suspicious death. The medical superintendent Dr Alexander Robertson felt that large monumental barrack style asylums of which Kew was a prime example were not suited to patient recovery as they became overcrowded. The cottage style accommodation, as was found at Yarra Bend, was considered a better design. The Inquiry was also informed about the inadequate supply of fresh water, poor sanitation and overcrowded bedrooms in which it was difficult to get pure air to breathe.[20] By 1877 Kew Asylum was accommodating over 1000 patients yet had been built for only 600. Of these, over 90 per cent were judged incurable. Around a quarter were being secluded or restrained.[21]

I examined the first four volumes of the Kew Register of patients for the 16-year period from January 1873 until December 1888. The 423 admissions aged 60 years and over, excluding twelve transfers from other lunatic asylums, were analysed. Over two-thirds of admissions were males and while a similar proportion of males and females were married, most unmarried males were single and unmarried females were widows, which largely reflects the demographics of the Victorian colony at the time. On average, there were only two admissions per year from a benevolent asylum. The majority of patients were given a dementia diagnosis though from the case registers it is not possible to determine how closely that relates to twenty-first century dementia diagnoses. Five per cent were judged to be unsuitable for admission to a lunatic asylum as they were 'not insane' or 'mentally feeble'. Around 27 per cent of older patients were discharged, which is lower than the overall recovery rate for Kew Asylum of 37.8 per cent for 1871–1888 as documented in the 1888 Inspector General Annual Report. Over sixty per cent of older admissions died in care and over a quarter of deaths were within three months of admission suggesting that many of these admissions were for a nineteenth-century version of palliative care as was noted in Tasmania. Deaths within a month of admission were not uncommon and as was the case in Tasmania, it is likely many of these cases had terminal delirium.[22,23]

Older admissions to Victorian lunatic asylums increased throughout the second half of the nineteenth century but particularly from the late 1870s. Ballarat asylum opened in 1877 with a specific focus on 'idiots and imbeciles' and while some older patients were transferred there, its main focus was on intellectual disability.[24] The 1878 Inspector General report drew attention to the increase in admissions aged 50 years and over since 1875 and within that there had been a doubling of admissions aged 60 years and over. Deaths were increasingly being attributed to old age.[25] It was during this period in 1876–1877 that the 'Vagabond Papers' appeared in Melbourne newspapers under the pseudonym 'Julian Thomas' and were later compiled into a book. They were the work of American reporter Stanley James who worked as an attendant at Kew and Yarra Bend asylums. He commented:

> 'I see ... a number of poor, harmless men, who, imbecile to a certain extent, their minds having fallen into second childishness before the decay of their bodies, are certainly not, according to the ideas of the old world, fit inmates of a lunatic asylum.'[26]

The opening of Sunbury Asylum in 1879 helped reduce overcrowding but the transfers were mainly younger patients. In 1879, the report from Ararat Asylum noted that 'the majority of patients have been in a very weak state from old age or advanced brain disease, and many of these have died not very many days after admission'.[27] Reading these annual reports gives the impression of numerous older admissions that were inappropriate and could have been avoided, but lost in that overview is the personal struggles that many families endured. In April 1879 the *Camperdown Chronicle* reported on the lunacy hearing of an old man from Camperdown, who suffered from unsoundness of mind of varying degrees, but his family had not noted any serious consequences and so had not taken any action until the previous Friday when 'the symptoms took a turn for the worse' and a strict watch was necessary. On the Saturday he became violent and needed a straitjacket, 'while this was being put on, the struggles of the unfortunate man were something fearful and the assistance of no fewer than five men were put into requisition'. This deterioration into 'acute mania' resulted in his admission to Kew asylum.[28]

In his 1880 report, Paley listed all of the admissions from benevolent asylums, gaols and hospitals and comments that most of those aged 40 and over were in advanced stages of bodily disease, although only eleven were aged 60 years and over. The main deficit related to the inadequacy of resources to care for those with severe physical disabilities and any suggestion of lunacy opened the door to access institutional care ill-designed for the purpose but better than the alternatives.[29]

In the 1881 Inspector General Report, the report from Yarra Bend gave the most specific, insightful, and detailed summary of concerns about the admission of older patients:

> 'A considerable number of patients were admitted suffering from chronic disease and the impairment of mind consequent of old age, and who hardly required the restraint of an asylum for the insane, but were more suitable as inmates of a benevolent home. These patients for the most part being incurable, and having no friends able to assist them, become a burden on the asylum until relieved by death .... patients of this class being feeble and helpless, and frequently uncleanly in their habits, absorb much time and care from the attendants in our hospital wards, and they might with advantage be cared for in a benevolent asylum at much less cost to the State.'[30]

While Paley is probably correct in stating that that many of these patients did not require psychiatric care and identifies the level of physical care such older patients require, his solution that they be cared for in a benevolent asylum, which in that era had less capacity to provide such care, was clearly impractical.

Paley continued his campaign in his 1882 report in which he describes a 65-year-old man, admitted to Ararat from Ballarat around 100 kilometres away, who had large bedsores and was unable to walk on admission and died a week later. Paley comments:

> 'To send such a man in such a condition to a lunatic asylum is, in my opinion, unnecessary and wholly unjustifiable ... I think it would be well if magistrates were counselled before ordering the conveyance of a feeble person to an asylum to obtain from one of the certifying medical men a written statement that the patient is in a fit condition of bodily health to bear removal to his destination.'[31]

These observations about the appropriateness of psychiatric admission and the importance of ensuring that an older person's physical health needs are considered before embarking on a long transfer remain pertinent today.

Despite the large investment over the previous two decades with the opening of five new asylums, there was concern that the number of patients continued to grow and that there were ongoing complaints. The 1884 Royal Commission chaired by Ephraim Zox (the Zox Commission) sat for two years and was given a broad remit to enquire into the public and private asylums for the insane and inebriates including their management, processes of classification, remedial treatments, staffing and their qualifications and policies regarding large metropolitan asylums.[32] A key recommendation of the Zox Commission was to increase the powers of the medical superintendents of asylums and the setting up of receiving houses to facilitate medical assessments.[33] It recommended closing both Yarra Bend and Kew Asylums and favoured the cottage style accommodation of Yarra Bend but the economic depression that followed a few years later stymied that.[34] It was also critical of Paley, who had retired, regarding his conflicts of interest in tendering processes and being the inspector of lunatic asylums while being the superintendent of an asylum.[35]

While the Zox Commission was sitting, the 1885 Inspector General Report continued the theme about older patients and extended it:

> 'A considerable number of persons advanced in years have been admitted into the asylums … Many of these were feeble and helpless, their mental weakness having supervened upon bodily decay. This class of patients could be cared for outside of an asylum, as could a considerable proportion of the older population accumulated in these institutions.'[36]

Here the report clearly identifies that there were two populations of older patients in the asylums – those admitted in late life and those who grew old in the asylums, and that they could be accommodated elsewhere 'at a reduced cost'. The 1885 Inspector General Report later states:

> 'Many of these persons … are not insane in the strict or commonly accepted sense of the word, but rather in their dotage. Their presence in the asylums is objectionable, inasmuch as they occupy space which can ill be spared, and divert the attention of a skilled and expensive staff from their legitimate duty of attending upon patients who have a prospect of recovery.' [37]

Putting aside the reasonable observation that frail and cognitively impaired older people might not be best suited for care in a lunatic asylum, the inherent ageism of the tone in these comments stands out. Their presence is 'objectionable', their care needs are implied to be 'not a legitimate concern' of the 'skilled and expensive staff', and it bemoans the impact of their deaths in the statistics. During this period the Kew patient register records comments such as 'He is only kept in this asylum as no other place to send him to',[38] 'doubtful case for a lunatic asylum',[39] and 'I do not think present condition is a fit case for a lunatic asylum'.[40]

The Kew patient registers from January 1873 to December 1888 indicated that there were 272 patients who were admitted under the age of 60 but were over the age of 60 at discharge, transfer or death. The mean age of admission was 45 years and although the majority were male (56%), this was lower than for the older admissions. The spread of diagnoses was broader than in the older admissions with fewer cases of dementia and more cases of delusional insanity and mania. Only ten per cent were discharged, the majority died (56.3%). These patients spent an average of nearly 23 years at Kew and as nearly a third were transferred to another asylum after the age of 60, the overall average length of stay was longer. On average these patients spent nearly nine years at Kew when they were aged over 60 years, which again underestimates the total time spent. There were 32 patients who resided at Kew for over 40 years, the longest being for 61 years. While few of the males had partners, it is interesting to note that over half of the females were married, a similar observation to that at Tasmania's New Norfolk Asylum.[41]

The late 1880s continued the twin trends of increasing admissions of older people and the ageing of the long-stay population. The number of admissions aged 60 years and over topped ten per cent of admissions by 1886 and numbered over 100 per year by 1888.[42,43] Again in the 1890 annual report attention was drawn to the lack of alternative accommodation for those who were harmless and had incurable conditions often related to old age and yet were being certified as insane.[44] This situation is exemplified by a report in the *Mount Alexander Mail* from the Castlemaine police court in October 1887 when an old man was brought forward on a charge of lunacy. Dr Barr stated that he was suffering from senile dementia and although:

'he did not seem very bad, but still seemed unfit to take care of himself or be at large' and 'as there was no one to take charge of him in a comfortable home, he recommended that he be removed to the Kew asylum, and to that institution the bench committed him'.[45]

Over the 1890s admissions of older people remained a concern, peaking in 1893 when there were 164 admissions aged 60 years and over representing 18.3 per cent of admissions that year.[46] This was when the depression of the early 1890s was at its height and over the latter half of the decade the numbers reduced but still hovered around 15 per cent of admissions at a time when the proportion of people aged 60 years and over in Victoria was around half that. The number of ageing long-stay patients grew rapidly in this decade from 565 aged 60 years and over in 1891 to 910 in 1900, representing around 20 per cent of the long-stay population and with the proportion of female patients increasing over the decade.[47, 48]

The extraordinary growth of Victoria's lunatic asylums in the second half of the nineteenth century likely contributed to overcrowded gaol-like accommodation, poor sanitation, custodial-style care, overuse of restraints, and institutional design that for the most part would be likely to accentuate behavioural disturbances in older people with dementia. End of life care and the nursing management of the bedridden patient was likely to be well below what would be expected today as implied in this report of an inquest into the 1892 death of an old male patient with dementia and delusions at Beechworth Lunatic Asylum. Bedridden from paralysis and a foot abscess, the medical evidence was that he had bed sores for a month. The post-mortem reported a bed sore over the sacrum that was six inches in diameter.[49] This aspect of the evidence raised no concerns at the inquest much in contrast to the allegations of neglect that would likely occur today.

While it was recognised that it was best to separate acutely disturbed patients from those with chronic disorders characterised by apathy and impaired cognition, this was not seen as an age issue. The long-term effects of institutionalisation were becoming apparent yet it was not conceptualised that the chronic withdrawn behaviour was likely the result of institutional care rather than indicative of the need for such care. Alternative solutions were other types of institutions, though in the 1890s a boarding out scheme was trialled without much success.[50]

The extent to which GPI was responsible for dementia in the younger population in this era is not clear. Although only four out of 314 admissions to Kew Asylum in 1887 were diagnosed with GPI, the post-mortem summary in the 1888 Annual Report of the Inspector General listed GPI as being the cause of death in about ten per cent of cases suggesting many were not being clinically diagnosed on admission.[51, 52] It may well be that as the course of illness became clearer in the asylums that clinicians reformulated their admission diagnoses but this was not being formally captured in the casebooks or registers.

A well-known case of GPI was that of Dr Walter Richardson, who was a patient at Yarra Bend in 1878 before his wife took him home to die. He was the father of novelist Henry Handel Richardson who fictionalised her father's life and decline into dementia in his early 50s in *Ultima Thule*, the final volume of her trilogy *The Fortunes of Richard Mahony* that was published some forty years later. In this novel Richardson provides perhaps the best fictional description of the evolution of dementia and its impact upon the person, starkly describes the poor care being provided in the public asylum and the difficulties encountered by relatives trying to visit family members in the asylum. Richardson based her novel on the experiences her mother had with the care of her father and her own observations as a child of her father's cognitive decline and the impact that had on her and the family.[53]

## Benevolent Asylums

During the 1840s about twenty Benevolent and Friendly Societies were established in Melbourne but by the end of the decade it became clear that something more organised was required. The Melbourne Benevolent Asylum opened in 1850 in North Melbourne under the management of the Victorian Benevolent Society. In the early days there were relatively few older people which largely reflected the population demographics of the fledgling colony. The asylum very quickly had funding problems and by 1854 was in debt.[54,55] A report in *The Argus* in 1856 noted dirty utensils, a lack of towels and coldness due to windows and doors being left open at the insistence of the matron. Leaking roofs and inadequate drainage had been a problem from the beginning. The medical care was also criticised. There were also concerns about restrictive regulations, such as the forbidding of personal belongings in the dormitories.[56]

By the end of the 1850s, as increasing numbers of older inmates were admitted, the triple-storey building design with steep staircases was felt to be inappropriate for their needs as many could not walk properly. The most debilitated inmates had to be housed on the ground floor even though most of the wards were on the second and third floors. The asylum increasingly became a geriatric home particularly after the 1860s. By 1870 most deaths were of people aged 60 years and over,[57] with the average age at death increasing from 57 in 1870–1872 to 75 in 1912.[58] In the 1870s and 1880s the majority of inmates were male, approximately double the number of females.[59] Asylum policy was for married couples to be separated as there were male and female dormitories.[60] As the inmates aged and became more infirm their capacity to work diminished yet even in 1898–1899 the vegetable garden was still being maintained by inmates alone.[61]

Other benevolent asylums opened across regional Victoria, some were linked with district hospitals and others were stand alone. The number of benevolent asylum inmates that had dementia is unknown, but it is clear from lunatic asylum records and newspaper reports that it was expected that the benevolent asylum would care for older people with dementia, particularly if the dementia was mild. In 1875 the *Geelong Advertiser* reported that a man, who was remanded on a charge of lunacy, was represented to be:

> 'perfectly harmless, but was getting silly and helpless from natural causes. A woman who knew him appeared in court with a ticket for his admission to the Benevolent Asylum…….as it was evident that he was not such a subject for treatment in a Lunatic asylum as the Act contemplated.'[62]

Despite the likelihood that dementia was prevalent in the benevolent asylums, surprisingly few were transferred to the lunatic asylums. Yet when eight benevolent asylums contributed to the Victorian Royal Commission on old age pensions in 1898, not one mentioned mental disability as a cause of destitution.[63]

The benevolent asylums were not intended to restrict the freedom of the inmates. So it is not surprising that some with dementia wandered away or would not stay. In 1888 the *Mount Alexander Mail* reported the lunacy hearing of a man who, according to medical evidence, suffered from dementia with delusions, loss of memory and inability to care for himself. He had wandered away, become lost and was discovered in a water hole. He had no property and no one to look after him. He had been sent to the benevolent asylum twice but refused to stay. He was committed to Kew Asylum.[64] Here the lunatic asylum became the default form of care as the Lunacy Act provided the legal grounds to hold the person against their will.

## General Hospitals

Victoria was the best-served of the colonies with bed numbers, having one bed for every 395 persons.[65] Hospitals were intended to focus on the acute care of individuals that were expected to recover. This became an issue of public concern when hospitals refused to admit acutely unwell patients who were incurable. This included terminal cancer as well as conditions such as dementia. In 1882 a complaint was made to the Melbourne Hospital Management Committee for refusing to admit a man who was vomiting blood. According to *The Age*, 'Dr Miller stated that he refused the man admission as he was suffering from senile dementia. He could not recover and to all appearance there was no reason why he should not live for months.' Dr Miller then came to the crux of the issue 'there were patients in the institution who had been suffering from that malady, and occupying beds to the exclusion of acute cases, for six months.'[66] He went on to say 'if he admitted all cases of the kind he would soon have the hospital full. As it was the institution resembled a poor house too much already and when cases like that of (G) were admitted, it was very difficult to get rid of them.' The Committee were informed that Dr Miller had been given instructions to keep such patients out of the hospital and accepted his explanation.[67] Dr Miller implied that the patient was in a stable condition when his admission was refused, and presuming that was the case, then perhaps his decision was similar to current practice. But the big difference is that Dr Miller did not appear to regard it as his responsibility to consider what alternative forms of care were required for such a patient. The other issue is that even in the early 1880s Melbourne Hospital was starting to accumulate long-stay patients with dementia resulting in bed management problems.

Another case occurred in 1875 at Maryborough hospital when an old man 'suffering from softening of the brain and senile dementia, and as no lunatic ward was attached to the Maryborough hospital, the presence of (the patient) in the general wards was considered injurious to other patients.' Dr Dunn, the resident surgeon, took the patient from the hospital and placed him on the public street adjoining the watch house with the expectation that the police would arrest him and send him to the lunatic asylum. The police did not believe that he was a lunatic, refused to arrest him, and left him on the footpath where he remained for some time exposed to the weather. The hospital refused to re-admit him, he was taken care of by local residents before being sent to Kew asylum where he died within days. A Government board of inquiry found Dr Dunn to be guilty of a grave error of judgement and regretted that neither Dr Dunn nor the police had followed the course laid out in the Lunacy Statute.[68] This case demonstrates a second type of concern regarding people with dementia in general hospitals that still resonates in the twenty-first century – anxiety about how to safely manage behavioural disturbances in the ward. Yet very few such patients were transferred to lunatic asylums.

## The Community

Evidence that there were older people living in the community with serious mental disorders can be gleaned from a few newspaper reports. In 1886, a 66-year-old blind newspaper salesman who sat on the corner of Bourke and Swanston Streets in Melbourne, was admitted to hospital after drinking hard for some time suffering the long-term effects of alcoholism and pneumonia, dying two days later.[69] In 1895, an 85-year-old widow 'declining in her dotage', died after wandering six miles from her son's home in Traralgon in order to see her late husband at Echuca as she didn't recognise that he was dead.[70]

Suicidal behaviour is another indicator of mental disorders in the community. Simon Cooke examined coroner's inquests on suicide in 154 persons aged 60 years and over in Victoria in the period 1841 to 1921. He presented data on suicide rates in Victoria between 1869 and 1913 that show the male rates to be much higher than female rates across the age range but particularly so after the age of 60. Throughout the period male suicide rates peaked in those aged

60 years and over, being highest in the period 1879–1883 when they reached around 80 per 100,000, and 1889–1993 when they were over 70 per 100,000. In contrast female rates peaked at around 10 per 100,000. In comparing the older suicides in his sample with the younger cohort, Cooke notes that older people were less likely to be found insane in the coroner's verdicts, for example, only 42 per cent of the older men were described as insane, while 58 per cent of the younger cohort were found insane.[71]

Two of the three themes that Cooke found in his examination of the coroner's reports are similar to the themes found in the current examination of late life suicide.[72] The first theme was illness and insanity, which included the effects of chronic pain. The second theme, dependency and welfare, emphasised the mix of requiring financial assistance due to the physical inability to work. The third theme, loneliness and isolation, was one Cooke expected to find and one prevalent in current late life suicide but was absent and not mentioned in the inquests or suicide notes. Only four suicides were in institutional settings. However, one pertinent observation was that of the 28 male suicides that lived alone, all but two lived in rural Victoria. Cooke described the suicide of a 93-year-old man in 1896 that caused much discussion in the Victorian press after Coroner Greene found that he committed self-murder, or *felo de se*, which meant that he was in a sound state of mind, the consequence being in Victorian law at the time that he be buried at night. Much discussion occurred in Parliament which led to repealing of the law condemning suicides to night burial.[73]

The suicide of prominent pastoralist Thomas Chirnside, a single man aged 72, in June 1887 exemplifies a number of the themes identified by Cooke. Thomas and his brother Andrew established extensive properties with sheep runs in western Victoria from the 1840s. Thomas Chirnside was the first pastoralist in the district to employ Aboriginal men as station hands. He was a breeder of Hereford cattle and horses, a director of the National Bank of Australasia. A religious man, he was popular in his local community. From 1884 he was plagued by sickness becoming morbidly depressed. He had transferred most of his estate to his family but, believing himself bankrupt, shot himself, leaving an estate valued at over £100,000.[74] In the weeks leading up to his death he had been drinking heavily, 'during which he frequently exhibited suicidal tendencies' and was placed under treatment. He had suffered 'depression of spirits' at intervals for some months.[75] On the day of his suicide, he insisted on having alcohol after lunch, but was refused it by his relatives and a little later they heard the gunshot.[76] What is highlighted by Chirnside's suicide and not mentioned in Cooke's study is the role of alcohol. Here the abuse of alcohol appeared to accentuate his depressed mood and suicidal tendencies and the efforts of the family to control its use were unsuccessful.

At the end of the nineteenth century, Victoria had the largest population of older people in Australia and the number of older people institutionalised in lunatic and benevolent asylums was increasing. There was little assistance available in the community for older people who were unable to work and required support, particularly those without families. After much debate, a restricted old age pension scheme for those who were deemed to be deserving commenced in 1899 but this would hardly provide viable community support. It was little wonder that institutional care proliferated.

Chapter 7

# Nineteenth Century South Australia, Western Australia and Queensland

## South Australia

South Australia was founded as a free colony in 1836 with a system of colonisation proposed by Edward Gibbon Wakefield which envisaged a low number of dependents and thus there was little planning to support the sick, the poor, and those with mental illness.[1] The early efforts to care for lunatics in the colony followed the practice in other colonies and the Adelaide Gaol was used. By 1849 it was overcrowded.[2] The first mention of an older patient is in Bostock's *Dawn of Australian Psychiatry*. A 60-year-old patient with delusions of persecution accused a keeper of brutally assaulting him and that there was a conspiracy between Colonial Surgeon Nash, the keepers, and his son-in-law. Dr Nash's report to the Colonial Secretary noted that the injuries were imagined and at times the patient was violent and required restraint.[3]

The Adelaide Lunatic Asylum was built at the eastern end of North Terrace and opened in 1852. Within two years it was overcrowded and part of Adelaide Gaol was modified and declared a lunatic asylum in 1854. Continual overcrowding and poor design of the Adelaide Asylum did not allow for sufficient patient classification, remaining an issue through the 1850s and 60s.[4] Relatively few older patients were admitted to the lunatic asylums in this period partly because senile older people were admitted to the Destitute Asylum. The older patients were those unmanageable in the Destitute Asylum or long-stay patients that had grown old in the asylum.[5] In October 1859 William Whitridge addressed the Adelaide Philosophical Society and provided details of the first 412 lunacy admissions to Adelaide Lunatic Asylum and its predecessor from 1846 to 1859 and found that only nine were aged 60 years and over.[6] Whitridge appreciated that an age-related understanding of the prevalence in the community is required to interpret these data. In the 1861 Census 1.7 per cent of the South Australian population was aged 60 years and over,[7] but even these low admission numbers represented over two per cent of admissions.[8]

There were relatively few long-stay patients in the lunatic asylum as there were no legal requirements for the Adelaide Lunatic Asylum to admit such patients under the *1847 Lunacy Act* and the Destitute Asylum provided an alternative form of care.[9,10] This meant that recovery rates were high in the period 1858–1866 and that the medical superintendent Robert Waters Moore was able to use moral treatment as the preferred model of care. The use of the Destitute Asylum gradually declined from the mid-1850s when 25 per cent of the Destitute Asylum adult inmates were classified as 'idiots and imbeciles' in 1856 to thirteen per cent in 1868, by which time the *1864 Lunacy Act* and its revisions were in place.[11] The *1864 Lunacy Act* gave provisions for the admission of 'lunatics wandering at large, not being properly taken care of, or being cruelly treated' to be admitted to the lunatic asylum.[12] This of course would include the 'idiots and imbeciles', in essence, those with chronic mental disorders where cognition was affected that included chronic psychoses, dementia and intellectual disability, who had been previously housed in the Destitute Asylum.

After the mid-1860s there was a move away from moral treatment, with its greater attribution of psychological factors in causation of lunacy, towards a medicalised focus, with its greater attribution of neurobiological factors in causation, as had been happening in Europe and North America. This coincided with the new Lunacy Act and the appointment of Colonial Surgeon Alexander Paterson. Moral treatments such as activity programs, which tended to improve quality of life, were used less frequently and there was a restorative approach with rest and diet, improving health, and a greater reliance on restraints, sedating drugs such as chloral hydrate, and seclusion rooms for treatment of behavioural issues. Recovery rates declined. Evelyn Shlomowitz and Stephen Garton speculate that it was the change in treatment focus and greater reliance on custodial aspects of care that reduced the recovery rates. Day to day decisions about the use of these interventions was left in the hands of the attendants many of whom were untrained.[13] While this was a likely factor, Paterson notes in his 1870 Annual Report, as reproduced in the *South Australia Chronicle and Weekly Mail*, that the lower recovery rate that year (41.8 per cent) was likely due to the increase in senile dementia and GPI admissions and still compared favourably with Scottish asylums.[14]

The Parkside Asylum opened in 1870 but only one of its three pavilions had been built. There was insufficient day space and the airing courts construction did not commence until 1877. Parkside was incomplete until well into the 1880s; the patients were limited to the airing courts for exercise until 1883 as there were no boundary walls. Overcrowding continued and the number of patients in the lunatic asylums progressively increased.[15] In 1870 there were 307 patients,[16] by 1900 there were 978 patients remaining in the two asylums with the ageing of the long-stay patients being commented on.[17] Thus, while it had been intended for Parkside Asylum to replace Adelaide Asylum, the latter remained open until 1902 with small additions including a bathroom for feeble and aged women being completed in 1886.[18] An 'eyewitness' visiting the Adelaide Asylum in 1878 observed that the male patients with dementia, which he described reasonably based on the work of Esquirol, were housed in the ground floor 'A' ward for dirty patients, who were not all elderly, and were categorised as refractory.[19]

After a series of complaints and letters in the press documenting cruelty and violent acts towards patients by the attendants, a Royal Commission was held in 1884. One problem identified was poor patient classification by Paterson, who was using social distinction rather than behavioural risk to classify patients, which often resulted in violent patients being mixed with the quiet and harmless patients. The overcrowding accentuated the problems and the Royal Commission concluded that the 'attendants had used undue violence to control the behaviour in consequence of their close proximity'.[20] The Royal Commission also reported the lack of activities and patient boredom as being a major problem.

In his 1886 Annual Report on Hospitals for the Insane, Dr Paterson provides some details of patients aged 60 years and over. Of the 122 discharges for the year, six were aged 60 years and over. A review of deaths from the previous decade revealed that 25 per cent were in patients aged 60 years and over.[21] The 1900 Annual Report was summarised in the *Adelaide Observer* where it was noted that the majority of deaths from senile decay were in patients who had been recently admitted and that 'it is sad to reflect that these aged persons could not have managed to end their days in their own homes. As a matter of fact, however, their mental condition rendered them unconscious of this deprivation'. [22] As far back as 1871 Paterson had commented in his Annual report that many patients were dying due to old age or bodily exhaustion that could scarcely be regarded as insanity. He felt that they were in a lunatic asylum due to the lack of a hospital for people suffering incurable disease and the challenges for friends and neighbours to care for them at home. Paterson acknowledged that at least they had the benefits of medical and nursing care in the asylum which was when all was considered perhaps the best and easiest option available. [23] Yet the level of concern about older admissions did not reach those expressed in NSW, Tasmania and Victoria.

The Adelaide Destitute Asylum opened in 1852 and from the outset, unlike the other benevolent asylums in colonial Australia, it conceived its role as being primarily medical in providing long-term care for those with chronic illnesses, hence its willingness to admit people with chronic mental disorders. [24] At the time South Australia had the lowest number of hospital beds per capita amongst the colonies which might have influenced this approach. [25] The Destitute Asylum developed an aged care focus with ageing single male labourers being the main admissions by the late 1860s. [26] In June 1885 the asylum was overcrowded, the average age of male inmates was 70 years and female inmates 64 years. [27] According to Pat Jalland, the average inmate was far more debilitated than the inmates of benevolent asylums in NSW and Victoria. Jalland observes that in 1887–88 three quarters of the 223 admissions were older migrants with no relatives in Australia, or none willing to support them. Many of the older inmates were transferred from the hospital with chronic incurable conditions and up to 75 per cent were expected to die in the asylum. [28] In June 1900, 295 persons were aged over 61 years, with 96 admissions in the previous financial year on the grounds of old age and infirmity. [29]

The number of older inmates with dementia is unknown and transfer to a hospital for the insane would tend to occur when the inmate's behaviour became a challenge. For example, the 1886 Annual Report on Hospitals for the Insane noted that five older patients were admitted from the Destitute Asylum, four with dementia and one with alcohol related problems.[30] But it is also clear that there were inmates with severe dementia provided with high level end of life care at the Destitute Asylum as noted from this 1894 response to a letter received by the *Adelaide Observer* that questioned the medical care at the asylum. The death of an 83-year-old man from 'senile decay' was described in some detail. Dr Clindening was reported to state '(he) had a reticent incoherent manner and eventually got into the condition of senile dementia, becoming quite imbecile. For months he had to be handfed. He was paid every possible attention, I can assure you. His diet was changed from full diet to sick diet for several months.' Other staff who were interviewed agreed with this summation.[31]

Despite having a good reputation, the Destitute Asylum still had restrictive institutional practices such as separating married couples, the wearing of asylum clothing, and strict rules.[32] Pejorative attitudes towards it were present in the community, for example, the *South Australian Advertiser* published reports from the Destitute Board in a column headed 'Social Evils'.[33] A report in the *Adelaide Advertiser* in May 1898 commented on the 'apparent aimlessness and joyless nature of the lives of the male inmates' who took no interest in the library and games provided but 'were sitting in rows on benches, to all appearances without any occupation but their own thoughts'.[34] Later in 1898 a more positive view was expressed in a report in the *Weekly Herald* that observed high quality care from nurses and attendants who enjoyed their work despite the overcrowded conditions and the pressing demands of changing the linen of bedridden incontinent senile inmates.[35]

Several suicides and suicide attempts in older Destitute Asylum inmates were reported. In 1880, a 74-year-old man, described as quiet and sensible, cut his throat. He had been despondent about his daughter's failed business. He had been living in the asylum for 9 months despite being in good health and having a son and daughter.[36] A 72-year-old man, had been an inmate of the Destitute Asylum on and off for 22 years when he cut his throat with a knife in 1889. He had a previous suicide attempt by the same method two years earlier and had been in the lunatic asylum for seven months. He was described as a morose man in good health but having to go around on crutches. Dr Clindening from the Destitute Asylum felt he should have been kept in the lunatic asylum as he still seemed to harbour suicidal tendencies.[37]

As in Australia today, for some older people the thought of having to move to an institution for the rest of their days could precipitate suicide. A bushman in his mid-60s died of a strychnine overdose in 1875 at the Bushmen's Club in Adelaide. After he had taken the overdose, he told William Smith, who found him that he wanted to die as he dreaded the Destitute Asylum. According to Smith, who had known him for about a decade, 'his habits were steady, and I never saw him 'the worse of liquor', but he was old and feeble, and sometimes childish. I think his mind was a little light occasionally'. While a number of witnesses deputed that he had not noticed any suggestion of insanity, the inquest jury determined that he had 'committed suicide while in a despondent state of mind produced by physical weakness and straitened circumstances.'[38]

In contrast to the other colonies, the South Australian government through the Destitute Board provided a large amount of outdoor relief. While not primarily directed towards the aged and infirm, they were a group in receipt of support with one advantage being that it was provided where they lived whether in town or country. Throughout the second half of the nineteenth century South Australian newspaper reports illustrated that there were older people with mental disorders residing in their own homes. An 1873 lunacy hearing of a 64-year-old farmer demonstrated a high level of appropriate concern of his well-being by the Primary Judge in Equity, Mr Justice Gwynne, who relocated the hearing from the Supreme Court in Adelaide to the Strathalbyn Local Courthouse in the neighbourhood to which the farmer lived and where all the witnesses resided to reduce expense and inconvenience. The hearing was precipitated by difficulties encountered in the attempted sale of the farm. According to his oldest daughter, there was about a three-year history of her father having various delusions that included that he was 'Our Saviour', at other times an angel, at other times Napoleon Bonaparte. His conversational skills had diminished and although he had neglected his farm he was under the false impression that it was prospering. Neighbours and a local labourer also described his delusions which led to him refusing payment for work done. The auctioneer instructed to sell the farm became concerned when the farmer called him the Prophet Daniel. None of the witnesses expressed concern about his memory, a point identified by Justice Gwynne who commented after medical evidence, that he did not think the malady was senile dementia. The jury concluded that he was of unsound mind and incapable of managing his affairs. Apart from the detailed account of a late life psychosis, this report indicates that there was no attempt to commit him to a lunatic asylum, the entire hearing was about his competency to manage his affairs. In other words the expectation was that his family would look after him at home.[39]

## Western Australia

Slow population growth in the early days of the colony meant that the few mentally ill patients were cared for in temporary accommodation including the first prison, the Fremantle Round House and when convict transportation commenced in 1850, in the Colonial Hospital.[40] In the 1850s and 1860s the colony was struggling under an economic recession and the effects of isolation and poverty which fuelled alcohol abuse and despair. The population of Western Australia increased fivefold between 1850 and 1870 through convicts and free settlers, few were elderly, many were poor, with limited education and without extended families.[41]

The arrival of convicts from 1850 onwards increased the number requiring care in an asylum. A temporary lunatic asylum located in Scott's warehouse in 1857 was an unsatisfactory solution being dismal and fetid.[42,43] The Fremantle Lunatic Asylum was built out of local limestone in Dutch Colonial style with convict labour, commencing construction in 1861, opening in 1864, and being completed in 1869.[44, 45] It was designed to house 32 patients but on opening it took 45 patients which exemplified the overcrowding that dogged it throughout and prevented effective patient classification.[46, 47] Most of the patients were male convicts and the management approach was penal in style with the former gaol warders being assisted by convict constables and orderlies whose main role was to subdue and restrain.[48] There are no specific records of older patients for this early period but it is unlikely that there were many as in the 1861 census only 308 persons aged 60 years and over (2 per cent) were recorded in the colony, increasing to 684 persons (2.9 per cent) in 1870.[49]

Throughout the nineteenth century there was lack of psychiatric expertise in the medical staff. The first medical practitioner in the colony to have psychiatric training was Dr Sydney Montgomery who arrived in 1901.[50] The first Lunacy Act, proclaimed in 1871, was inspired by the British Act of 1845 and provided better legal safeguards, record keeping and supervision with a Board of Visitors and a Board of Inquiry to guard against irregularities of admission and discharge, and the ill-treatment of patients.[51]

With the perennial overcrowding, the Fremantle Asylum had to use all available space for dormitories which meant there were no recreation areas. Patients were kept outside most of the day in bare areas. At night the darkly painted rooms were dimly lit and patients had to use a bucket in the middle of the dormitory as a toilet. With the incontinent patients this meant that there was a perpetual foul odour. The barred windows were small which hindered ventilation. In addition there were restrictions on bathing with only one bath allowed per week, with the water shared between three people.[52] Repeated complaints about the conditions and overcrowding featured regularly in the annual reports of the medical superintendent Dr Henry Barnett from 1873 onwards but without much impact.[53] A series of extensions were built between 1886 and 1896, but a Parliamentary Select Committee was informed in 1891 that the building could never comply with hospital standards.[54] Roger Virtue observed that the lack of knowledge about contemporary views on the treatment of mental illness from Europe, North America or even from other Australian colonies hindered the Committee in its desire for reform. The lack of medical expertise meant that the approach to manage insanity was still based on legal rather than medical principles.[55] Overcrowding increased in the 1890s after the gold rushes resulting in the reorganisation of facilities and planning for a new asylum.[56] In this period there was high mortality in part due to endemic typhoid and medical superintendent Barnett had to discharge patients prematurely and at times refuse admissions.[57]

A complaint about nurse cruelty in the female section of the Fremantle asylum in 1898 led to the removal of one nurse after an investigation requested by F.C.B. Vosper MLA, who was also editor of the *Sunday Times*, and prompted his concern about mental illness as a social problem. As federation approached, comparisons with the lunatic asylums and mental health systems in other colonies, particularly Victoria and NSW, emphasised how poor the development was in Western Australia.[58] In October 1900, two letters in the press, one from the husband of a woman who died in the asylum, the other from a former patient, described the poor physical conditions, use of restraints, and poor medical treatment in the asylum and led to a parliamentary debate. A parliamentary select committee inquiry with Vosper as chair tabled its report in November 1900, which recommended the demolition of the Fremantle asylum and construction of a new asylum. The need for some experienced attendants was stressed (the inquiry heard that only one of the seventeen attendants had any prior asylum experience) and it recommended the appointment of a medical officer whose sole duties would be to administer to the insane. Parliament was prorogued in December 1900 leaving a number of issues including the response to this inquiry up in the air.[59]

In 1896 there were still eighteen male ex-convict patients who on average had been in the asylum for 30 years. Colonial women were the other group of long-stay patients, particularly those who were widows or those sent there by disgruntled husbands who accused them of neglect of domestic duties.[60] I examined the register of patients remaining in Fremantle Asylum in 1901 which indicated that by 1900, when the Fremantle Asylum held 277 patients, there were at least 35 patients (12.6%) aged 60 years and over, of whom fourteen had been admitted at the age of 60 years or over. Around two-thirds of those admitted in late life were given a dementia diagnosis with 'old age' and 'alcohol' identified as the main causes. Two had been transferred from the old men's home or invalid depot.[61]

Perhaps the most notorious older patient of the Fremantle Asylum was Joseph Bolitho Johns, otherwise known as the bushranger Moondyne Joe. He was transported to the colony for larceny arriving in May 1853, granted a conditional pardon in 1855 but was arrested for horse stealing in 1861 having worked from an isolated gorge on the Avon River known as Moondyne Springs. Subsequently, he escaped, was recaptured and served three years' imprisonment, but after release was sentenced in 1865 to ten years for killing an ox with the intent of stealing the carcass. Over the period from late 1865 until early 1867 Moondyne Joe escaped three times. Despite being locked in irons in solitary confinement, he managed to escape again during an exercise period, remaining free for two years. After recapture he was released again in 1871 and became a respectable stockman and timber-feller. His wife died in 1893 and in 1900, when in his early 70s, he was found wandering the streets in a confused state and ordered to the Mount Eliza Invalid Depot. He managed to escape from there and because of increasing senility was committed to the Fremantle asylum with dementia where he died in

August 1900. Moondyne Joe is regarded as Western Australia's only bushranger of note capturing the public imagination with his frequent escapes.[62, 63]

The gold rush era in the 1890s witnessed a spate of suicidal behaviour in older people reported in the media with the main themes of difficult marital relationships and alcohol abuse as exemplified with this report. In 1894, an 84-year-old man who ran a boarding house, shot himself after an argument with his young second wife about money that had gone missing. Their relationship had been troubled for some time and they had recently been separated for two months. He had accused her of living with another man which she denied. She had repeatedly been charged in the police court with being drunk and disorderly. On the day of the suicide they had been summoned to court over a charge that she had assaulted him but as they were walking to the court, he said that he did not want to press charges and they went to the hotel to drink together. After a drink, he went home to sleep. She returned in the afternoon with a carter to take her luggage. He then went to the hotel with the carter, had five or six drinks but was said not to be drunk. It was at this point he claimed money was missing from his wallet and accused his wife of taking it. She denied it, he went looking for a revolver, said it was missing but shortly after a shot was heard. His wife claimed that he frequently threatened to shoot her and kill himself.[64, 65]

In 1869 the Mt Eliza convict depot became an invalid depot that housed destitute and invalid males and continued to be financed by the British government.[66] At the outset there were 83 mainly old and invalid ex-convict males and over time it became a home for the aged and infirm as there were many ageing ex-convict males without family support. The Poor House for Women was a much younger population in this era and included children.[67] During the 1870s and 1880s the population of Western Australia aged rapidly to the extent that amongst the colonies in the 1881 census it had the second highest proportion of persons aged 60 years and over (5.3 per cent) with the number of older persons more than doubling in the previous decade. As in Tasmania, this was driven by the ageing of the convicts and their being relatively few younger immigrants. By 1901 only 3.3 per cent of its population was aged 60 years and over due to the influx of younger immigrants in the gold rush.[68]

In 1877, regulations for the government poor houses were proclaimed which made them akin to gaols. The regulations gave the inmates little freedom as their privacy and independence was lost and there were few conveniences. Mt Eliza was often overcrowded but plans to rebuild in the mid-1870s were not followed through. An 1878 Commission of Inquiry reported that many of the invalid males were ex-convicts who had attained a great age and were unfit for work. There were few staff in the depot, for example, in 1886 under the Officer in charge, William Dale, there was a Master, a cook and one orderly who between them had to manage over 120 men, many of whom were aged and infirm.[69] An unfulfilled proposal to unite the Invalid Depot with the Fremantle Convict depot and move them to Freshwater Bay commented about the mental infirmity of the older inmates drawing attention to a recent drowning suicide of an inmate and that prevention was possible by not having a river frontage – a suggestion ahead of its time in recognising that suicide prevention includes removing access to means.[70]

## Queensland

Until Queensland became a self-governing colony in December 1859 it was administered from NSW and patients with serious mental disorders were transferred to Tarban Creek Asylum, those with chronic disease who were in hospital for more than two months were transferred to Parramatta Invalid and Lunatic Asylum.[71] There were often long delays as the process required a warrant to be sent to Sydney and returned by ship before the patient was transported to Sydney. Patients often died before the warrants were returned and the Brisbane Hospital Committee in 1854 resolved to refuse admissions of lunatics.[72] The transfer to Sydney could also be a challenging process as noted in this case history taken from the medical casebooks of Gladesville Hospital. A married man in his 60s was transferred to Tarban Creek from Wide Bay, 200 kilometres north of Brisbane, with a diagnosis of senile mania and delusions that had been present for ten months following a robbery that had caused him great shock. On the voyage to Sydney he attempted to throw himself overboard. Subsequently he threatened his wife's life. At Tarban Creek he was noted to be in great fear and that his 'memory is quite gone'.[73]

After 1859 patients were kept in the Brisbane Gaol or the hospital. This quickly became untenable with the gaol rapidly filling with cases of insanity, many relating to alcohol. The 'lunatic' cases received little in the way of treatment in the gaol with the 'hard labour punishments' for the criminals including 'looking after the lunatics', while the turnkeys brutalised them. Conditions were overcrowded, with open drains to cesspools creating a foul stench, poor ventilation, and enclosures with lack of shade from the sun running the risk of sunstroke.[74]

The first Queensland lunatic asylum, Woogaroo Lunatic Asylum, was opened at Wacol on the south bank of the Brisbane River midway between Brisbane and Ipswich in 1865. It was later renamed Goodna Asylum in 1880.[75] Although touted to have been built on the best model procurable, Colonial Architect Charles Tiffin told an 1869 inquiry that 'not a tithe' of his plans had been followed in the design.[76] Dr Kearsey Cannan, who had provided the medical care to the lunatics in the gaol, was appointed as the first medical superintendent but was dismissed for 'gross mismanagement' and 'unfitness' after an inquiry by a joint select committee of parliament in 1869.[77, 78] The inquiry found that conditions in the asylum resembled a gaol; fifty-four women were confined to bedboards in the corridor, there was no bath, no drainage, exercise yards were ankle deep in mud, all the patient's clothes were soiled, and there was an intolerable stench. It was reported that at night, ten to twelve dirty patients were placed in the sick ward with the dying and locked in until the morning, with those that died doing so unattended and often being buried before being seen by a doctor. One man had actually been buried alive.[79]

Cannan's replacement, Henry Challinor, introduced recreational activities, proper record keeping, and improved sanitation but had to resign in 1872 due to typhoid fever acquired from the poor asylum conditions. His repeated requests to get conditions improved were largely ignored. *The Lunacy Act of 1869* established reception houses, which were subsequently opened in Brisbane, Townsville, Rockhampton and Maryborough, where disturbed patients could be committed by magistrates for up to a month instead of the asylum.[80] These, however, provided little treatment and were more akin to gaols where the patients were treated in a punitive way.[81]

John Jaap became the medical superintendent in 1872 and noted that there was a sense that the patients had been sent to Woogaroo for punishment rather than comfort or treatment. He abolished the wooden cages that had housed violent patients in the exercise yard. He drew attention to the poorly ventilated conditions in the male division which he regarded as not fit for human habitation. Staff were untrained and often illiterate, many feared the patients and treated them insensitively and in an intimidatory manner.[82] In 1877 a Royal Commission into Woogaroo Asylum and the reception houses heard reports of outdated treatments including patients being strapped to a bathroom door and having cold water directed from above onto their head and shoulders, use of physical restraints, and chloral hydrate for sedation.[83] The Commission heard that due to overcrowding, classification of the patients could only be imperfectly carried out.[84] The report recommended that there be proper medical supervision of interventions such as physical restraints and use of chloral hydrate which had often been used indiscriminately by warders.[85] *The Insanity Act (1884)* included the appointment of an Inspector of Asylums for the Insane, with Dr Richard Scholes being appointed as the first Inspector in 1885.[86]

Due to overcrowding at Woogaroo, asylums were opened at Ipswich in 1878 and Toowoomba in 1890 with little impact and by 1899 there were 1111 patients at Goodna.[87] How many were aged 60 years and over is not clear as specific age-related information is not available. While Queensland had the lowest proportion of its population aged 60 years and over for most of the second half of the nineteenth century, there was a 64-fold increase between 1861 and 1901.[88] Around eight to ten per cent of admissions in the 1890s are likely to have been aged 60 years and over if a similar pattern to other colonies occurred. The *Gympie Times and Mary River Mining Gazette* reported the admission of a 65-year-old widow who had never really recovered from the disappearance of her infant son from a frontier outstation followed by the unrelated death of her husband a quarter of a century earlier. Despite remarrying, she had never ceased hoping her child would return.[89] Reports of older suicides featured in the newspapers with issues such as unrelieved pain, alcohol abuse and family troubles being mentioned. One example from 1888 involved a 60-year-old labourer who shot himself in the Maryborough Botanic Gardens. He had recently had a serious family dispute and had been drinking heavily for a few days. He had also frequently threatened to commit suicide.[90]

After self-government in December 1859 the Brisbane hospital was no longer able to send its incurable cases to Sydney and within a year was requesting a

Benevolent Asylum building. The *1861 Benevolent Asylum Wards Bill* established rules and regulations about work expectations and behaviour that did not appear to reflect the limitations imposed by their chronic disabilities and ill health. The Bill allowed inmates to be sent to gaol and kept there on bread and water for up to a month for such 'crimes' as wilfully wasting goods, disobedience, or insubordination. Government funding to support disabled paupers was inadequate, the belief being that private benevolence should contribute, and often these were aged ex-convict men completely unfit to work and frequently bedridden.[91]

The removal of the Benevolent Asylum inmates to the empty Quarantine Station at Dunwich located on remote Stradbroke Island commenced in May 1865. The view prevailed that alcohol was the main cause of the inmates' chronic disabilities and thus sending them to an isolated location would alleviate temptation. There was a sense in Parliamentary debate that Dunwich would be an institution primarily for discipline and restraint although some, such as Dr Sachse from Toowoomba Hospital, disagreed and pointed out that it was hard to distinguish paupers from those with incurable chronic medical disorders and listed categories that included old age.[92] The first sixty inmates transferred to the Dunwich Asylum were placed under the care of Dr Jonathan Labatt, an alcoholic who had previously been admitted to the lunatic asylum in controversial circumstances. In 1864 a Select Parliamentary Committee found that while he had been excitable and eccentric, in all likelihood he had not been insane. While no formal compensation was given, the appointment to Dunwich the following year might be regarded as a gesture by the government.[93] Labatt was in the late stages of the ravages of alcohol abuse. He was excitable in manner and had the habits of frequently repeating the same phrase and at times disagreeably interfering in conversations.[94] Over the following year there were reports of Labatt being intoxicated and in 1866 he was relieved of his duties after an episode of delirium tremens while attending a penal establishment on nearby island St Helena. One of his reports beforehand indicated that he believed that the many inmates had 'senile infirmities and diseases'. As in other Benevolent Asylums around the country, the more able-bodied served as wardsmen to the more disabled for a small remuneration and this process continued unchecked for the next 50 years.[95]

Labatt was replaced by the first of a series of laymen supervisors whose approach to care was one of discipline. Conditions were poor, the buildings were cold with ill-fitting windows and lack of fireplaces. The buildings were dirty and not well-maintained. The food ration skimpy, deplorable and at times rotten. The inmates were unhappy and their insubordinate behaviour reflected that. The 1884 Legislative Council Inquiry heard how violence was part of the asylum management with one witness reporting on how he saw an old demented man being knocked down with a broom and receiving head lacerations, while a 70-year-old female inmate described being physically assaulted by the matron for not taking medication that disagreed with her.[96]

Certain types of chronic disabilities were not admitted to Dunwich with those individuals that were regarded as 'imbecile' or 'epileptic' being redirected to Goodna. Although Dunwich Asylum was intended for 'incurable' cases, the 1884 Inquiry heard that the committal procedures were lax, allowing persons requiring treatment to be admitted without any specific instructions. In 1885, when there were 258 admissions, around a half were over the age of 60, with old age/senility the most common reason. The hospital wards were shunned by many of the inmates as they were regarded as wards for dying people where no treatment could be expected and where the attendants lacked experience. Few changes occurred after the 1884 Inquiry. Dr Patrick Smith, formerly the medical superintendent at Goodna, was appointed medical officer, but overall conditions including food rations and recommended building renovations remained an issue. Over the next decade the number of inmates at Dunwich increased from 397 in 1886 to 877 in 1895. All beds were occupied by 1893 and the overflow was placed in tents.[97] By the 1890s there were repeated reports of the neglect of the inmates' medical needs and how they were ignored for weeks before their death. According to Pat Jalland, in the second half of the nineteenth century Dunwich Asylum was probably the worst asylum of all in Australia.[98]

# Chapter 8

# From Federation to the Second World War

At the time of Federation in 1901 there were over 230 thousand people aged 60 years and over in Australia, which represented 6.2 per cent of the population. Sex ratios had changed with near parity in the younger populations but male predominance remained in the older populations where there were about 128 males to 100 females aged 60 years and over. In the first half of the twentieth century there was a near fourfold increase from just over 233 thousand to over 880 thousand aged 60 years and over, representing an approximate doubling of the proportion in the population to 11.9 per cent in 1945. The other major demographic change occurred in 1934 when the number of women aged 60 years and over outnumbered the number of men for the first time and this has remained the pattern. Life expectancy at birth increased for men from 55.2 years in 1901 to nearly 65 years in 1950 and for women from 58.8 years in 1901 to around 70 years in 1950.[1]

The main policy change that affected older people in this period was the introduction of Commonwealth means tested old age pensions in 1908. These were based on the NSW *Old Age Pensions Act* of 1900 at least in part because of the political impossibility that Prime Minister Alfred Deakin faced if he were try to wind back the pensions in NSW that established the rights of older people to independence and dignity. The exclusions of the NSW Act regarding race, Australian residency, and moral character were retained in the Commonwealth Act. Pensions were available from the age of 65 years for men and 60 years for women.[2] The introduction of old age pensions became a marker of retirement. In accepting an old age pension, it was tacitly understood that the older person should retire from business. Although many continued to work part time, this was not well-received by others and this practice gradually petered out. Those who had jobs held on to them as long as they could as the age pension was inadequate in comparison. There was a steady rise in older people taking the pension. In 1911, only 28 per cent of males aged 65–69 years were classified as dependent and this increased to 52 per cent by 1939. Retirement for some became a process of exclusion from useful activity and loss of self-esteem with all of the implications for mental health.[3]

With Federation, the States were left with the responsibility of running health care including the hospitals for the insane and state hospitals for the aged and infirm. For older people with mental disorders and dementia this meant that from a public health service perspective, acute and long-term residential care were under the same jurisdiction and this remained the case until the 1960s. Thus for the period until the Second World War, dementia was by default a State responsibility, not that this was clearly articulated anywhere. Of course within each State jurisdiction there was concern that increased over the first half of the twentieth century about whether older people with senile mental disorders should be primarily a responsibility of the hospitals for the insane, State-run hospitals for the aged and infirm, or the Government subsidised benevolent asylums.

The pressures upon the State hospitals can be understood by examining the estimates of dementia prevalence in this period. Using the same method described in Chapter 3, the estimated number of persons with dementia in Australia increased by over fourfold from just over nine thousand to nearly 39 thousand between 1901 and 1945, outstripping the growth in the number of older people. Throughout the nineteenth century dementia had been more prevalent in males than females but by 1921 this changed with the estimated number of females with dementia being greater than the number of males, a situation that has not changed over the last century. A large increase in estimated dementia cases (around ten thousand) during the 1930s coupled with the Great Depression provides the backdrop to understanding the large increase in older admissions experienced by the mental hospitals[4], for example, in NSW between 1934–35 and 1940–41, for the 60 years and over age group, there was a 21 per cent increase in admissions and 30 per cent increase in those under care.[5,6]

Before the First World War there was one last growth spurt of mental hospitals in Australia with the opening of six new facilities including Kenmore, Claremont, Mont Park, and Royal Park hospitals and the closure of Adelaide and Fremantle Asylums. The admission of voluntary patients commenced in this period with Eric Sinclair opening a small 'mental ward' attached to the Darlinghurst Reception House for non-certified males in 1908 (even though there was no legislation for voluntary patients in NSW) and in 1914 the introduction of voluntary patients in Victoria.[7] This move was related to the commencement of outpatient clinics which were seen as the setting for early interventions and, as noted by Stephen Garton, the view was that the majority of cases had a hereditary or biological predisposition that became incurable unless treated early. Mental hospitals became regarded as repositories for the incurable.[8]

Across the country older people continued to be admitted to the mental hospitals at rates disproportionate to general population prevalence. Admissions to Fremantle Asylum between 1901 and 1906 before its closure in 1909 reveal that 8.1 per cent were aged 60 years and over at a time when the 60 years and over population in Western Australia was less than four per cent.[9] Over 70 per cent of older admissions were male and 37 per cent were single; over ten per cent were transfers from invalid depots and old people's homes. As with previous research from the nineteenth century in Tasmania and New South Wales, 'old age/senile decay/senility' and 'alcohol' were the two main 'causes' of the insanity assigned by clinicians, although the majority had no cause identified. Where there was information available from thirty-eight completed admissions, the average length of stay was about nine months. However, nearly half of the admissions remained in hospital and their length of incomplete admissions was already two and a quarter years.[10]

Transfer of patients to the new Claremont Mental Hospital commenced in 1908 and while precise details of the number of older admissions is lacking, the Annual Report of the Inspector General of the Insane for 1913, as reported in the *West Australian*, indicates twenty-four patients were diagnosed with senile dementia, senile mania, or senile melancholia.[11] As around 40 per cent of older admissions had another type of diagnosis in the 1901–1906 period, it is likely that there were as many as sixty admissions aged 60 years and over in 1913, a steep increase since 1901. In 1919 over twelve per cent of admissions were aged 60 years and over which was double the proportion of older people in the State population.[12] In the first decade of the new century it soon became apparent that the dying out of the old convicts would not solve the problem of care for the aged and infirm in Western Australia as the overall number continued to rise. In the latter part of the decade all of the old Poor Houses had been closed and new Government homes for old and invalid men and women had been opened at Fremantle (Claremont old men's home at Freshwater Bay) and Geraldton. The old men's home at Claremont was built in 1906 based on a military model design for 400 men who were moved from the Mt Eliza Invalid's Depot.[13] That these developments did not resolve the issues of quality of care is hardly a surprise and in 1916 an inquiry was held into the old men's home at Claremont after allegations of vermin in the wards, staff insubordination, and the victimisation of a staff member by management.[14] The allegations were largely substantiated with the blame being attributed to management,[15] although the Australian Labour Federation claimed that there were insufficient staff.[16] The manager, Master Rust, was initially suspended and then to the disappointment of inmates reappointed by under-secretary North.[17]

In Victoria, while the number of older admissions declined by nearly 18 per cent between 1901 and 1907, in the same period there was a 23 per cent increase in the number of patients aged 60 years and over that remained in the mental hospitals and from 1901 onwards these were predominantly female.[18,19] In 1905 James McCreery, the Inspector General of the Insane, in his last annual report listed the extensive defects in the design and maintenance of the Victorian mental hospitals. While none of the defects were specific for older patients some, such as problems with heating and bathrooms, would have been keenly felt by them.[20]

The period to the end of the First World War in NSW saw the number of admissions aged 60 years and over more than triple, increasing from around nine per cent of admissions in 1901 to over 17 per cent in 1918. This is reflected in an over threefold increase of 'senile' diagnoses during the period, particularly those of senile dementia. While the number of older patients under care steadily increased, this was at about the same rate as other age groups. Discharges of older patients changed little over the period but deaths of older patients more than doubled largely due to ageing long-stay patients.[21,22] It was during this period that Inspector General Eric Sinclair created separate acute and chronic mental hospitals, the latter including Parramatta and Rydalmere, which resulted in a rationalisation of staff and resources to the detriment of the chronic patients, most of whom were older, where staff/patient ratios were around half that in the acute wards increasing the likelihood of custodial care.[23] In his 1913 Annual Report, Sinclair examined admission rates for the previous thirty years, comparing admissions aged 51 years and over with those up to the age of 50. Throughout the period, the proportion of admissions per population were consistently higher in the older population particularly in the period 1903 to 1913.[24] Aftercare, under the leadership of Emily Paterson, began in 1907 as an outreach service for those leaving Gladesville Hospital to assist with employment, temporary accommodation, and provision of support. While it tended to focus on the young, between 1914 and 1922 around fourteen per cent of its clients were elderly, a proportion consistent with the proportion of older discharges.[25]

The hope that the introduction of old age pensions in NSW would solve the problem of the increasing numbers of old people in State Hospitals for the Aged and Infirm were soon dashed. After some decline in numbers in 1902 and 1903, older people found that the meagre ten shillings per week pension was inadequate to sustain them and they drifted back to the State Hospitals.[26] The Rookwood Asylum was placed under medical administration in 1906 and renamed Lidcombe State Hospital and Home. By 1913 there were clinical departments with wards specialising in categories such as chronic neuromuscular diseases.[27]

Royal Commissions were a feature of the period in Tasmania, South Australia and Queensland. Tasmania had by this time become used to Royal Commissions into their institutions and so the 1904 Royal Commission was no surprise and nor were most of the recommendations about New Norfolk. The Official Visitors and Medical Superintendent were recommended to have expanded powers, training of nursing staff to be improved, trial leave for patients increased, and the building of suitable structures to improve patient classification and reduce the use of mechanical restraints. The level of use of restraints and seclusion was compared unfavourably with Victorian and international facilities. The number of older patients at New Norfolk remained higher than the general population. In 1916 sixteen per cent on the patient register were aged 60 years and over with most of the older admissions from the New Town Infirmary.[28]

The Royal Commission of 1909 into Adelaide's Parkside Asylum was principally focused on criminal lunatics but had broader recommendations including the establishment of a receiving house, better patient classification, more medical staff, merit-based grading of attendants, the purchase of an estate for a hospital with larger grounds, and the name to be changed to Parkside Mental Hospital.[29] The purchase of land for a new hospital was postponed due to financial constraints. The passing of the *Mentally Defectives Act* of 1913 saw the official change from 'lunatic' to 'mentally defective' which encompassed both mental illness and mental retardation and the Act included the establishment of a receiving house.[30]

The ageing of the patients at Parkside continued. In his 1911 Annual Report, Dr Cleland noted that there had been a large increase in senile admissions and that

'it is well known that one of the features of senility is the development of restlessness which makes the patient difficult to manage. It seems a pity that these cases of natural decay should have to be sent to a hospital for the insane.'

He recommended a cottage-type home with suitable accommodation and 'extensive and secure pleasure grounds' would be more acceptable to relatives and friends.[31]

By 1915 over 40 per cent of the deaths were aged 65 years and over, some being sent for admission in a weakened state.[32] The Inspector's Annual Report for 1916 noted that there were fifty-three admissions (17.7 per cent) aged 60 years and over.[33] The Adelaide Destitute Asylum closed in 1917 with the inmates being transferred to the Old People's Home at Magill.[34]

In Queensland, by 1908 there were over two thousand patients in the lunatic asylums and in 1910 over twelve hundred in Goodna Asylum alone.[35,36] Conditions had not improved in the asylums since the mid-nineteenth century with allegations of neglect and ill-treatment by inadequately trained staff responsible for the 'mental torture' of patients, overcrowded grossly inadequate facilities, and poor sanitation.[37,38] Dr Henry Ellerton, appointed to the dual post of Inspector of Asylums for the Insane and Medical Superintendent of Goodna Asylum in 1909,[39] had predicted that unless these issues were addressed, there would be an outcry for an inquiry and this occurred as a reaction to newspaper reports in 1915 when Labor Premier T.J. Ryan appointed a Royal Commission.[40] The Royal Commission found most of the criticism was unjustified, although the overcrowding and the need for more staff training were accepted.[41] Between 1915 and 1919 new dormitories and a hospital block were built and more nursing staff were trained.[42] One development that in the long term had a positive impact on old age mental health was the opening of a psychiatric ward in Brisbane General Hospital in 1918.[43] Little information is available about the older patients, though in Ellerton's Annual Report for 1916 he notes that there were fifty-three admissions with senile dementia.[44] Dunwich Asylum continued to be a 'dumping ground' for incurable cases despite the opening of Diamantina Hospital in 1901 for that purpose. Dunwich had few trained staff, adverse conditions were concealed by the authorities, and segregation along racial lines was practised. However, between 1908 and 1919 the number of residents at Dunwich declined by about ten per cent, despite which in 1919 over 250 residents remained living under canvas without sewerage and electricity.[45]

In this period before the First World War, Alfred Deakin, Australia's second prime minister, developed dementia at a young age. Before entering politics in Victoria, Deakin was a barrister and journalist, professions he maintained through most of his political career. He was prominent in the spiritualist movement and in 1877 became president of the Victorian Association of Spiritualists. Politically a Liberal, he was adept at compromise and served as Liberal leader in a coalition Victorian Government in the 1880s. In the late 1880s he became interested in federalism and by the late 1890s was chairman of the Federation League of Victoria and the central figure of the cause in the colony. He formed the National Liberal Organization in 1901 and became the attorney-general and leader of the House in Edmond Barton's cabinet. When Barton retired to the High Court in September 2003, Deakin became prime minister but this was for little more than six months. His second term as prime minister from July 1905 to November 1908 was the most productive and included the Commonwealth's old age pensions. It was during this term that the earliest symptoms of dementia became apparent in his late 40s and early 50s. Upon return from the 1907 Imperial Conference in London and under political pressure, not sleeping well, feeling stressed and exhausted with bouts of giddiness, his journals reveal his subjective concerns about his deteriorating memory. His speech faltered and observers described him as having a 'nervous breakdown'.[46] Young onset dementia often presents in this way with a mix of psychological and cognitive symptoms revealed through life stress.[47] Seven months after losing support of his Labor coalition partner, Deakin was back for his third term as prime minister in June 1909 in a fusion coalition of disparate parties which caused much confusion and that many thought represented a naked grab for power. It may have also represented a loss of judgement and decision-making capacity associated with his evolving dementia. It lasted ten months before being routed in the April 1910 election.[48] After serving as opposition leader, he retired in January 1913 by which time his 'once magnificent memory was virtually non-existent'.[49] In February 1915, he led an Australian Commission to the International Exposition in San Francisco, held to celebrate the opening of the Panama Canal, but with his declining memory, progressive ill health and disputes with the Labor minister of external affairs, he resigned.[50] From there on his notebooks became increasingly introspective revealing loneliness and concern, 'my memory is but a little fiction'.[51] After 1916 he lived as a recluse supported by his wife, family and friends, his memory further deteriorated and he became increasingly dysphasic before his death in October 1919.[52] There is some dispute about the type of dementia that Deakin had with vascular dementia, Alzheimer's disease, vitamin $B^{12}$ deficiency (Deakin was a strict vegetarian) and even neurosyphilis (without good evidence) being suggested.[53] This will likely never be fully resolved. It is almost certain, however, that Deakin had mild dementia during his third term as prime minister and joins the list of international leaders, such as his contemporary Woodrow Wilson, who had dementia in office and whose performance at the 1919 Paris Peace Conference showed him to be erratic, forgetful and irascible.[54]

Older people have been characterised by Pat Jalland as the 'Forgotten People' in the period between the wars as concerns of charities and relief agencies were mainly focused on the unemployed with young families. There were few developments to improve services for older people and this was certainly the case for people with dementia and mental disorders.[55] In the mental hospitals older patients continued to accumulate as the long-stay patients aged. A report in the *Adelaide Mail* in December 1920 highlighted the longevity of some of the patients who had resided at Parkside Mental Hospital for over fifty years. The superintendent Colonel Downey attributed the healthy ageing to a mix of diet, useful occupation, regular bathing, and medical care.[56]

Two prominent older Australians died by suicide in the early 1920s – the playwright George Darrell at the age of 79 in 1921 and the pastoralist and politician William Abbott at the age of 70 in 1924. Both had become depressed in late life in the context of physical illness, with Darrell having the added worries of financial difficulties and the departure of his son Rupert to the United States.[57,58] Darrell's best known work is *The Sunny South* first produced in Melbourne in 1883 and later becoming the first production of the Sydney Theatre Company in 1980.[59] Abbott had been president of the Pastoralist's Union in the late 1890s and the first decade of the twentieth century, the period in which the shearers' dispute over poor working conditions and the use of non-unionised labour that resulted in the 1891 shearers' strike, was resolved. Abbott would not negotiate with the Australian Workers' Union over its refusal to accept non-unionised labour working alongside unionised labour.[60]

Ongoing concerns from the previous twenty years about the *1898 NSW Lunacy Act* and its administration along with conditions in the mental hospitals particularly related to overcrowding, staff attitudes, staff shortages and inadequate treatment regimens led to a Royal Commission in NSW in 1923. The outcome was disappointing despite numerous recommendations that largely tinkered at the edges, none were specifically about older people, with perhaps the most obvious change being the building of a mental hospital at Orange to relieve overcrowding.[61]

During the 1920s in NSW, the number of admissions of older patients gradually increased to around nineteen per cent of admissions in the mid-1920s and then remained stable as a proportion of overall admissions until the Second World War. What did increase considerably between the wars was the number of patients aged 60 years and over remaining under care with nearly 73 per cent increase in numbers to 3329 in 1939/40.[62] The 1927/28 Annual Report returned to the theme espoused in the late nineteenth century by recommending that many senile cases would be better suited for infirmaries such as Newington rather than mental hospitals and drew attention to a Report on the Provision of Mental Hospital Accommodation in England and the Tooting Bec Hospital as the type of institution that would be more appropriate. It was repeated almost word for word in the Annual Reports for the next decade. Clearly it was being ignored by the political decision-makers.[63]

Perhaps the 1928 scandals at Newington and Lidcombe State Hospitals played a role in the failure to consider State Hospital options for older people with dementia.[64] A series of newspaper articles with headlines such as 'Newington's Cold Charity' in the *Truth* and 'Pitiful Scenes Lidcombe Hospital' in the *Sydney Morning Herald* documented the overcrowded conditions, around fifteen hundred men at Lidcombe of whom a thousand were hospital cases and six hundred and eighty women at Newington of whom two hundred and fifty were hospital cases.[65,66]

At Lidcombe more than one hundred and fifty old men with senile dementia were housed in one ward with mattresses arranged between beds and on verandas. There was little room for recreation, the atmosphere was gloomy, not helped by the hospital being located next to the large Rookwood Cemetery, and the patients were described as 'depressingly rubbing their hands in the sun or with their heads buried in their hands, unhappy, despondent, alone'.[67] Both hospitals were understaffed with few doctors, nurses, and ancillary staff. Allegations of neglect were made by families of some patients who died, one with senile dementia, shortly after transfer from Newington to Rydalmere Mental Hospital. The Minister for Health was forced to respond, tubercular patients were transferred to Randwick and Waterfall, vacated wards refurbished and extra staff employed but relief was short lived. During the Great Depression patient numbers increased at Lidcombe Hospital to nearly nineteen hundred men by 1938, with over half being hospital cases, and staff shortages continued.[68]

The other trend in the 1920s in NSW was the regular admission of patients with a diagnosis of dementia *a potu* (alcohol-related dementia) such that the number of cases remaining in the hospital increased from seven in 1920 to ninety-two in June 1930. Oddly, when a new diagnostic system was introduced for the 1930/31 reports onwards, there was no equivalent diagnosis and these cases must have been subsumed into another category.[69]

Older people did not attract much comment in the Annual Mental Hospital Reports in the other states during the 1920s. For the three years between 1925 and 1927, the *Medical Journal of Australia* published articles that summarised the main issues highlighted in the various State Annual Reports and there is no mention of older people.[70,71,72] In Victoria, Yarra Bend Asylum was finally closed in 1925 with the remaining patients transferred to the new Mont Park Hospital for the Insane but this did not solve problems of chronic overcrowding that prompted newspaper correspondence.[73] In South Australia, Northfield Mental Hospital (later renamed Hillcrest Hospital) opened in 1929.[74]

The 1930s and early 1940s witnessed some important new developments in the treatment and care of mental patients. Legislation to allow voluntary patients was passed in NSW in 1934 and in Queensland in 1938 and generally there was a move towards outpatient treatment across the country. Social Workers and occupational therapists started to appear in mental hospitals in small numbers but mainly for the younger patients. New treatments appeared that showed modest effectiveness in treating serious mental disorders. Malaria therapy was used to treat GPI with some success until antibiotics appeared in the 1940s. Cardiazol and insulin therapy were introduced in the late 1930s for the schizophrenic and depressive psychoses. Cardiazol was a forerunner of electroconvulsive therapy (ECT) being administered intravenously to cause a convulsion. While effective in treating depressive psychoses that had previously had to run their natural course, it was also a dangerous and uncomfortable drug to administer and was phased out when the more effective and safer ECT was introduced in the 1940s.[75]

Concerns about the number of older people in the mental hospitals were expressed during the Great Depression in the 1930s. Admissions of older people, particularly those with senile dementia, increased in NSW in the second half of the decade. Throughout the 1930s the Annual Inspector-General Reports in NSW commented on the inappropriateness of caring for many of the older patients with dementia in a mental hospital. While acknowledging their mental infirmity, the reports stress that most were not insane and that there was stigma attached to being cared for in a mental hospital.[76] The report for the year ending June 1940 bemoaned the need to use highly trained staff to nurse these older patients and that staff time would be better spent with recoverable patients. Such views, if not ageist, certainly appear ignorant of the challenges of nursing older people with dementia. But there was at least some acknowledgement that 'there is a proportion of cases of senile mania and persecutory delusional cases, which are often, despite their age, very difficult to control and can only be cared for properly as certified patients in a Mental Hospital ward.'[77] The overcrowded understaffed Rydalmere Hospital, where many of these patients were housed alongside those with chronic psychoses, was run-down, dingy and antiquated, and smelled of urine, faeces and body odour, being reminiscent of nineteenth-century neglect. Patient clothing was drab and shapeless. The staff were shocked by the conditions.[78,79] And yet the Annual Inspector General Report for the year ending June 1938 reported that the conditions at Rydalmere were 'very good'![80]

In the report for the year ending June 1937, it was noted that elderly infirm male patients had been occupying a building in the female division at Gladesville Hospital which meant having female nurses, an arrangement appreciated by patients and their relatives.[81] This was still the era where the norm was for male nurses to look after male patients, female nurses the female patients and for the sexes to be housed in separate wards. Ruth Ford presented the case of Harcourt (Annie) Payne whose admission to Orange Mental Hospital in 1939 put the issue of gender identity into sharp focus. Payne was a 64-year-old recently widowed invalid pensioner who collapsed in the street and was taken to Lidcombe Hospital for old men where Payne was found to be a woman dressed as a man. After transfer to Newington State Hospital for Women and a police investigation, Payne was remanded to Darlinghurst Reception House before being certified insane and transferred to Orange Mental Hospital. According to Ford, the grounds for certified insanity were based entirely on Payne's choice of male gender identity, although there is an absence of case notes to confirm that. Payne was nursed in a female ward in female clothing despite having lived her life for over fifty years as a male including two marriages to women. This provoked much discussion in the press where concerns were expressed about how Payne might seduce other female patients although it was also acknowledged that a male ward would be inappropriate too. Payne died a year after admission.[82] While later Mental Health Acts excluded gender identity as a specific cause of mental illness, issues faced by older lesbian, gay, bisexual, transgender, intersex (LGBTI) persons in mental hospitals and aged care facilities have not been addressed in a meaningful way until more recent years.[83,84] The separation of the sexes in mental hospitals had largely ended by the 1980s and indeed in the past decade due to concerns about sexual assaults in younger adults, there has been move back towards separate wards.

In Victoria, the *Weekly Times* reported that Dr Ernest Jones, the Director of Mental Hygiene, expressed concerns about the number of admissions of ageing patients in his report for 1935. Like his NSW counterpart, he believed that the curative work in the mental hospitals was being inhibited by having to observe older people in 'the terminal stages of their existence'. He cited the success of the boarding out of patients to Castlemaine Benevolent Home as a model to follow.[85] As reported in *The Age*, similar views were expressed in the 1936 report and overcrowding at Kew Mental Hospital which also drew attention to the lack of response to repeated concerns about admissions of older patients in previous reports.[86] In the 1937 report, the new Director of Mental Hygiene, Dr Catarinich observed that the rates of insanity were increasing and that it 'will go on increasing, as insanity is mainly a disease of middle and advanced age'.[87] This has a shift in emphasis as Dr Catarinich seemed to be accepting that cases of dementia are forms of insanity.

The Annual Reports of the Inspector for the Hospitals for the Insane in Queensland had limited information about the older patients. However, the reports from 1937/38 through to 1941/42 show that around ten per cent of admissions had a diagnosis of senile dementia and between four to five per cent other types of dementia, while around twenty per cent of deaths were attributed to senile dementia or decay.[88] Dunwich Asylum continued throughout the 1930s into the 1940s although plans to abandon it and build a new home for older people in the Greater Brisbane area were under consideration in 1938.[89] Many of the older hospital cases had dementia.[90] By 1940 the number of inmates at Dunwich had dropped to less than seven hundred but by 1944 had increased back to 770 after the army had taken over the Dalby home as a maternity home for servicewomen.[91,92] In 1944 the suicide of a 68-year-old man who jumped from the Story Bridge brought Dunwich back into the headlines with the contents of the suicide letter. He was a former professional footballer and a bush poet who wrote under the name 'The Lone Swaggie'. A self-admitted 'slave to alcohol', he had been in and out of Dunwich which he described as 'earthly purgatory' with many inmates 'so broken in spirit they have lost courage to speak for right treatment'. With concerns that he was losing his sight and might end up back in Dunwich, he killed himself while intoxicated. A ministerial inquiry was ordered.[93]

In South Australia concerns were regularly expressed about older admissions to the mental hospitals.[94] By 1940, with Parkside Mental Hospital overcrowded thus preventing proper patient classification, a quarter of the admissions were aged 65 years and older with the cause of the mental disorder put down to senile decay, and it was these patients who were identified by Dr Jeffries the Director-General of Medical Services as being better placed in an infirmary.[95] Although in 1937 the Chief Secretary said that a home for aged patients was under consideration, this did not eventuate until the 1960s.[96] The Old Folk's Home at Magill continued but was short-staffed and by 1943 could only admit people who could look after themselves which would have excluded people with moderate to severe dementia.[97]

In Western Australia, the old men's home at Claremont housed up to 750 men in the Great Depression. In 1943 it was renamed Sunset Home.[98] Although the annual reports of the Inspector General of the Insane of Western Australia did not provide information about patient age, it is clear from the diagnoses and causes of insanity that older admissions increased over the 1930s. In 1932 around twelve per cent of presentations to Heathcote Reception House, which kept patients for 6 months or longer, were due to senility, while over twelve per cent of admissions to the mental hospitals were diagnosed with senile dementia and a further nine per cent another type of dementia such as due to epilepsy or GPI.[99] By 1940, while senility was still felt to cause twelve per cent of presentations to Heathcote, senile dementia now accounted for twenty per cent of mental hospital admissions and other types of dementia a further fifteen per cent.[100] This high proportion of admissions with dementia did not appear to prompt any specific concerns despite Claremont Hospital being overcrowded. It is also unclear whether there was any separation of the older patients with dementia from the other patients. Similarly in Tasmania there was no mention of concerns about older patients during this period despite patient numbers increasing.

During the first half of the century, overall numbers of Aboriginal people increased.[101,102] Policies of separation of Aboriginal children from their parents were at their height with State Aboriginal Protection Boards or those of Church Missions administering institutions to raise the children, a policy that has had long lasting impacts into late life for Aboriginal people in the second half of the century.[103] In the 1920s occurred the last recorded massacres of Aboriginal people at Forrest River in Western Australia and Coniston Station in the Northern Territory. European diseases and lifestyles were still having a disproportionate impact on Aboriginal populations including those with known deleterious effects on mental function such as syphilis and alcohol at the forefront especially in institutionalised settings.[104] This was also the period that witnessed the birth of self-determination with the formation of the Australian Aboriginal Progressive Association a short-lived forerunner of similar organisations.[105]

There is little information about older Aboriginal people with mental disorders in the first half of the twentieth century but undoubtedly they occurred as noted in the following examples. The register of the Fremantle Asylum reveals that there was one 60-year-old Aboriginal woman admitted with a diagnosis of mania in 1906 who died a month later.[106] A depressed Aboriginal man in his 70s from Cape Barren Island who had been hospitalised at Launceston Public Hospital after cutting his throat in a suicide attempt, died of a head injury after falling about ten metres from a hospital balcony in 1932. He was described as being a quiet man who was frightened of being arrested by the police. The death was determined by the coroner to be accidental.[107]

Chapter 9

# International influences in the Twentieth Century

Although most of the international influences on the development of old age mental health and dementia services in Australia occurred after the Second World War, there were some key discoveries early in the century involving the neuropathology of dementia, further refined in the 1960s and 70s, and the confirmation that syphilis was the underlying cause of GPI, which had a long-term impact upon service delivery. These discoveries contributed to the fine tuning of Emil Kraepelin's classification of mental disorders that had first been published in the 1899 edition of his book but really did not have much impact until the 1904 edition. Kraepelin's classification, in part based upon prognosis, had worldwide impact and despite now having some obvious limitations, still underpins aspects of current classifications.[1] Further work by Martin Roth and colleagues in the UK in the 1950s and 1960s focused on older people and most importantly indicated that some disorders such as late life depression had a good prognosis and were responsive to treatments.[2] Population ageing and its impact upon health and social service needs, while mounting in the first half of the century, had its first notable responses from clinicians and policy makers in the UK in the 1940s.[3] While the journey of service development and policy responses in the UK for those who were ageing with various physical and mental disabilities was not a smooth one, from mid-century until the 1990s it was the world leader for geriatric medical and old age mental health services and had a large impact on developments in Australia. International organisations such as the World Health Organisation (WHO) issued important statements in the second half of the century which also witnessed the emergence of organisations that focussed on dementia and old age mental health such as Alzheimer's Disease

International and the International Psychogeriatric Association. This chapter will examine these influences and the impacts that they had in Australia.

## Research into the neuropathology of dementia

In the 1890s, European neuropathologists, armed with new stains that improved the visualisation of neural tissue under the microscope, were able to distinguish various types of neuronal degeneration from cerebral arteriosclerosis and GPI. One of the new stains, the Bielschowsky silver staining technique, enabled neuropathologists Oskar Fischer in Prague and Alois Alzheimer in Munich to describe neuritic plaques and neurofibrillary tangles in their research on dementia.[4] In a 1906 clinico-pathological conference presentation that was published in 1907, Alzheimer described the case of a 51-year-old woman, Auguste D, who had symptoms of hallucinations, disorientation and memory loss that progressed over some years till her death at the age of 55 years. In his post-mortem examination of the cerebral cortex, Alzheimer identified the plaques and tangles that characterised what became known as Alzheimer's disease, an eponym conferred by his colleague Emil Kraepelin.[5] This represented the first steps towards recognising senile dementia as a disease. Around the same time in 1907, Fischer published a series of twelve senile dementia cases in which he described the neuritic plaques.[6] Initially Alzheimer's disease was regarded as a type of pre-senile dementia occurring before old age, although Kraepelin acknowledged that there were similarities to senile dementia. This led to debate through the first half of the twentieth century about the relationship between senile dementia and Alzheimer's disease and it gradually became clear that most cases of senile dementia had the same brain changes as Alzheimer's disease.[7] The work of John (Nick) Corsellis, Gary Blessed and Bernard Tomlinson in the UK in the 1960s and of Robert Katzman and Robert Terry in the US in the 1970s was largely responsible for the removal of the age criterion and the eventual emergence of what was initially named 'Senile Dementia of the Alzheimer-type' but later the word 'senile' was dropped.[8,9] In effect, this formalised the scientific transition of senile dementia from being a part of the ageing process to being a degenerative brain disease associated with ageing and paved the way for it to become more formally regarded as a health condition.

## Syphilis and the Cure of General Paralysis of the Insane

In the early twentieth century GPI was an invariably fatal disease that was prevalent in asylums worldwide and was one of the main causes for male admissions in mid-life. In 1904 alone, there were 1795 deaths from GPI in Scottish asylums and around 2250 deaths in English asylums.[10] Of interest, Alzheimer had completed his post-doctoral research on the histology of GPI before his study of neurodegeneration and was acknowledged, along with Nissl who had provided him the Bielschowsky silver staining technique, to have accurately recorded the microscopic features in the cerebral cortex in 1904. In 1905, Fritz Schaudinn and Erich Hoffmann identified the bacterium *Treponema pallidum* as being the cause of syphilis but the debate on whether syphilis was the underlying cause of GPI continued until 1913 when Hideyo Noguchi and J.W. Moore were able to demonstrate the presence of *Treponema pallidum* in the brains of patients with GPI. This did not result in any immediate changes in the treatment of GPI but did herald the commencement of rational therapeutic trials. Malaria therapy, a form of pyrotherapy in which fevers were used as therapy, was introduced by Julius Wagner-Jauregg in 1917, and proved to be effective in the treatment of GPI, although the treatment was complex and had contraindications. However, it was effective enough for Wagner-Jauregg to be awarded the Nobel Prize in Medicine in 1927, the first psychiatrist to do so. It was not until the introduction of penicillin in 1943 that an effective cure for GPI became available and over the next few decades GPI became uncommon in mental hospitals.[11] At present, Alzheimer's disease and other dementias remain in the phase of undergoing rational therapeutic trials but once disease altering therapies become available there will be an expected change in the need for institutional care.

## Classification of Mental Disorders and their Treatment

As was noted in Chapter 1, before Emil Kraepelin first published his classification of mental disorders in 1899, there was a diverse range of diagnostic categories in use with little agreement between them. Without a reliable classification system that could clearly indicate the nature of a person's mental disorder, researchers were hindered in communicating their findings and investigating new treatments, while clinicians had limited capacity to prescribe the most appropriate therapy and give an accurate prognosis. This was amply demonstrated in Chapter 4 where the 'mania' diagnosis translated into many twenty-first-century diagnoses. Kraepelin had painstakingly observed and recorded the presenting symptoms and outcomes of numerous patients. By including the longitudinal course of the illness in his systematic observations, he was able to demonstrate that diverse entities such as hebephrenia, catatonia, mania, folie circulaire and many others could be reduced to two broad categories, Dementia Praecox (twenty-first-century schizophrenia) and Manic Depressive Psychosis (twenty-first-century bipolar disorder).[12] Dementia Praecox had a relatively poor prognosis while Manic Depressive Psychosis had a better prognosis but was prone to relapse. Subsequent research over the past century has shown that this separation was neither as clear cut, nor the prognoses as different as first thought but at the time it was a major step forward.[13]

Kraepelin's classification embraced the full range of psychiatric disorders including those in which there was overt evidence of neuropathological changes in the brain, the 'organic brain syndromes' that included senile dementia, GPI, and epileptic psychoses. As new neuropathological findings were reported from his Munich laboratory and others, Kraepelin updated his classification, for example, Alzheimer's disease first appeared in the 1910 edition of his textbook as a presenile dementia.[14] Despite these advances that by 1932 were reflected in the diagnostic terminology used in the annual reports of the NSW Inspector-General of Mental Hospitals,[15] there was little impact upon how mental disorders in late life were regarded. The sense was that they were as a result of the ageing process and therefore untreatable with an almost universally poor prognosis.[16]

This viewpoint was not challenged until 1955 with the pioneering work of Martin Roth, who undertook a retrospective examination of 472 older patients admitted to Graylingwell Hospital in Chichester, Sussex, during the 1930s and 1940s. He analysed the clinical history, symptoms and outcome of the patients and identified five diagnostic categories: affective psychosis, late paraphrenia, acute confusion, arteriosclerotic psychosis and senile psychosis. The twenty-first century equivalent diagnoses are the mood disorders (major depression and bipolar disorder), late onset schizophrenia, delirium, vascular dementia and Alzheimer's-type dementia. What was most important was that the prognosis of each was different and in particular, the outcomes of those with affective psychoses, late paraphrenia and acute confusion was much better than that of arteriosclerotic psychosis and senile psychosis and just as importantly they did not inevitably lead to dementia.[17] These were treatable conditions. In an era that pre-dated antipsychotic and antidepressant medication perhaps the main issue was one of attitudes towards the management of the patients. The one effective treatment for severe mood disorders and psychoses that had been introduced by this time was electroconvulsive therapy (ECT). Mayer-Gross in 1945 had already demonstrated in a large study that included 76 patients over the age of 60 that older patients had benefits similar to younger patients, although the older patients were more prone to adverse effects particularly acute confusion and memory changes, understandable in an era where unmodified bilateral application of ECT was the standard.[18] Later, in a study from Newcastle-upon-Tyne where Roth was now based and led by David Kay, who moved to Tasmania in the 1970s, the prevalence of mental disorders in people over the age of 65 was determined for community and institutional settings. It showed that 31 per cent of older people had functional mental disorders, mainly mild-moderate mood disorders and neuroses, the vast majority of whom lived in the community. In addition over 80 per cent of those with dementia lived in the community.[19] They emphasised the importance of social factors and community interventions.[20] These studies clearly indicated that a significant proportion of older patients had treatable disorders but the implications of these studies from the perspective of service development took more than a decade to have an impact in the UK.

Leslie Kiloh from the University of Durham, Newcastle, who later became the foundation Chair of the School of Psychiatry at the University of NSW in Sydney, published an important review of pseudo-dementia in 1961, which pointed out that there were likely to be older people with severe forms of depression languishing in mental hospitals misdiagnosed with dementia at a time when effective treatments with antidepressant medication and ECT were available. His work was influential in reminding clinicians to exclude severe depression when diagnosing dementia and he advocated for therapeutic trials of antidepressant therapy if there were any doubts.[21]

As new antidepressant and antipsychotic drugs became available from the mid-1950s onwards, the exclusion of older people from most clinical trials meant that many drugs were approved for marketing before adequate numbers of older people had been exposed to them. This is exemplified by a Cochrane Collaboration review of the use of antidepressants to treat depression in late life in which the earliest placebo-controlled trial identified that focused on older people was published in 1980.[22] Similar issues are apparent in the use of psychological therapies in treating depression with the earliest study identified that qualified to be included in a systematic review being published in 1982.[23] Sigmund Freud's pessimism about using psychoanalysis in older people, which for him began at around the age of fifty, influenced generations of psychotherapists even though other prominent therapists including Karl Abraham did not share his views.[24] Thus through to the 1980s when there were relatively few old age psychiatrists and psychologists working with older people worldwide, there was also little research on therapeutics in older people to guide general psychiatrists and other clinicians. This changed during the 1980s with a rapid increase in controlled trials using a broad range of therapies for various mental disorders in older people.

In 1980 the American Psychiatric Association released the third edition of its *Diagnostic and Statistical Manual of Mental Disorders* (DSM III) which for the first time used operationalised diagnostic criteria to improve reliability.[25] The most recent fifth edition (DSM 5) released in 2013 removed the diagnosis of dementia and replaced it with 'major neurocognitive disorder' due to concerns about the stigma attached to the term 'dementia'.[26] The change does not seem to have had much impact as yet outside of research settings. To aid in the clinical diagnosis of Alzheimer's disease, in 1984 a work group under the auspices of the US Department of Health and Human Services Task Force on Alzheimer's disease published diagnostic criteria for Alzheimer's disease that built on the 1980 DSM III criteria and emphasised that it was a clinical diagnosis and that laboratory tests were to eliminate other possible causes of dementia as at this point there were no laboratory tests that could detect the underlying neuropathology.[27] These criteria were revised in 2011 to accommodate the use of emerging laboratory tests (biomarkers) to improve diagnostic accuracy and to include pre-dementia syndromes.[28] In the past decade as biomarkers for Alzheimer's disease have improved, the potential to accurately diagnosis Alzheimer's disease during life and even before the person has dementia is on the horizon.[29]

In the treatment of dementia, the two main developments occurred in the same period. The introduction of cognitive enhancing drugs, such as donepezil, rivastigmine and galantamine, for the treatment of Alzheimer's disease in the late 1990s and early 2000s, while having only a modest benefit, did have the important symbolic role of emphasising that dementia was a health condition that could be treated. In the UK significant limitations were placed on their use in the National Health Service (NHS) by the National Institute for Health and Care Excellence in 2009 that was inconsistent with other guidances,[30] but after much complaint by advocacy groups and the introduction of the Equality Act in 2010, the guidance was revised in 2011.[31] The other development was in the use of antipsychotic drugs to treat agitation, aggression and psychosis associated with dementia. For many years these drugs had been used with very limited research to support it. Well-designed studies in the late 1990s and early 2000s confirmed modest benefit but also revealed hitherto unexpected harms with increased risk of strokes and mortality that was first noticed in a trial based in Australia.[32] These adverse effects were confirmed in reanalysis of previously completed trials resulting in the US Food and Drug Administration (FDA), along with other authorities, issuing black box warnings about the risks. Despite these concerns and recommendations to use non-drug treatments first, antipsychotic drugs are still overprescribed to people with dementia in nursing homes worldwide.[33]

The increased and better quality research into the treatment of dementia and other mental disorders in older people over the last forty years has emphasised that older people do not necessarily respond to treatments in the same way as younger people, yet can still obtain benefit. In 2004, a WHO Health Evidence Network review that I led emphasised the important therapeutic role of specialised older people's mental health services in effective treatment.[34]

## The impact of population ageing in the UK on service development

The first half of the century witnessed significant increases in the number of older people in Western countries, yet very little change in the way health and social services were organised. The UK, representative of an 'old world' country, saw the proportion of persons aged 65 years and over increase from 5 per cent in 1901 to 11 per cent in 1951.[35] By comparison, 'new world' immigrant countries, such as the US, had less increase in those aged 65 years and over from 4.1 per cent in

1900 to 8.1 per cent in 1950,[36] change that was similar to the four per cent to 7.8 per cent increase in the same age group in Australia.[37] Life expectancy at birth was similar in the US and the UK, increasing by over twenty years between 1900 and 1950 so that in 1950, in the US it had reached 68, while in the UK it was over 65 in men and over 70 in women.[38, 39]

Concerns about the ageing population had been expressed in the UK since 1940 when the proportion of persons aged 65 years and over was more than ten per cent of the population. Falling birth rates and rising life expectancy contributed to this. Out of a meeting of individuals, voluntary organisations, and government in 1940, the Old People's Welfare Committee was born and this became the National Old People's Welfare Committee in 1944, the forerunner of Age Concern which became Age UK in 2010.[40] In 1941 the government appointed Sir William Beveridge to lead an inquiry into Social Insurance and Allied Services. The Beveridge report of 1942 strongly influenced post-war legislation. While much of the report dealt with social security issues across the age range, there was a specific section on the 'problem of age'.[41]

Post-war innovations in the UK regarding the health and social needs of an ageing population had the greatest influence on developments in Australia. Population ageing occurred earlier and put pressures on health and social welfare systems over thirty years before such effects were felt in Australia. For example, in 1980 when the proportion of persons in Australia aged 65 years and over was still under ten per cent,[42] in the UK it had reached fifteen per cent.[43] Thus Australia was able to benefit from the UK experience, which was enhanced by the common phenomenon for Australians in the 1950s through to the 1980s to undertake postgraduate studies and work in healthcare professions there.

In health care, the emergence of geriatric medicine was a key issue. The term 'geriatrics' was coined by American Ignatz Nascher in 1909. He was concerned about the neglect of older people by the medical profession.[44] Although having its origins in the US with the formation of the American Geriatrics Society in 1942, the momentum for the development of geriatric medicine as a medical subspecialty came from the UK where the British Geriatrics Society was formed in 1947.[45] The integration of Poor Laws hospitals with other medical services after 1929 revealed large numbers of old disabled long-stay hospital patients in poor quality accommodation who were receiving little and poor quality medical care and no access to rehabilitation that could have enabled them to live at home. This led to a focus on rehabilitation in older people by clinicians such as Marjorie Warren at West Middlesex County Hospital, which was further facilitated by the introduction of the NHS in 1948 and the expansion of geriatric medicine.[46,47] There were 70,000 hospital beds in England occupied by chronic old disabled patients and according to Charles Webster, historian of the NHS, this was seen as an impediment to its embryonic development.[48] By improving the quality of health care through modern medical interventions, geriatricians and their multidisciplinary teams were able to change expectations about the outcome of chronic disorders in older people by discharging many, increasing bed turnover, and reducing bed requirements significantly. The Ministry of Health supported this approach and took measures to improve recruitment, establish geriatric units in general hospitals, and develop a range of community services.[49] In Scotland, the introduction of the NHS had an initial deleterious impact on older people's access to acute hospital beds. To address this, by the mid-1950s geriatrician William Ferguson Anderson developed specialised geriatric units in each of the five hospital districts in Scotland and in the process established sound principles of geriatric medicine that remain relevant today. These include that people become ill due to illness and not age, accurate diagnosis is essential, the home environment should be assessed, and that there is immense potential for recovery.[50]

These service developments with their principles of care provided a template for the development of psychogeriatric services in the UK but changes were slow for a number of reasons. Perhaps the key issue was the seeming inability to increase bed turnover in the way that geriatric medicine had been able to thereby attracting political attention. Claire Hilton noted that the evidence that started to accumulate in the 1940s through to the 1960s that depression and other functional mental disorders were distinguishable from dementia and were treatable had limited impact. Yet almost one-third of mental hospital inpatients in England and Wales was over the age of 65 in 1955.[51] Until the 1970s, there were few psychiatrists specialising in the treatment of older people (then commonly called psychogeriatricians) and in 1969 there were less than ten old age mental health services in the country. Psychiatrists generally had a pessimistic view on the potential for older people to improve as they regarded most of their older patients to inevitably deteriorate, while policy makers could see no benefits on bed turnover in period in which austerity dominated thinking.[52] There were, however, two Australian connections in this early period.

Aubrey Lewis, an Australian psychiatrist born and educated in Adelaide, was appointed as the inaugural Chair of Psychiatry at the Institute of Psychiatry, Maudsley Hospital at Denmark Hill in South London in 1946, a position he held for twenty years building an impressive reputation for the quality of medical education and psychiatric research. He was knighted in 1959.[53] Lewis was keenly aware of the dearth of research on older people with mental disorders. Earlier, working with Helen Goldschmidt, he had demonstrated the importance of social factors in the admission of older people with mental disorders. Lewis set up a 'geriatric unit' at the Maudsley Hospital and in 1949 appointed Felix Post, who had published a study on depression in old age in 1944, to lead it. It was a research ward that focussed on older patients without dementia, mainly depression and late life psychoses. It was not at all representative of the older patients admitted to mental hospitals in the UK, most of whom had dementia and were admitted for long-term care, often bypassing the assessment wards in the process. Thus, although Felix Post was able to produce some high-quality research from the geriatric unit at the Maudsley in the 1950s, it had little impact on service delivery.[54]

Eric Cunningham Dax, who had been working at Netherne Hospital in Surrey, was appointed as the inaugural Chair of the newly established Mental Hygiene Authority in Victoria in 1952 and during his sixteen-year tenure he oversaw a major transformation of mental health services in Victoria, including those in psychogeriatrics that will be discussed in Chapter 11.[55] In the year of his appointment, Dax along with lead author Leslie Cook and colleague Walter Maclay, published a study in the *Lancet* of older admissions to six psychiatric hospitals in which they concluded that many admissions related to social factors. They were concerned about the mounting number of older people in the mental hospital and were keen to identify how that could be addressed. They also reported that 20 per cent died within six weeks of admission, an outcome little different from 50 years earlier, and that 40 per cent were eventually discharged, outcomes which were far worse than younger patients.[56]

In the early 1970s a 'coffee house' group of psychogeriatricians began to meet informally to exchange views about developing mental health services for older people which became the forerunner to the Section of Psychiatry of Old Age that was established in the Royal College of Psychiatrists in 1978.[57] The group included Tom Arie who was to have a major impact on the development of older people's mental health services in Australia in the 1980s and 1990s. Arie commenced a mental health service for older people at Goodmayes Hospital in Essex in 1969 based on the principles of a low hierarchical service structure, prompt assessments which were preferably undertaken in the patient's home and often by a consultant, and the fostering of an enthusiastic multidisciplinary team. The first year of service had impressive results with an increase in admissions and discharges, a reduction in deaths, and the vacating of forty beds on the long-stay wards.[58] Importantly, these results were noticed by influential people in the Department of Health including Chief Medical Officer George Godber.[59] These developments contributed to a 1972 Department of Health and Social Security (DHSS) memorandum 'Services for Mental Illness Related to Old Age' (otherwise known as HM(72) 71) which outlined a blueprint for comprehensive service development.[60] This included acute and long-stay inpatient beds, day hospital care and continuing care in the community provided by a trained multidisciplinary team interacting with other agencies. Of significance, a survey undertaken by the Health Care Evaluation Team at the University of Southampton in 1974 found that no locality had all of the components required for a comprehensive service.[61] Indeed, throughout the 1970s there was evidence of resistance to change, with general psychiatrists sceptical about the need for psychogeriatricians and the Royal College of Psychiatrists being reluctant to increase training posts in the field.[62]

One of the challenges faced in service development in this period related to the division between health and social care. In a review of the NHS in 1956 the Guillebaud Committee redefined the boundaries between health and social care and much of the continuing care of older and disabled people which had been provided by the NHS became social care and the responsibility of local authorities.[63] This included community and 'low care' residential care. One major difference was that the NHS was free but social care had to be paid for with a means tested approach. The boundaries between health and social care were grey and coordination between health and social services poor.[64] This of course meant that the long-term residential care for people with dementia in mental hospitals was free. Moreover, closure of mental hospitals that had long been recommended was hindered as the extra social care required was in a different budget and savings from hospital closure would not necessarily flow to that purpose. The HM(72) 71 memorandum had indicated that local authorities were responsible for developing 'low care' residential homes that would have been suitable for patients with mild dementia but development was slow and standards were poor.[65] This divide in administrative responsibility for components of treatment and care for older people with mental disorders and dementia has also been an issue for service development in Australia. It was the Thatcher government's introduction of Supplementary Benefits Regulations in 1980 which enabled people entering private residential care to obtain public financial support that changed the configuration of long-term care in the UK. This was a similar arrangement to that which had existed in Australia for nearly twenty years and it had the same predictable outcome with a rapid growth of private sector residential places in the 1980s to the extent that growth outstripped demand. Subsequently in the 1990s there was a steady reduction in long-stay hospital beds and local authority homes by around 50 per cent. The regulation of private nursing homes lagged behind the public sector but in 2001 National Minimum Standards were enacted alongside a National Service Framework for Older People that acknowledged person-centred care as an essential standard.[66]

Tom Arie understood the importance of active collaboration with geriatricians in general hospitals and working with geriatrician colleague Tom Dunn developed a four-bed 'Do-it-yourself' joint assessment unit in a general hospital without additional resources. Again impressive results were published in the *Lancet* in 1973 showing short length of stay and the majority of patients returning home.[67] Proposals to develop such joint psychiatric-geriatric units in the UK had existed since the late 1940s but they never became widespread. There were many reasons for this that included different administrative service boundaries, resource limitations, lack of government support and the personalities of the individuals involved.[68] Indeed, as noted by Arie and Dunn in their report, 'we tend to see eye-to-eye'.[69] Later, in 1977 Arie was appointed professor of a joint geriatric-psychiatric clinical and academic position in the newly created 'Department of Health Care of the Elderly' at Nottingham.[70] From Nottingham, during the 1980s Arie led courses on psychogeriatrics for international participants that were sponsored by the British Council and attended by key Australians including Ed

Chiu, Henry Brodaty and John Snowdon, before bringing the course to Australia and other countries.[71]

One of the difficulties confronting UK psychogeriatricians in the 1970s and 1980s was the difficulty in obtaining accurate data. As psychogeriatrics was not a subspecialty recognised by the DHSS there was no impetus to collect information about services. A survey led by John Wattis showed that the development of psychogeriatric services was rapid during the late 1970s with the number of psychogeriatricians in the UK increasing from twelve in 1970 working at least 17.5 hours per week with older people, to 120 in 1980, but there was considerable geographical variation with a predominance in the south-east of England. Most of the beds were located in mental hospitals.[72] Further development in the 1980s was enhanced by *The Rising Tide* initiative which grew out of a workshop sponsored by the Hospital Advisory Service (an agency that inspected hospitals) which brought together for the first time key stakeholders including the DHSS, hospitals, social services, voluntary organisations and general practice to discuss what was needed to improve services for older people with dementia and mental disorders. *The Rising Tide* report proposed expanding recognised good practice including comprehensive multi-disciplinary and multi-agency teamwork, short-term and continuing care in hospital and community locations. Perhaps the spur to further development was the allocation of £6 million start-up money for 'demonstration districts' proposed by Norman Fowler, Secretary of State for Social Services. While there was much disagreement about how that would be best spent, ultimately it proved a catalyst for service development as exemplified by the increase in the number of psychogeriatricians in the UK to 405 in 1993.[73] These developments were accompanied by the DHSS recognition of psychogeriatrics as a medical subspecialty in 1989.[74]

The 1988 Griffiths Report on community care that led to the *National Health Service and Community Care Act 1990* contained several key reforms that were later taken up in Australia. These were that the State should be an 'enabler' rather than a provider of care, that the care purchaser and care provider roles should be separated, and the devolution of budgets and budgetary control. This meant that independent non-government organisations were the main care providers. It attempted to bring clarity to the boundaries of health and social care but this remained a problem.[75]

The opening of the Dementia Services Development Centre at Stirling University under the leadership of social worker Mary Marshall in 1989 provided a model for research and development that has influenced the establishment of similar centres in the UK as well as in Australia, notably the Wicking Dementia Research and Education Centre that was established at the University of Tasmania in 2008. Marshall was at the forefront of championing dementia-friendly principles in design for residential care and health facilities which influenced the work of Richard Fleming in his examination of the influence of the physical environment in dementia care.[76] This in turn became the foundation for the comprehensive World Alzheimer Report 2020 on dementia-related design and the built environment including the concept of the dementia-friendly society.[77]

The 'Dignity in Care' movement evolved out of concerns within older people's services in the late 1990s that later permeated the entire health and social care system in the UK,[78] being exemplified by the abuses of patients documented in the Mid Staffordshire NHS Foundation Trust in the Francis Report of the public inquiry in 2013.[79] It reflects consumer concerns that there had been an erosion in standards of care although it may also represent in a historical context an evolution of the dignity construct to be inclusive of each individual, mirroring person-centred approaches to care.[80] In the Australian dementia context, the ten 'Dignity in Care' principles were included in the Australian Clinical Practice Guidelines for Dementia in 2016.[81]

Counselling for older people with psychological disorders often accompanying physical illness was not readily available in the UK.[82] The challenges of providing adequate access to psychological therapies led to an initiative in 2007 that followed an economic model which skewed access towards younger people although eventually the program was adjusted.[83] Similar difficulties occurred in Australia where access to psychological therapies for older people living in residential aged care facilities was not covered by Medicare until 2018 when a new program allowed access via a Primary Health Network.[84]

In 2013 the Joint Commissioning Panel for Mental Health issued a guidance for NHS Commissioners on older people's mental health services, in part as a reaction to the Francis Report, and also due to concern that age discrimination was increasing in the NHS with some NHS trusts merging their adult and older people's mental health service. It provided ten key messages to NHS

Commissioners about the number of older people, the target group for services (which in the UK includes people of any age with dementia), their complex mental health needs and the challenges for service providers.[85]

## International Organisations

WHO first identified mental health problems of ageing in a 1959 report which espoused sensible basic principles including the need for short-term assessment admissions, active treatment, rehabilitation, and maintaining people in their own homes.[86] As noted in a subsequent WHO report in 1972, the 1959 report had little impact on service development and it again emphasised the need for widespread services based on 'epidemiology, origin, prevention, development and treatment' of mental disorders in old age. It also stressed the need to go beyond rhetoric with reference to community care.[87] This report had some impact in the UK being contemporaneous with the HM(72) 71 memorandum. In 1998, WHO and the Geriatric Psychiatry section of the World Psychiatric Association issued a technical consensus statement on the organisation of care in old age mental health which provided guidance for service development.[88] In Australia, the latter report was very useful as a resource document for lobbying policymakers in advocating for new services.

The two international organisations that have had the greatest impact on the field in Australia are Alzheimer's Disease International (ADI) and the International Psychogeriatric Association (IPA). ADI is a federation of over one hundred not-for-profit dementia associations from around the world that was founded in 1984 by an initiative of Alzheimer associations in the UK, USA, Australia and Canada.[89] The individual organisations were founded in Canada in 1978, the UK in 1979, and the US in 1980, with these consumer led advocacy organisations influencing the development of individual state organisations in Australia in the early 1980s. ADI has become very influential with a range of initiatives including: the Alzheimer University that is a series of workshops for national associations; annual World Alzheimer Reports on a range of topics including dementia prevalence, costs and dementia prevention; the 10/66 project that has been researching dementia in developing countries; collaborating on reports with WHO; advocating for national public health responses to dementia;

and biennial international conferences.[90] Australians have been very active in ADI with Henry Brodaty a past president and Glen Rees, former CEO of Alzheimer's Australia (the forerunner of Dementia Australia), is the current Chair of ADI. Dementia Australia has been able to utilise the various products from ADI in its advocacy work in Australia.

IPA traces its origins to the first Arie course in Nottingham in July 1980 when course members decided to former an association and was officially established at its first international congress held in Cairo in November 1982.[91] Membership of IPA comprises of individuals from multidisciplinary professional backgrounds who are involved in clinical and academic work with older people with mental disorders as well as affiliated national organisations, such as in Australia, the Faculty of Psychiatry of Old Age of the Royal Australian and New Zealand College of Psychiatrists. Other affiliate organisations include the American Association for Geriatric Psychiatry (established in 1978), the Japanese Psychogeriatric Society (established in 1986) and the Canadian Academy of Geriatric Psychiatry (established in 1993). IPA runs annual congresses and other educational workshops and webinars, publishes its own academic journal *International Psychogeriatrics* and the benchmark *IPA Complete Guide to Behavioral and Psychological Symptoms of Dementia (BPSD)*, and has organised taskforces to examine issues such as suicide in late life, residential aged care, and mental health service delivery. Australians have been very active in IPA having a high number of members, two past presidents (Ed Chiu and Henry Brodaty), numerous board members, and two past editors of both *International Psychogeriatrics* and the *IPA Complete Guide to Behavioral and Psychological Symptoms of Dementia (BPSD)*. There have also been three IPA congresses held in Australia. Due to this high level of engagement, IPA has been very influential with clinicians in Australia especially with the work on BPSD.

## Other US contributions that have influenced Australian service development

In 1975, a brief ten-minute, thirty-item cognitive screening test was published by Marshall Folstein and colleagues from Johns Hopkins University in Baltimore that could quantify cognitive impairment.[92] The Mini-Mental State Examination

(MMSE) became the tool for clinicians and researchers worldwide for assessing, measuring and communicating about cognitive impairment in people being assessed for dementia. The timing was exquisite. In the year of its publication, senile dementia was recognised as being due to Alzheimer's disease and the numbers of older people presenting to clinicians with concerns about memory, moods and behaviour were increasing. Before the MMSE, communication about dementia and its severity was hampered by lack of a common language. Now a simple score out of thirty provided a sense of the severity of cognitive change. While there are many other, and some arguably better, cognitive screening tools now available (for example two Australian tools, one developed for multicultural populations, the Rowland Universal Dementia Assessment Scale (RUDAS)[93] and the other for Indigenous populations, the Kimberley Indigenous Assessment Scale (KICA)[94]), the MMSE is still widely used and remains a gold standard against which other tools are matched. For the development of dementia services in Australia, the MMSE played an important role in quantifying cognitive change and allowed a range of clinicians at the coalface to improve the quality of their assessments. Undoubtedly the MMSE, and other cognitive screening tools, have also been misused in dementia diagnosis but the positive impact is likely to have outweighed the negative impact.[95]

Another publication from Johns Hopkins University that was published in 1981 has also had a major impact in Australia and worldwide. *The 36-Hour Day* written by Nancy Mace and Peter Rabins was written for carers of people with dementia and provides practical advice about living with a person with dementia. It brought to the forefront, along with the infant Alzheimer Societies carer support groups, the importance of supporting carers of people with dementia.[96] The numerous social factors identified in the research on admissions to psychiatric hospitals decades earlier were often related to the stresses that informal family carers experienced in supporting their relatives at home. By providing practical advice along with emotional support institutional care could be delayed.

# Chapter 10

# National Developments after the Second World War to 1980

There was a near doubling of the number of older people in Australia in the 25 years after the Second World War, but the impact of the baby boomer cohort meant that there was only a small increase in the proportion of people aged 65 years and over in the population (the age that became synonymous with retirement and old age in official reports from this period onwards), from 7.8 per cent (0.6 million) in 1945 to 8.3 per cent (1.1 million) in 1971. From the 1970s onwards both the numbers of older people and the population proportion steadily increased and by 1981, 9.7 per cent of the population (1.5 million) was aged 65 years and over.[1] The ageing of post-war immigrants, many of whom were refugees from Europe, fuelled the growth and meant that by 1980 the number of older people born overseas was increasing.

After the war there was a lack of infrastructure for older people including accommodation, hospitals, and long-term care and this was amplified by the post-war focus on returned soldiers and their families. Older people received fewer benefits than other groups in society in the post-war 'National Welfare Fund'. No concerted general community concern was expressed until the late 1940s at which time there was increased public concern being voiced about older people, particularly in Victoria. The Brotherhood of St Laurence and Oswald Barnett, a social reformer, were strongly advocating for the abolition of slums where many impoverished older people lived. The *Melbourne Herald* and *Argus* newspapers took up a campaign supporting the work of the Brotherhood of St Laurence and the Salvation Army with the elderly and warning the public of the demographic 'time bomb' of the ageing population and the lack of resources.[2] This culminated with a 1950 banner headline 'Is old age a crime?' over a *Herald* story by the journalist John Hetherington.[3] There was a crisis in accommodation, particularly for the frail aged. The shortage of beds in benevolent homes led to Ben Chifley reluctantly agreeing to loan five wards of Caulfield Repatriation Hospital in 1949. In the late 1940s, 11 per cent of older people in Victoria had to share a room in a boarding house. The acute housing shortage coupled with increased rents and high living costs challenged even those with otherwise modest means.[4]

## Voluntary Organisations

Developments in the UK influenced post-war changes in Australia. Kate Ogilvie, senior social worker at Sydney Hospital, was one of many Australians who visited the UK to study the aged care reform in the early years of the welfare state. In 1951 she wrote an article about these innovations in the Bulletin of the Council of Social Service in NSW. It was in Victoria where the newspaper campaigns and public concern about the plight of older people led to changes that started to appear. In April 1951 the Older People's Welfare Council (OPWC) was launched. It was based on the English model and came out of an initiative by the National Council of Women in Victoria. By the end of the 1950s each state had its own OPWC, with OPWC NSW being formed in 1956. There was also a National OPWC under the presidency of Sir Giles Chippindall from 1958 to 1969. These OPWCs eventually became Councils of the Ageing (COTA) in the 1960s, with COTA Australia, a federation of state COTAs, being founded in 1979. In the 1950s, OPWC in Victoria focused its efforts on lobbying local councils to establish recreational clubs for older people, meals on wheels, home helps, home visiting and nursing. Each of the state OPWCs took the same community care focus. The Victorian OPWC was particularly concerned to concentrate on voluntary effort for home and community care rather than activities more appropriate for state action. However, OPWC Victoria did receive generous subsidies from the Victorian government which was in contrast to the experiences in NSW.[5] The Australian Association of Gerontology, with the involvement of Sir Giles Chippindall from the National OPWC, Dr Sidney Sax and Dr David

Wallace, was established in 1964 and grew out of the Gerontological Society of NSW that had formed in 1962.[6]

The Melbourne Rotary Club funded a survey of older people in Victoria in the early 1950s and brought Bertram Hutchinson, a young social investigator from London University, to Melbourne to investigate the 'Problem of the Aged'.[7] This resulted in the Hutchinson Report of 1954, *Old People in a Modern Australian Community* which, while flawed in its attempts to impose theory based upon British experience upon empirical data that was inconsistent with the theory, provided the first detailed description of the demographic and economic foundations of older people in Australia. Hutchinson argued that older people were being neglected by their families but his data showed families often lived close by and provided meals and other support to ageing parents.[8] Alan Stoller, the chief clinical officer of Victoria's Mental Hygiene Authority, was particularly critical and pointed out that 25 per cent of older people were single or childless and had no relatives to care for them.[9] The empirical data involved interviews with over 1300 people aged 55 years and over randomly extracted from Victorian electoral rolls, smaller scale investigations in four inner Melbourne districts, and visits to 45 homes for the aged. One important finding was that extreme poverty and distress of older people was largely limited to slum areas of inner Melbourne suburbs where many lived alone. Other noteworthy issues covered in the report were the gendered nature of ageing alone with women predominating, the inadequacy of the old age pension rate, the need for community amenities, poor physical health and lack of adequate health services including severe shortage of hospital beds.[10]

## Geriatric Medicine

Despite the increasing number of older people, the first half of the century saw little change in health service responses. Sick older people were treated in hospitals in acute episodes of care in the same fashion as younger people with the number having chronic disability and associated social and psychological needs being relatively low.[11] Geriatric medical services had their beginnings in Australia in the 1950s, although for many years the distribution was sporadic. Due to this, and the fact that the states were responsible for running hospitals, there were different pathways to their establishment around the country. Perhaps the most well-known and influential early example was the so-called 'Newcastle Experiment' led by the physician Dr Richard (Dick) Gibson from 1954 at the Royal Newcastle Hospital, NSW. This was the first service in Australia to offer a comprehensive multidisciplinary (physician, social worker, occupational therapist, nurse) rehabilitation service that included hospital, half-way house and home care by domiciliary nurses. Home based assessments were encouraged as Gibson believed that most geriatric health problems could be managed in the older person's home in collaboration with their general practitioner. The William Lyne Block, located just over 6 kilometres from the Royal Newcastle Hospital, was opened in 1957 and was the site of inpatient geriatric rehabilitation.[12, 13] In 1994, Sidney Sax commented that the Newcastle service attracted visitors from all over Australia and 'probably was the strongest influence on the evolution of our current systems of assessment and rehabilitation of disabled and dependent elderly persons'.[14] Perhaps the most obvious influence was on the transformation of Lidcombe Hospital in NSW in the 1960s from a former home for aged and infirm destitute men to a modern geriatric hospital with comprehensive rehabilitation services, albeit with a greater hospital focus than Newcastle. Successive NSW Director-Generals of Public Health, Cyril Cummins and Sidney Sax, wanted to use the Newcastle Experiment as the basis of statewide rehabilitation reform. Dr Gary Andrews became the medical superintendent after a period working in Glasgow with prominent Scottish geriatrician Fergus Anderson. Andrews was instrumental in promoting modern approaches to geriatric medicine which included changing expectations about outcomes by treating acute exacerbations of chronic conditions and facilitating recovery with multidisciplinary rehabilitation input that allowed many older people to be discharged back home.[15,16]

In Victoria, from the mid-1950s to the mid-1960s, the state-subsidised benevolent homes were reclassified as geriatric hospitals but their focus remained on long-term residential care, albeit with a change from the charity custodial model of care to a medical model of restorative treatment, in order to maintain people as active healthy functional members of community. Only at Ballarat was a domiciliary service established to keep people in the community. The Sir Herbert Olney geriatric assessment and retraining unit was established at Mount

Royal Hospital at Parkville in 1957 with Dr Robert Butterworth as director and was replaced by a purpose built 76-bed unit in the early 1960s.[17,18] But overall in the 1950s and 60s in Victoria the barriers to establishing comprehensive geriatric medical services proved insurmountable. The institutional focus of the medical staff, barriers to training of nurse aides and the limited power of the Hospitals and Charities Commission (HCC) to enforce change contributed to this.[19] In Queensland, a Division of Geriatrics in the Department of Health was established in 1961 and the Director of Geriatrics, Peter Livingstone established a geriatric unit at Brisbane's Princess Alexandra Hospital in 1963.[20] Western Australia established geriatric services within the Public Health Department in 1963 with Dr Richard (Dick) Lefroy as director. Although Lefroy believed that geriatric services should be based in a teaching hospital, this was not achieved until 1967.[21,22] The development of geriatric medical services across the country was piecemeal in this era, but the growing interest in geriatric medicine led to the formation of the Australian Geriatrics Society (AGS) in 1972 with Gary Andrews as foundation president.[23] Physician geriatricians were first mentioned in a Commonwealth publication in 1977. The AGS commenced a training program in the late 1970s with the first locally trained geriatricians qualifying in the early 1980s.[24]

## Mental health

Much like the lack of aged care infrastructure after the Second World War, mental health services across the country had endured decades of neglect and lack of investment. A series of reports in the *Melbourne Herald* in 1946 about Victorian mental hospitals epitomized the poor conditions present nationwide. The article about Kew Mental Hospital under the heading 'Kew conditions horrifying' focused on older people and noted that new female admissions were often aged over 70. It painted a bleak picture.[25]

> 'They are old, querulous and senile (and to that extent insane) and they come to Kew because their families don't want them any more, and the benevolent institutions are full (and also, perhaps, because benevolent institution inmates receive pensions and mental hospital inmates do not). Their new environment with its total lack of privacy

and comfort, the awful airing yards, the cold drab green walls, the constant association with the insane quickly turns senility into dementia. There is no hope or warmth in the cold walls of this asylum, only the dreadful certainty of months and years in cold passages, of confinement for refractory behaviour in the cells, of long days without books or friends in the airing yards where there are few seats and nauseating filth.'[26]

Other issues raised in the article included that there were few baths, taps having handles removed forcing patients to drink water coming down walls or in drains, bad smells, cells euphemistically described as single rooms, and an overall appearance more like a gaol. Contrast was made with the better conditions in admission wards.[27]

In 1947, concerns about the aged and those with senile dementia in the mental hospitals led the fledgling Australasian Association of Psychiatrists, the forerunner organisation to the Royal Australian and New Zealand College of Psychiatrists, to request that their South Australian branch prepare a report about the issue. However, if such a report were prepared there are no records of it.[28] In October 1950 the officers in charge of Mental Hygiene Divisions of each State met for the first time in Melbourne. Two major problems were identified across the Commonwealth; a shortage of female nurses and shortage of accommodation for patients. With the latter, Basil Stafford from Queensland reported that

'on analysis it was found that each State was confronted with an increasing problem, the care of the aged. Mental Hospitals were admitting and caring for ever larger numbers of patients whose affliction was senility. They were people who had lived as useful and productive units of society until sixty and more years of age, and who until aged were capable of filling important posts in every and any sphere of communal activity. The Directors in Melbourne felt that these patients constituted a very special class and could be more appropriately and in time more skilfully cared for in a special institution. They are folk who are not able to care for themselves or to assume full legal responsibility so that a Home has to be devised whereby the law would provide sufficient protection for their person and their assets'.[29]

No comment was made about the poor conditions that the older patients had in the overcrowded mental hospitals.

Not much changed and a further newspaper exposure of conditions in Kew cottages in 1954 led to one of the few Commonwealth interventions into mental health in this era largely because Kew was in the electorate of Prime Minister Robert Menzies.[30] He authorized Alan Stoller to undertake the first national survey of mental hospitals in Australia. The Stoller report was comprehensive and highly critical of the conditions in the mental hospitals and the overall standard of psychiatric services in Australia. Apart from the overcrowding of the hospitals, which Stoller felt required a massive building program to remedy, he noted that adequate maintenance of the existing stock in the following decade would cost £108.5 million (or $4.13 billion in 2022 dollars).[31,32] While the report recognised the deficiencies of community and general hospital psychiatry, it failed to appreciate that overcrowding could be better addressed by other approaches. Perhaps the timing of the report which coincided with the introduction of various psychotropic drugs and the concern about the overall low standard of psychiatric care in the country influenced this. With regard to older people, Stoller noted that they comprised up to a third of admissions, about double the population proportion. Solutions were implied:

'the problem of the senile has been a severe burden to all Mental Hygiene Departments and was roughly parallel for all states … we had observed that many senile patients crowded into mental hospitals, were similar to those held in Old People's Homes …'[33]

Nothing was specifically recommended, nor a process suggested to remedy the issue. Again, perhaps the timing of the report which occurred in the same year as Martin Roth's research about classification and outcomes of mental disorders in late life, meant that the potential impact of better quality assessment and management was not appreciated.[34] Not all older patients were senile with an inevitable and untreatable decline. Alternative long-term residential care options for those with dementia was not the only reform required.

One important outcome of the Stoller Report was the acceptance by the Commonwealth of some financial responsibility to provide assistance to the States in renovating and providing modern accommodation in mental hospitals.[35] Otherwise Commonwealth funding of mental health largely focused on the repatriation population. The 1961 Royal Commission at Callan Park provided a stark contrast between the good quality conditions and food in the repatriation wards and that available to civil wards. According to the Deputy Commissioner of Repatriation, 'whenever money is needed for any amenity in the Repatriation Wards, it is made available.'[36] The implication here was that if adequate funding were to be provided for the civil patients, conditions would improve. In another context, the Commonwealth was reluctant to pay older hospitalised mental patients their pension; this only changed in 1971 for those in open wards and in 1980 for those in locked wards.[37]

Despite the concerns graphically described in the Stoller Report, there were significant improvements occurring in mental health services across the country from the 1950s onwards. 'Open door' policies that appeared in England earlier in the decade were introduced in the mental hospitals.[38] The deinstitutionalisation process commenced in the 1950s in part related to the resocialisation policies to assist the military to return to the community, although for older people this usually meant transfer from one type of institution to another.[39] The introduction of antipsychotic drugs such as Largactil (chlorpromazine) and antidepressants such as Tofranil (imipramine) from the mid-1950s onward facilitated recovery, discharge and outpatient treatment. Together with electroconvulsive therapy (ECT) there were now some effective treatment options. Voluntary admissions increased as did discharges which were assisted by the expansion of half-way houses largely run by non-government voluntary organisations.[40]

General hospital psychiatry started to flourish particularly through the 1960s and 70s. Victoria, under the leadership of E. Cunningham Dax, led the way in developing community treatments which were mainly based in outpatient departments. It took the Whitlam government in the early 1970s to set up the first community mental health centres, although a change of government in the late 1970s curtailed their development. Professional training started to improve. After the Second World War, it became commonplace for those who were seeking post-graduate training in psychiatry to travel to the UK and the US. There were

Diplomas of Psychological Medicine in various states such as the one offered by the University of Queensland from 1948 but it was not until the 1960s that nationwide accredited training in psychiatry commenced. The Australasian Association of Psychiatrists was established in 1946, became a College in 1963, the Australian and New Zealand College of Psychiatrists, and then the 'Royal' College (RANZCP) in 1978. From 1965 College membership became the basic psychiatric qualification and it became a 5-year training program in 1977. Academic psychiatry started to become independent of the UK in the 1980s.[41]

There were new challenges too. Indigenous mental health that had largely been ignored, became recognised for its unique elements that were entwined in the rights of Aboriginal and Torres Strait Islander people that required a different approach to mental health care, one that remains a struggle to achieve to this day. The post-war immigrant boom which included refugees from Europe and then from the 1970s onwards from wars and persecution in South East Asia, the Middle East and Latin America had a significant impact on mental health services, not the least in the care of the often non-English speaking and poorly educated older migrants.[42] From an old age perspective the early moves towards developing specific mental health services for older people that went beyond custodial care started to emerge in Victoria in the 1950s and NSW in the 1960s and this is covered in more detail in the next chapter. At a national level, Bruce Peterson in his October 1972 RANZCP Presidential address at Hobart entitled *The Age of Ageing*, gave the first indication that psychiatry and the College in particular needed to do more for older people. Without using the term 'ageism' that had only just been coined by Robert Butler, he wondered if stereotypical attitudes towards older people that were inconsistent with facts about ageing contributed towards psychiatrists' lack of interest in older patients. Apart from working more closely with geriatric medicine, Peterson had no specific suggestions as to how the psychiatry could improve its care of older people.[43]

## The Commonwealth Government and aged care services

The involvement of the Commonwealth in funding long-term care developed in piecemeal fashion over many years. Some degree of Commonwealth support for residential aged care occurred at an early stage. From 1910 under the

Commonwealth *Old Age Pensions Act, 1908*, pensioner residents of benevolent asylums were not entitled to receive the pension but 'act of grace' payments were made to the institution instead and this continued until 1963. In 1943 the Commonwealth government started to provide support for nursing home care in an indirect way by paying a 'wife's allowance' to wives of invalid or age pensioners resident in benevolent asylums or psychiatric hospitals.[44] The first major involvement of the Commonwealth in residential aged care occurred with the Menzies government in 1954 as a response to the accommodation crisis for older people that had worsened post-war. The *Aged Persons Homes Act* committed the Commonwealth to match the contributions of approved religious and charitable organisations to build hostel style accommodation for older people in need and led to a massive expansion of residential care.[45,46]

The start of Commonwealth government involvement in recurrent funding of nursing homes occurred in 1963 when a daily payment for patients in approved nursing homes was introduced to assist about 15 thousand chronically ill older people with their fees, as the rules of private health insurance organisations excluded them from private health coverage. This resulted in the unintended rapid growth in the industry over the next five years with 220 new homes (20 per cent increase) and nearly 12,500 extra beds (48 per cent increase). This was further enhanced in 1966 when the Holt government started providing capital subsidies towards accommodation for 'residents requiring continuous nursing care'. Because nursing homes were reluctant to admit severely disabled immobile people, further daily supplementary benefits for patients requiring intensive nursing care were introduced in 1968.[47]

The growth in nursing homes chiefly occurred in the private sector where the Commonwealth subsidies provided financial incentives to speculators to build unregulated nursing homes at relatively low risk resulting in uncontrolled growth in the number of nursing homes.[48] State mental health services took advantage of the situation and transferred many older patients with a range of mental disorders as part of their deinstitutionalisation process. This in effect was cost shifting from the States to the Commonwealth. Cecily Hunter noted that the lack of follow up care provided to these patients and the lack of skills and training of nursing home staff meant that there was a lack of specialist mental health care being provided.[49] A study of residents aged 60 years and over in Perth nursing homes by Peter

Burvill in 1967 found high rates of mental disorders. Approved nursing homes that met certain State medical requirements thus qualifying for State subsidies had 40 per cent of their residents having dementia and overall 69 per cent with a mental disorder. The non-approved nursing homes had many residents with schizophrenia and intellectual disability. Burvill noted that the nursing homes were not well-equipped to deal with the residents with their low nurse patient ratios with staff lacking psychiatric training.[50]

Many older people who were admitted to nursing homes did not require that level of care. This first came to attention in NSW after the 1965 Committee chaired by Sidney Sax reported on *The Care of the Aged* (The Sax Report) and recommended over £4.5 million state capital expenditure on nursing homes over the next ten years.[51] In June 1966, this was rejected by NSW Director of Health, Louis Wisenholt, who estimated that 30 to 40 per cent of nursing home residents did not need to be there as they only required personal care. He noted that the certification required for nursing home admission was easy to obtain and there were even residents who went out to work.[52] As pointed out by Dick Lefroy in the *Medical Journal of Australia* in 1969, the Commonwealth only recognised two types of living arrangements for older people – independent living in the community or nursing home care. Yet the reality was that there were stages of dependency that required different levels of support.[53]

In the 1969 election campaign, the Gorton government provided a range of uncoordinated small subsidies to various voluntary community groups that in time came to be known as the Commonwealth Home Care Program that was administered by two departments, health and social services, and were cost shared. The Department of Social Services had three programs that included provision of home help, provision of aged care welfare officers, and construction subsidies for senior citizens centres. The Department of Health offered salary subsidies for paramedical staff such as podiatrists and physiotherapists. The take up by the states of these programs was quite varied, for example, half of the welfare officers were employed in Victoria while most of the paramedical staff went to South Australia.[54]

At the end of the 1960s there was no coherent national aged care policy and a lack of coordination between the States and the Commonwealth. The quality of care in many nursing homes, particularly those in the private sector, was substandard but often these were the only homes with vacancies. Yet costs had risen substantially such that by 1972 Commonwealth expenditure on nursing homes was almost three times that of Commonwealth hospital benefits for insured patients and most of this came in the private sector. The combination of spiraling costs and the acceptance that around 25 per cent of nursing home residents did not need to be there on medical grounds resulted in the McMahon government passing legislation in 1972 to provide control of nursing home admissions, the growth of nursing home accommodation, and nursing home fees.[55] There was also encouragement for the provision of hostel level of care and a domiciliary nursing care benefit for accepting the responsibility of the care of a person at home. These measures did curb the growth of nursing home accommodation and this was further encouraged by the Whitlam government's focus on encouraging community alternatives to nursing home admission by making more funds available for home care. Under the Fraser government costs exploded again with a substantial increase of nursing home beds but community programs such as home help were grossly under-resourced with only 22 home helpers per 100,000 population compared with 265 in Great Britain.[56,57]

In 1980 there was no clear understanding as to where the responsibility of the care of people with dementia lay.[58] Jan Carter listed six areas of divided responsibility: between mental health and aged care; between institutional and community care; between specialist and generalist services; between private families and the state; between formal and informal care; and between State and Commonwealth governments.[59] The federal government had no defined responsibility for dementia care even though research in NSW and Victoria had shown that the main reason for admission to a nursing home was due to a 'confusional state/senility'. Tom Arie spoke at an Australian Association of Gerontology meeting in 1979, the first at which psychogeriatrics was a topic, and used the term 'confused elderly' that rang true to those who were there.[60] This set the scene for the major changes that commenced in the 1980s.

# Chapter 11

# State Developments after the Second World War to 1980

Eric Cunningham Dax, in his book *Asylum to Community* that documented the first decade of reforms under the Mental Hygiene Authority in Victoria, observed that 'very little money had been spent on mental hospitals before the war and by the time it ended they were in a bad way, more particularly because of the acute staff shortage.'[1] In the first decade after the Second World War not much changed in the mental hospitals across Australia apart from the number of patients continuing to accumulate and the proportion of older admissions increasing in each State. For example, in Queensland the number of admissions aged 60 years and over more than doubled between 1944/45 and 1954/55, increasing from a quarter of admissions to nearly a third,[2,3] and in NSW the doubling of older admissions occurred between 1944/45 and 1955/56, increasing from over 26 per cent to just over a third.[4,5] Certain mental hospitals became the repository of older senile patients, such as Rydalmere in NSW and Kew in Victoria, and overall the focus was on care rather than treatment.

There is some evidence that treatment was not completely neglected. The introduction of electroconvulsive therapy (ECT) in the 1940s saw it being used in a wide range of disorders including dementia until it became clear that its main benefits were restricted to the severe mood disorders and acute psychoses. For five years after the Second World War, the Inspector General Reports from NSW contained statistics on the use of ECT by diagnosis and hospital (not by age). By aggregating the data from these five years, 140 patients who were in a 'demented state' (the term used in the reports) received ECT in NSW, with nine patients (6.4 per cent) recovering, forty-one (29.3 per cent) being 'relieved', and ninety (64.3 per cent) not improving. No one died. The poor outcomes are not surprising and it is likely that the few who benefited either had depression rather than dementia (the ones that recovered) or depression superimposed on dementia (the ones who obtained some relief). Another diagnostic category that was likely to have included mainly older patients was 'confusional states' and here the outcomes were much better and many more patients were treated. Of the 443 'confusional state' patients treated with ECT, 287 (64.8 per cent) recovered, 104 (22.6 per cent) relieved, fifty-one (11.5 per cent) showed no improvement, and one died (0.2 pe rcent). Confusional states can include an array of conditions and in contemporary thinking would mainly be associated with delirium due to an acute physical illness but it is likely that most of these cases were forms of agitated confusion associated with depression, mania, or psychoses. [6,7,8,9,10]

As noted in the previous chapter, the Stoller report in 1955, while documenting the rise in older mental hospital admissions at a rate disproportionate to that in the general population, had little in the way of solutions beyond suggesting other types of residential options. In reporting the situation in Victoria, where improvements in general aged care service provision had commenced in the early 1950s, Stoller noted that the boarding out of patients to various benevolent homes in regional Victoria demonstrated that 'a number of milder senile mental patients could be handled at this level. It was realised that provision of extra-mural services for the community, including social provisions (such as housing, prepared meals, social workers), and psychiatric outpatient services would help keep people at home.'[11]

Improvements in old age mental health service delivery commenced in Victoria but not in any significant way until after the Stoller Report.

After repeated concerns about the conditions in Victorian mental hospitals, two government enquiries recommended the establishment of a Mental Hygiene Authority which was formed in 1952 under the auspices of the *1950 Mental Hygiene Authority Act* with Eric Cunningham Dax from England as the foundation chair. As noted in Chapter 9, Dax was co-author of a study published in *Lancet* in 1952 that had focused on the 'geriatric problem in mental hospitals', and so he was well aware of the issue.[12] But his initial focus was on the broader problems in the mental hospitals. He noted that staff in mental hospitals were disillusioned, frustrated by insufficient funds, lack of public interest, and depleted medical and nursing staff. The mental hospitals had appalling conditions that were dirty, unsanitary and abominably smelly, maintenance was grossly inadequate, and the food and its presentation revolting. There was considerable overcrowding with many sleeping on mattresses on the floor. Even when funds were available for maintenance and renovations, the Public Works department had trouble in getting contractors to work in the hospitals. The Victorian Mental Hygiene Authority was fortunate to be able to commence reforms with sufficient funds as well as public, government, and departmental support for reform.[13] Thus at the time of the Stoller Report in early 1955, while some inroads had been made into improving the mental hospitals as recognised by the Report, work had not commenced on addressing the 'geriatric problem'.

The appointment of Herbert Bower as the Medical Superintendent of Kew Mental Hospital in 1955 was an important turning point. Of Jewish background, Bower grew up in Vienna and studied medicine there, having to complete his studies at the University of Basel after escaping the Nazi takeover of Austria in 1938. He was on the last ship to Australia when war broke out in 1939. During the war he worked as a medical officer for Chinese tungsten miners in the Northern Territory and also had a period on Dunk Island with a private patient who had schizophrenia. Despite this, after the war he still had to complete four years of further medical training at the University of Melbourne. He later obtained his Diploma of Psychological Medicine in 1953 while working as a medical officer in the Mental Hygiene Department. Before moving to Kew Hospital, he had been the Psychiatrist Superintendent at Beechworth Hospital.[14]

At the time of his appointment, Kew Mental Hospital was already predominantly a geriatric mental hospital and in the last annual report of his predecessor Dr Brady, the overcrowding, poor facilities particularly in the infirmary were seen as contributory to the general health of the patients with problems such as diarrhoea, ringworm and scabies, while falls leading to femur and wrist fractures were common.[15] In 1956, Bower's first full year in charge, there were over eleven hundred patients with the average age of admissions 64 years. During that year Bower reports that there were 271 deaths (average age 72 years) of whom 141 had been admitted in 1956 with the majority dying within a few days or weeks of admission, some being moribund on admission.[16] Bower commented that when he was appointed to Kew, he did not have any particular views on the overall problem of ageing, but 'was primarily interested in providing a favourable *milieu* for the recovery or rehabilitation of my elderly patients'.[17] In contrast to the lack of direction from the Stoller Report, Bower was taking his cues from the restorative approach that was being attempted in the recently rebadged geriatric hospitals in Victoria. Bower was not prepared to sit back and let things drift. From a personal standpoint, he ensured that he fully educated himself about gerontology, late life mental disorders, and provision of services to older people. This included undertaking a worldwide survey of psychogeriatric services in 1961 with site visits in Europe and North America. The breadth of his research and self-education are readily apparent in his Beattie-Smith lectures for 1963 on the topic of 'Old Age in Western Society'.[18,19] From the standpoint of improving conditions at Kew Mental Hospital and the outcomes of the older patients, Bower had the support of Dax who was well aware of the overall direction and improvement in the care of older people in the community through organisations such as the Old People's Welfare Council, the upgrading of the Benevolent Homes with their rebadging as geriatric hospitals, the pilot geriatric units in general hospitals, and the efforts of local authorities. Bower and Dax saw that as the future direction for old age mental health, but first it was essential to upgrade the facilities at Kew including developing a geriatric admission unit that bypassed the receiving house, support and train the staff, ensure that there were stimulating activities for the patients, engage with visitors and volunteer organisations, and commence work on developing outpatient and follow-up services.[20]

Cecily Hunter, in her thesis on the social history of geriatric medicine in Victoria, was critical of the approach taken by Dax at this time. Dax had been vocal about the importance of prioritising the development of acute geriatric medical units. The geriatric hospitals were intermediate and long-stay facilities, while general hospitals were reluctant to admit confused older people, leaving only the mental hospitals as institutions prepared to admit older people with confusional states that were often due to a mix of acute physical disorders and varying degrees of dementia. Dax believed that many of these cases should be initially admitted to an acute geriatric medical unit. Hunter took the view that Dax, as Chair of the Mental Hygiene Authority, failed to adequately address long-term care by developing relationships with voluntary organisations that were involved in long-term care and was following a model of care too biological, with his dogged adherence to desiring that acute medical care be fixed first, preventing the development of appropriate long-term care. The criticism appears harsh and seems to over-interpret a presentation he gave in a 1961 geriatrics conference and ignore his broader biopsychosocial approach to mental health service development. Yet there is a kernel of truth in it too as the quality of long-term dementia care was not given the same attention as other elements of mental health reform. There was also limited interaction between psychiatry and the emerging discipline of geriatric medicine. One factor that contributed to this was the bureaucratic divide between the Hospitals and Charities Commission that was responsible for the geriatric and general hospitals and the Mental Hygiene Authority.[21] For general practitioners (GPs), this divide contributed to their uncertainty about where to refer patients. In a 1968 study of those misreferred to Mt Royal geriatric hospital, around 50 per cent of older patients were misreferred to either geriatric hospitals or mental hospitals, with GPs and relatives citing stigma as a reason for not going to a mental hospital.[22]

In the 1957 Kew hospital section of the Mental Hygiene Authority annual report, Bower described the efforts made to develop occupational therapy programs of meaningful activities in the hospital maintenance and laundry departments (mainly for the younger patients) including the challenges of creating a program for the broad spectrum of geriatric patients – some frail, some confused. He noted the range of entertainments available but conceded that there was a preponderance of passive entertainment and 'attempts to correct this state of affairs will be made in the future'.[23] The extensive building program was outlined in the report including the contributions of numerous voluntary organisations in the process. By the end of 1957 there were no more 'floor beds' in the hospital. An important component to Bower's approach to service development was his commitment to describing and evaluating his work in medical journal publications and conference presentations and his 1957 report noted that he was already preparing an article for publication about the resocialisation program for patients with chronic psychosis.

Bower mentioned 'stimulation therapy' for the first time in the 1958 report and stated that it was 'aiming to alter the behaviour of withdrawn and passive patients, and results, particularly with geriatric cases who suffer from somatic disuse atrophy, have been encouraging'.[24] He also mentioned the deliberate policy of getting patients out of bed and the benefits to patients of improved appetites, prevention of illness, and easier ward management. In 1959 Bower commented that the female geriatric patients had much improved function being able to feed and toilet themselves, being more mobile, less lethargic and more aware of reality.[25] Eventually Bower described the sensory stimulation program in more detail in a 1967 article in the *Medical Journal of Australia* in which he provided data from a non-blind controlled six month study involving patients with dementia that indicated benefit for the stimulation program. From a methodological perspective the study was deeply flawed with the comparison group already hospitalised for an average of four years at baseline and much frailer than the newly admitted treatment group. But the stimulation therapy was described and involved four and a half hours structured nurse supervised stimulation per day, five days per week including exercise, daily living and social activities, entertainment and games on an open, pleasantly furnished ward.[26] Despite the flaws in the research, there had been few previous reports of this approach to dementia care with Bower acknowledging the work of the geriatrician Lionel Cosin at Oxford as being one exception. This work carried out in the late 1950s and early 1960s in Melbourne was at the cutting edge of dementia care and it is likely that in an era when research published in antipodean journals had limited exposure, that it was largely unheard of in Europe and North America.

Bower was well aware of the importance of developing community mental health and dementia services. The Mental Health Act 1959 had provided for easier admission and discharge and gave the renamed Mental Health Authority more power to facilitate provision of community services.[27] The day hospital was another initiative pioneered by Lionel Cosin in Oxford. The first psychogeriatric day centre in Victoria was based at Kew hospital and had a long genesis from the 1956 discovery of a ramshackle abandoned building that formerly housed patients with schizophrenia to its emergence after a decade of gradual renovation, largely through the input of voluntary organisations, to be opened as the Janet H Bowen Day Centre in November 1966, at about which time Kew Hospital was renamed The Willsmere Hospital (there is no 'official' date recorded for this change). Bower described that after overcoming the initial difficulty of obtaining referrals, within a year it was thriving and was needing expansion. It was designed for mobile, continent, GP referred patients aged 65 years and over with a psychiatric disorder (dementia and other disorders) not severe enough to warrant admission and living within a defined distance from the hospital to enable transport. Before acceptance into the day centre, the patient was assessed by a psychiatrist and the social worker interviewed the family. Activities at the day centre were similar to the sensory stimulation program in the hospital.[28] After suffering a massive heart attack in 1965, Bower resigned his position as superintendent at Kew but continued work in old age mental health with the Victorian Mental Health Authority until 1970 during which time he also became President of the Victorian Society of Gerontology in 1968. He continued to work in a lesser capacity in psychiatry of old age through the 1970s including the provision of a consultative service at Mount Royal Hospital as he expanded his work in gender dysphoria and postgraduate training in mental health.[29] In 1995, Bower received an International Psychogeriatric Association Award for Service to Psychogeriatrics.[30]

Overcrowding at Kew (Willsmere) hospital remained a problem through the 1960s and 1970s. The 1962 annual report of the Mental Health Authority comments on the increase in numbers of older people seeking admission to the mental hospitals despite there being more alternatives available in private nursing homes and geriatric hospitals. It was observed that geriatric hospitals were reluctant to take admissions from mental hospitals despite the patients being similar in type and the increased finances that the geriatric hospitals had received compared with the overcrowded mental hospitals that were 'bearing the brunt of the geriatric problems'.[31] This observation was confirmed in a 1965 study by G. Vernon Davies at Mont Park where in just over a quarter of admissions, the degree of physical impairment was similar to or worse than the degree of mental impairment. He noted that some patients presented with acute confusion (delirium) and recovered yet were still refused admission from the mental hospital.[32] In a related study of female admissions to Mont Park, Davies reported that in 18 per cent of cases admissions were prompted by 'objections of other institutions (mainly private hospitals)'.[33]

The overcrowding at Willsmere Hospital was accentuated in 1968 when a tragic fire caused by an older woman smoking in bed resulted in the death of six patients. The fibro and timber building dated from the beginning of the century. As a consequence, three similar buildings housing thirty patients were vacated adding to the overcrowding.[34] It was noted in 1972 that there were at least two hundred older patients at Willsmere who could be more appropriately placed in the community if facilities were available.[35] There was little change over the next few years with Mont Park also affected with each hospital having its capacity to assess new admissions curtailed. A pilot project to determine whether patients with mild to moderate dementia could be managed in supervised hostel (low level care) accommodation in the community was established at Camberwell in 1975 with Arthur Harrison, consultant psychiatrist from nearby Willsmere Hospital providing a psychiatric assessment in the mental health clinic of those the social worker felt had not been adequately assessed before referral. In many ways this was the forerunner of assessments by an Aged Care Assessment Team that were introduced over a decade later. Seventy-five per cent of those who had the social worker and psychiatrist assessments settled and remained in the hostel for over fifteen months, demonstrating that admission to a long-stay ward in a mental hospital could be avoided for many cases.[36] The study also demonstrated that Willsmere remained at the cutting edge of old age mental health service developments after the departure of Herbert Bower.

In parallel with the developments at Kew, Mont Park Hospital, with Dr Grantley Wright as psychiatrist superintendent, was also developing a geriatric service for females. Here the work of Dr (George) Vernon Davies featured in the annual reports of the Mental Health Authority between 1956 and 1965. Vernon Davies is a little known pioneer of old age mental health in Australia. His work in psychiatry started late in career after the Second World War. He obtained his medical degree at Melbourne University in 1916 before serving as Captain in the Australian Medical Corps in the First World War where he was mentioned in dispatches and received the Distinguished Service Order (DSO). He completed his MD in 1920 before spending three years in the New Hebrides (Vanuatu) as a medical missionary in charge of Vila Hospital. On return to Australia, he moved to Wangaratta to work as a physician and was active in the local community particularly in the Returned Soldiers' League, the Presbyterian Church, and politics. By his mid-60s he had moved to Melbourne and was working as a psychiatrist at Mont Park Hospital. Perhaps his move was to be closer to his son Alan Fraser Davies, who on return from England had taken up a senior lectureship at the University of Melbourne in 1950 and over the course of the 1950s and 1960s became a prominent political scientist who drew on a range of influences including Freudian theories in his exploration of political behaviour.[37,38]

The 1956 Mental Hygiene Authority annual report notes that Davies was carrying out a pilot investigation on personality factors and social problems associated with geriatric admissions.[39] Further details were provided in the 1957 report about the 50 consecutive patients in the survey along with details of a study Davies had undertaken comparing niacin with reserpine in senile male patients. The report comments that 'intensive physical therapies (large doses of vitamins, tranquillizing drugs and physiotherapy) proved extraordinarily beneficial to our large population of elderly patients.' Music therapy was used with senile patients at Mont Park '…and many patients, hitherto considered quite immobile, have been encouraged to move about and even dance, with marked improvement in their physical and mental states.'[40]

In 1959 Davies published the first Australian overview on clinical advances in geriatric psychiatry in the *Medical Journal of Australia*. This detailed article is full of clinical wisdom and references to contemporary research such as the work of Martin Roth in England. Davies stressed the complexity of the multiple factors contributing to an older person's mental disorder including their various life experiences from childhood onwards to the mix of emotional and organic factors precipitating admission. He commented that it was easy to mistake cause for effect in symptoms. He notes how around a third of patients recover and are discharged along with the importance of conveying this prognosis to families at the outset, remembering that in this era there was little expectation that patients might be discharged. In terms of hospital treatment, he mentions that those with significant medical comorbidity being treated in the mental hospital infirmary and that the key factor there was to keep patients physically active. For the physically fit admissions, a full physical workup was still mandatory. The inpatient milieu with decorated wards, multidisciplinary activities and group therapies and involvement of the family was described. A brief overview of physical treatments available in 1959 was provided and some mention of prevention. For its time, this was very mature and practical article that espoused principles still relevant today, but it had little impact from either an academic perspective, with no citations recorded, or a clinical perspective where it is long forgotten.[41]

By 1959 Davies had extended his study of personality and social factors by obtaining two comparison groups involving 50 participants from Caulfield Geriatric Hospital and a further 50 females from an Old People's Club. Reorganisation of the Mont Park Hospital complex was under way at this time with the section that housed older long-stay patients divided from Mont Park and renamed Plenty Hospital, a process completed in 1963. Pleasant View located at Preston, formerly a receiving house that was an annex of Royal Park, had become a geriatric hospital for male patients with good prognosis likely to return home but it was in need of renovation.[42] Mont Park was struggling with the number of older admissions by 1961 and the proposed construction of two new female geriatric wards were hoped to remedy the problem along with the impact of the new geriatric admission ward at Kew.[43] It had been long noted by Davies that many of the older admissions had significant comorbid physical illnesses; he published an overview on the overlap of physical and mental illness in old age in the *Medical Journal of Australia* in 1961.[44] New admissions often had to be quickly transferred to the 'hospital' ward at Mont Park. To reduce the number of transfers required for older patients, from June 1962 all geriatric admissions to Mont Park were made through the hospital ward where treatment of physical ailments was more readily available. Two other initiatives involving direct admissions to Mont Park of those seeking voluntary admission and weekend sessions when the attending psychiatrist was able to interview relatives of the patients were hoped to increase the number of discharges.[45]

Vernon Davies' research into family relationships and social aspects of consecutive admissions to Mont Park eventually fulfilled the requirements for a doctoral thesis at Melbourne University when he was aged 79 in March 1968.[46] The work was published in the *Australian and New Zealand Journal of Psychiatry* in 1968 and 1969.[47,48] He retired in 1973 when he was 85 although even at that time he was still giving occasional lectures on psychogeriatrics.[49] After his retirement, Mont Park no longer had such a strong geriatric focus and in a 1975 Mental Health Authority annual report only Willsmere was listed as a psychogeriatric service in Victoria.[50]

During this period there were other Victorian mental hospitals admitting significant numbers of older patients including Larundel on the northern outskirts of Melbourne where Arthur Harrison in the late 1970s helped establish the first comprehensive psychogeriatric service in Victoria. The regional hospitals at Ballarat and Beechworth also admitted many older patients, with Ballarat developing a collaborative model of service interaction between geriatric medicine and psychiatry in the 1950s and by 1961 psychiatrists were visiting the benevolent home, there was a geriatrics outpatient clinic, and regular exchanges of patients between the mental hospital and the benevolent home occurred.[51] Two modern psychogeriatric wards to replace century-old wards were opened at Beechworth in 1976.[52] By the end of the 1970s, the promise of the early 1960s led by Dax, Bower and Davies had stalled and Victoria had two well-developed old age mental health services in Melbourne, albeit with a predominantly institutional focus. Few psychiatrists in Victoria were interested in old age mental health. Indeed Cecily Hunter believes that in the 1960s psychiatry was in a better position than geriatric medicine in Victoria to influence change but by the late 1970s this was no longer the case. However, the appointment of Derek Prinsley in 1976 as Foundation Professor of Gerontology and Geriatrics at Mt Royal Institute (later to be renamed the National Ageing Research Institute of Australia) that had been established as the first academic aged care unit in Australia in 1975 and at around the same time the linkage of Mt Royal with Royal Melbourne Hospital signalled the progress that had been made.[53]

The other state that took steps towards developing a modern older people's mental health service in this period was NSW. In 1953, there were over five hundred 'senile' admissions to the four Sydney mental hospitals – Callan Park (28 per cent of admissions), Gladesville (24 per cent), Parramatta (28 per cent) and Rydalmere (76 per cent).[54] Similar to Victoria, at the time of the Stoller Report in 1955 there had been little happening beyond accumulation of more long-stay patients. As noted in the Stoller Report, 'the senile problem' was being handled

> 'by herding old people together under appalling conditions. Old people require a special type of accommodation, and nurses need a special type of training. Much of this problem could be taken up through the extension of other old-people's homes.'[55]

NSW Inspector General of Mental Health, Donald Fraser, had been making similar remarks about alternative accommodation for the previous five years. In 1955 he authorised Dr D.M. Sommerville to undertake private postgraduate studies on the 'care and treatment of the aged who are mildly deranged'.[56] Some of the key findings in Sommerville's report included the need for earlier diagnosis and treatment in outpatient clinics that required 'tremendous expansion' to close the gap between institutional and private psychiatry. As far as possible, older patients should be admitted voluntarily into geriatric annexes bypassing the reception houses. The importance of social workers in investigating the social circumstances of the admissions and of notifying the GP about admissions and discharges including a discharge summary were stressed. Follow-up clinics were needed too. The Tooting Bec Hospital was cited as an example of how a voluntary system of alternative long-stay accommodation could work. These sensible recommendations came at a time in 1957 when the number of mental health patients aged 60 years and over topped five thousand and represented 31.5 per cent of mental health patients under care in NSW, clearly a time when service planning beyond alternative accommodation was required.[57]

The new NSW *Mental Health Act 1958* had more of a community focus than its predecessor, encouraged voluntary admissions and treatment rather than custody. Although there were no specific features relevant to older people, in the 1980s the definition of mental illness in the Act as it related to dementia became an issue and this is discussed in chapter 13.[58] The *Mental Health Act 1958* was a turning point that contributed to the rapid deinstitutionalisation of mental patients in the 1960s and early 1970s, dropping from the peak of around 14,500 in 1961 to just over 7,600 in 1974.[59,60]

At the beginning of 1961 the NSW Health Advisory Council was formed with the Director General of Public Health, Cyril Cummins, as Chair, its first project being a study of mental health services. The first report in June 1961 emphasised prevention, early intervention and long-term hospital and community services. For geriatric patients the focus remained on long-term accommodation, if not in alternative facilities external to mental hospitals, then special degazetted accommodation within mental hospitals and voluntary admissions.[61] Again, the lack of specific consideration beyond long-stay options is notable. In 1962, a Health Advisory Committee Report on the Aged resulted in the appointment of a State Director of Geriatrics within the Department of Public Health, the establishment of a geriatric unit as a pilot scheme in a metropolitan district hospital, a scheme to assist organisations to provide domiciliary nursing to aged or additional nursing to sick aged, and the appointment of a Consultative Committee involving health and welfare representatives and volunteer organisations to review the report and develop priorities for implementation. The report explicitly did not include the mentally infirm but noted that many of the initiatives would benefit them.[62]

The 1961 Callan Park Royal Commission handed down its findings after the Health Advisory Council mental health report. Commissioner McClemens commented on the geriatric patients and felt that it was 'an institution to which many people go to die'. Although some might be better off than in a nursing home, 'one is forced to the conclusion that the standards of treatment for the great majority of patients are far lower than they ought to be.' McClemens also minimised the nursing skills and time required to nurse those with advanced dementia. He felt that that they required 'no special nursing' and needed 'nothing more than to be kept warm, clean and comfortable and to be given that modicum of food and drink that a dying person needs.'[63]

In the early 1960s most developments for older patients focused on finding alternative accommodation for those with dementia and other chronic mental disorders, and of ways in preventing admissions. The NSW Association for Mental Health had a Standing Committee on 'Mental Health of the Aged' which during this period undertook a range of activities with the aim of reducing older admissions to the mental hospitals. It commenced in 1960 with a survey in conjunction with eighteen organisations working in the field,[64] followed by seminars in 1961 and 1962 for matrons of old people's homes and others working in the field,[65,66] and then in 1964 it prepared a booklet on the needs of old people and those looking after them in their homes. Subjects included diet, legal matters, occupations, hobbies, and social agencies that assist in the care of the aged.[67]

Allandale Hospital at Cessnock opened in February 1963 and in the first half of the year received 212 discharges from the State's mental hospitals. Choice of patients was based on them being chronologically and physiologically aged and no longer requiring continued psychiatric treatment. The importance of being discharged from the mental hospital was that it now made the majority of patients eligible for pensions.[68] The State Director of Psychiatry report for 1963–64 was the first to use the term 'psychogeriatric services' but still focused entirely on providing new and alternative accommodation for chronic cases noting that social workers, welfare officers and domiciliary nurses were able to facilitate the discharge of many older patients to nursing homes. The report noted the appointment of Sidney Sax as the Director of State Geriatrics in May 1964 and the hope that community services could prevent admissions to mental hospitals.[69]

The first report of the Consultative Committee for the Care of the Aged, which became known as *The Sax Report*, was submitted to the NSW Minister of Health in August 1965. It largely endorsed the Health Advisory Council Report and strongly recommended that the first priority should be given to the promotion of social well-being, preservation of independence and dignity, and the prevention of disability. *The Sax Report* made ten observations and recommendations about older people with mental disorders with the first being that the overall thrust of the services described to prevent disability would also prevent mental disorders and reduce the need for institutional care. It was stressed that a high proportion of mental disorders were curable but depended on proper diagnosis and assessment to get correct treatment. The GP was in the best position to do this but needed training, perhaps in geriatric units or psychiatry units. Outpatient clinics were required, geriatric or psychiatric, with an emphasis on the need for cooperation between physicians and psychiatrists. Community treatment was possible for many disturbed patients, providing community services were available. If hospital admission was required, in the first instance it should be for assessment and treatment, either in geriatric or psychiatric units depending on local circumstances and the patient's condition, with the expectation that many patients would be discharged home. For those requiring long-term residential care, most would be suitable for nursing homes with only those where severe disturbance with 'behaviour no longer acceptable to other patients or to the staff' remaining in non-gazetted special purpose nursing home accommodation. The need for such special purpose accommodation in any region would be assessed by regional committees and decisions reviewed at a State level to determine state priorities.[70]

From 1965 the State Director of Psychiatry reports contained admission diagnosis statistics by age group for the first time and used the age of 65 as the cut-off for old age. The importance of these data was that it was clearly demonstrated that dementia and other organic mental disorders were only accounting for around a half of older admissions with the rest being mainly due to depression, non-organic psychoses, alcohol-related mental disorders and psychiatric problems associated with physical disease.[71] Of course that such a wide range of mental disorders, many eminently treatable with antipsychotic and antidepressant medication as well as ECT, accounted for older admissions had been described by Martin Roth in England a decade earlier but that had seemingly escaped recognition in NSW despite being signalled in Dr Sommerville's report in the late 1950s. This further emphasised the points made in the Sax Report. Additionally, it was amplified in a survey of all admissions aged 65 years and over from Callan Park, North Ryde and Parramatta mental hospitals during the first six months of 1964 that was published in 1967. One of the main findings related to the much better treatment outcomes compared with those from a decade earlier; discharges rose from 27 per cent in 1954 to 68 per cent in 1964, deaths dropped from 40 per cent in 1954 to 18 per cent in 1964, and those remaining in hospital fell from 33 per cent in 1954 to 14 per cent in 1964. While the improved outcomes were in part explained by fewer dementia admissions, in the main it was improved physical and other treatments that seemed responsible for the change. Older people were no longer being admitted just for custodial care.[72]

Over the second half of the 1960s each of the major mental hospitals had defined psychogeriatric wards such as that by 1969, alongside Lidcombe Hospital, they were providing regional geriatric programs. It was noted in the 1968–69 annual report that in some regions community outreach programs were developing with domiciliary assessments.[73] The first comprehensive psychogeriatric service in NSW was developed by Miriam Merlin at Parramatta Mental Hospital and commenced in April 1968 although for some years prior to that there had been a more limited post-discharge service. It was a total care team that accepted all catchment area referrals of patients aged 65 years and over and younger patients with multiple disabilities. After a year of service, over 120 patients were receiving domiciliary care in the community. Merlin described the development of the service which included a six-month multidisciplinary planning period at which three aims were defined. The first was 'the provision of a comprehensive sophisticated diagnostic, assessment, treatment, management, and care service for the mentally ill aged'. The second aim related to provision of training to all members of the multidisciplinary team and the third aim was to provide evaluation and research facilities relevant to clinical care. At the outset the service had one sex-integrated admission ward (a development that caused some initial trepidation but ultimately caused no problems) and three long-stay wards.[74]

The decision to take all patients aged 65 years and over into the service meant that staff were able to see that many recovered and returned home, an important validation of the work they were doing that had a positive effect on morale and facilitated development of the multidisciplinary team. The internal evaluation of the service included follow-up studies that demonstrated many patients remaining well in the community for up to twelve years after admission. One fear that was expressed at the outset was that they would be inundated with 'inappropriate' referrals such as social problems or medical problems that other hospitals would not admit but this proved to be wrong as less than one per cent of referrals did not have a 'legitimate' psychiatric diagnosis. As was being shown in the annual reports of the State Director of Psychiatry at a Statewide level, referrals to the Parramatta team were due to dementia and other organic mental disorders in about 50 per cent of cases with the rest due to functional mental disorders. One important learning that the Parramatta team soon gleaned from their work was that the immediate post-discharge care was complex but critically important and needed to be comprehensive including medication management, embracing the social, financial and interpersonal needs of care with ideally day care too.[75]

From the early 1960s specialist physicians and surgeons commenced work in the mental hospitals. Fred Ehrlich, a surgeon who worked at North Ryde Mental Hospital during this period and who in the late 1980s became Professor of Geriatrics at St George Hospital, was firmly of the view that the mental hospitals were capable of providing good physical health care in addition to psychosocial care so long as adequate staff and resources were available. Although some medical psychogeriatric units were developed, such as the one in ward 16 at Callan Park that was an annex to the admission unit, Ehrlich's vision did not come to fruition.[76,77]

By 1971 the psychogeriatric units in the other mental hospitals were expanding their role. A day centre with transport was established at Callan Park while at Gladesville hospital, the psychogeriatric team was divided into two sub-teams each managing different metropolitan catchment areas that included Wollongong and the South Coast. The Gladesville psychogeriatric wards had acute admission and rehabilitation roles with a multidisciplinary therapeutic program. Consultant psychiatrist and domiciliary nurse home visits were preferred especially for initial assessments and fifteen geriatric day centres/hospitals, some run at the hospital and most at various church halls in the local communities, often provided an alternative to hospital admission. Consultation liaison work in general hospitals and to nursing homes was also provided.[78]

After this spurt of development, few changes occurred over the rest of the 1970s in NSW. Miriam Merlin had proposed a psychogeriatric service structure to the Mental Health Services Planning and Review Committee in 1977 but nothing came of it. According to Sid Williams in 1981, the psychogeriatric units were surviving because there was clearly a need, but survival was not enough. The psychogeriatric units in the mental hospitals lacked adequate access to high quality technical medical services and were to the most part geographically distant from their catchment areas. They also had difficulties in attracting staff, particularly with the lack of training programs across the disciplines. The only psychogeriatric service that developed in a general hospital occurred at Lidcombe hospital under the leadership of Sid Williams from 1974. This service was not formally administered by mental health, being a part of the geriatric neurology service at Lidcombe. During the late 1970s it had an institutional focus that was mainly acute and subacute care of people with dementia and other neuropsychiatric disorders without a formal catchment area or community outreach, although most admissions were from the local area and there were outpatient clinics.[79]

Although none of the other states and territories moved beyond the provision of acute and long-term institutional care for older patients during this period, there were some notable developments. Queensland led the way in finding alternatives to the mental hospitals for long-term residential care. Before that, Dunwich Asylum on Stradbroke Island was closed in October 1946 after a protracted period of secret political planning. The announcement and the move to Sandgate near Brighton as an Eventide home, occupying the huts on an old RAAF base surrounded by barbed wire, was sudden and took staff by surprise. At the time of the move there were 768 residents who were ferried to the mainland over two days. Conditions at Sandgate in the early days were worse than those at Dunwich, indeed it was not a move based on having a better alternative facility but one based at least in part on solving the political problem of Dunwich asylum brought on by the repeated scandals.[80]

In 1951 plans were announced to build a 500-bed Eventide home but this did not proceed as it was felt to be impractical.[81,82] What did appear to work well was having special accommodation in regional areas, Jubilee Hospital at Dalby and Mt Lofty Hospital at Toowoomba, which were administered by the local hospital boards. As Basil Stafford the Queensland Director of Mental Hygiene commented in 1954, 'this policy of caring for the aged in their own residential area, and amongst their own relatives and friends has much to commend it'.[83] Many of the residents had been discharged from Toowoomba mental hospital. The success of the Jubilee Hospital led to its expansion and the opening of other regional facilities at Wondai and Oakey as annexes to general hospitals. Discharges to these facilities increased such that in 1959/60 there were 354 senile patients discharged from the mental hospitals. Furthermore, admissions had reduced and by 1960/61, older patients only represented 22 per cent of admissions, a drop from around a third in the mid-1950s.[84] Contributing factors to this drop were the policy of retaining older patients in the general hospital area and the effects of Government policy in respect to Church Homes for the Aged meaning that more patients who would have otherwise been admitted to mental hospitals were accepted in the Eventide Homes.[85]

In 1962 Stafford felt that accommodation issues for dementia patients had been solved with the general hospital annexes and Eventide homes but he felt that the process of admitting patients to mental hospitals for assessment and then transfer elsewhere was unsatisfactory. He advocated for the development of a more active regime of medical and nursing care that was occurring in the recently opened Marjory Warren geriatric unit at Princess Alexandra hospital and felt a unit associated with a general hospital should be established. In June 1962, there had been 1356 patients transferred from mental hospitals to the annexes or Eventide homes.[86] A presentation given in 1961 by Dr H.N.

Noble from Brisbane about the assessment process stated that the patients were classified according to behaviour, treatment, and physical condition based on a system suggested by the World Health Organisation. He foreshadowed that in the near future some patients could be assessed in outpatient clinics, day hospitals or short-term admissions.[87] The Queensland *Mental Health Act 1962* encouraged voluntary admissions, the integration of mental health services with other health services and the treatment of the mentally ill in general hospitals.[88] Yet, for older people there were still concerns that patients being admitted to mental hospitals might have been better managed, at least initially, in a general hospital. A two-year review of older admissions to Brisbane Special Hospital (the former Goodna Mental Hospital) in 1968 found that 22 per cent died within a month of admission and that many were in a poor physical condition on admission.[89] A neuropsychiatric ward was built at Chermside (now Prince Charles) Hospital and opened in 1964, being renamed the Winston Noble Unit in 1977, while a nursing home ward opened at Prince Charles Hospital in 1978.[90]

In South Australia, after Bill Cramond became Director of Mental Health Services in 1961, classification of patients changed and by 1962 they were classified by age (as one criterion) and assigned to wards based upon the classification thus formally commencing psychogeriatric wards.[91] At Hillcrest Hospital, wards 9 and 10 became psychogeriatric wards in 1961. In 1975, Ward 8 was renamed Howard House and became the psychogeriatric admission and assessment ward. Wards 6 and 7 were added to the psychogeriatric service in 1978 but all the wards were substandard and did not provide adequate facilities for the aged who had added difficulties in negotiating the stairs with their limited mobility.[92] At Glenside Hospital, Downey House, a ward originally built for tuberculosis patients, was proclaimed a receiving house for geriatric patients in 1969.[93] In March 1979 Downey Grove, which was located near Downey House, was opened as a part of the redevelopment of Glenside Hospital, replacing substandard turn of the century buildings. It comprised four 32-bed psychogeriatric units spaced around open courtyards and each unit could be broken down to smaller sub-units.[94] Perhaps the major contribution from South Australia in this period was the establishment of Australia's first Guardianship Board in the 1977 Mental Health Act that was proclaimed in 1979. In 1993 it became an independent

Act. The South Australian Guardianship Board became the template for other Guardianship Boards that were established around the country from the mid-1980s onwards.[95] For people with dementia, guardianship provides a legal process that allowed for decision-making by an appointed guardian regarding medical, financial and welfare issues for a person who is incapacitated in any or all of these domains. In the absence of guardianship legislation, either Mental Health legislation or referral to Supreme Courts were the unsatisfactory legal alternatives.

At Claremont Hospital in Western Australia, which according to Philippa Martyr who researched the history of the hospital, 'was effectively used as a psycho-geriatric facility long before this was acknowledged as a separate discipline',[96] deinstitutionalisation with the discharge of many older and long-term patients to nursing homes and hostels increased after the appointment of Arch Ellis as the State Director of Mental Health Services in 1963.[97] In 1966, after representations by geriatrician Dick Lefroy, Sunset Home at Nedlands was renamed Sunset Hospital and provided restorative treatment for patients in the wards, with residents living in hostels on the grounds.[98]

There was little change regarding the organisation of care at Claremont Hospital until the early 1970s when the psychiatrist superintendent, Harry Blackmore reorganised the hospital into three divisions; a 'deficiency' division; a 'dementia' division; and a 'psychiatric' division. Claremont Hospital closed in 1972 and split into two hospitals – Graylands Hospital that treated acute psychiatric patients and Swanbourne Hospital that cared for the 'deficiency' and 'dementia' patients with Peter Reed as the psychiatrist superintendent.[99] Ellis, in his history of psychiatry in Western Australia, commented:

> 'when Claremont was replaced, it was predictable that the psychogeriatric hospital 'Swanbourne' would become the poor relation in respect to 'Graylands', as Claremont itself had done in respect to Heathcote. This happened and it is very difficult to recruit trained staff to nurse persons with long-term physical and intellectual handicaps.'[100]

Despite these difficulties, Peter Reed commenced the development of a psychogeriatric service based on contemporary British practice. Despite staff limitations, a domiciliary nursing and follow up service was established, with nursing home liaison. Admissions of patients living at home was prioritised over those in nursing homes.[101] In 1979, Swanbourne Hospital was severely criticised for its inadequacies in a report prepared by Dr Fred Bell, the Director of Mental Health Services and it was decided that it should be totally replaced, a process that commenced in the early 1980s.[102]

There were no specific psychogeriatric service developments in Tasmania during this period but the appointment of Scott Henderson as the Foundation Chair of Psychiatry at the University of Tasmania in 1970 led to important research in the 1980s. After moving to Canberra in 1974 to set up the Social Psychiatry Research Unit at the Australian National University, he was replaced in 1976 by David Kay who had collaborated with Martin Roth at Newcastle-upon-Tyne in the seminal research on the epidemiology of mental disorders in late life. Kay was also appointed as Chairman of the Tasmanian Mental Health Commission. General hospital psychiatry units opened at Launceston in 1964 and Hobart in 1970. Cunningham Dax, who had investigated mental health services in 1962, resulting in major changes at Lachlan Park Mental Hospital, was appointed Coordinator in Community Health services independent of the Mental Health Commission in 1969.[103]

By the end of the 1970s, despite the increasing older population, the early developments of psychogeriatric services in the late 1950s and 1960s in a few mental hospitals in Victoria and NSW had not progressed and were largely institutionally based with very little involvement of general hospitals and community services, while developments in the other states and territories were very limited. The high mortality within a month of admission signalled the need for closer relationships with geriatric medicine and acute psychogeriatric units located in general hospitals. The absence of any significant developments in community old age mental health apart from day hospitals was a major gap. The main change across the nation was the rise of private nursing homes, after the introduction of Commonwealth subsidies in 1963, to become the predominant site of long-term residential care in most states, with state mental hospitals 'deinstitutionalising' many long-term psychiatric patients and patients with dementia. By the end of the 1970s, the failure of the State mental institutions to provide adequate psychiatric liaison and support to these patients laid the foundations for the problems encountered in nursing homes in their management that has been ongoing. It seemed that it was largely a case of 'out of sight, out of mind'.

# Chapter 12

# National Developments in Dementia Services: 1980-2020

By 1981, 9.7 per cent of the population (1.5 million) were aged 65 years and over, increasing to 11.3 per cent (2.0 million) in 1991, 12.1 per cent (2.4 million) in 2001, 13.2 per cent (3.0 million) in 2011, and 16.4 per cent (4.2 million) in June 2020.[1,2] The ageing of post-war immigrants, many of whom were refugees from Europe, fuelled the growth.[3] The 1980s decade witnessed the first significant national steps in the development of comprehensive dementia services from policy, advocacy, and professional perspectives. Under the Fraser government, costs had again exploded with a substantial increase of nursing home beds but community programs, such as home help, were grossly under-resourced with only 22 home helpers per 100,000 population compared with 265 in Great Britain.[4,5] Following the 1980 federal election, the House of Representatives Standing Committee on Expenditure resolved to conduct an inquiry into 'Accommodation and Home Care programs for the Aged' and a sub-committee was formed led by Leo McLeay, with specialist advisors Bruce Ford and Anna Howe. The McLeay report in 1982 recommended the introduction of standardised assessment procedures prior to admission to a nursing home, reform of nursing home funding to control growth and expenditure, and an expansion of community-based services.[6] At the United Nations World Assembly on Ageing held in 1982, Australia had one of the highest rates of residential care for the aged in the world (140 beds per 1000 aged 75+) with only the United States and Denmark having more. A peculiarity was that most resided in high level care nursing homes rather than low level care hostels. When the Hawke government came into power in March 1983, ninety per cent of aged care funding went to the residential sector, and ninety per cent of residential sector funding went to nursing homes.[7]

The McLeay Report recommendations formed the basis of the Aged Care Reform Strategy of the Hawke government, and it was this report that first focused attention on the problem of dementia in nursing homes even though it had been a mounting issue for decades.[8] Scott Henderson, a psychiatric epidemiologist from the Australian National University, presented the keynote address at the RANZCP Annual Congress in Perth in 1982 on the 'Coming epidemic of dementia' in which he provided an overview of what was known about dementia and its causes, providing some estimates of projected increases in dementia numbers in Australia, and in a 'call for action' outlined the research imperatives particularly those related to social impacts and interventions.[9] Together with Anthony (Tony) Jorm, Henderson would subsequently publish the influential 1986 report for the Commonwealth Department of Community Services, 'The Problem of Dementia in Australia', which evolved over three revisions in the 1990s into 'Dementia in Australia'. These reports followed the same pattern as the 1982 address but with more detail about dementia assessment, management, and services. They became the main source of basic information about dementia for Australian policy makers, researchers, clinicians and advocacy groups in the late 1980s and through the 1990s.[10]

The first steps towards developing dementia-specific accommodation emerged from a 1985 Senate Select Committee into private nursing homes which recommended 'that special programs be set up within existing nursing homes for confused and psychiatrically ill elderly, including attention to the physical environment and staff training'.[11] The 1986 Nursing Homes and Hostels Review set out a strategy for the restructure of aged care programs along the lines of the McLeay Report and had a focus on community care. In residential care, limits were set on nursing homes and a greater emphasis was placed on hostel care.[12] The closures of State psychiatric wards for long-term dementia care continued throughout the 1980s leading to increasing numbers of persons with dementia being admitted to nursing homes and hostels. One recommendation of the Nursing Homes and Hostels Review was to establish recurrent funding for dementia care in hostels which led to the successful Hostel Dementia Grants Program and by

1991 it was estimated that half of hostel residents who could benefit from special dementia care were participating in programs.[13] The Nursing Homes and Hostels Review also recommended the establishment of uniform national nursing home standards of care. Previously each state had different standards and there was no check on them. A joint Commonwealth-State Working Party, after extensive consultations, came up with 31 outcome standards in seven categories: health care; social independence; freedom of choice; homelike environment; privacy and dignity; variety of experience; and safety. These were gazetted in 1987.[14] Outcome standards for hostels were introduced in 1991.[15]

Geriatric assessment services were announced in August 1986 to provide an evaluation of the care needs of an older person and such an assessment became mandatory for admission to residential care. These multidisciplinary Geriatric Assessment Teams were joint funded by the Commonwealth and the states. In 1992 the name was changed to Aged Care Assessment Teams (ACATs) due to community objection to the word 'geriatric'.[16] It was this innovation that facilitated the move of dementia assessment and management in public health services from mental health to geriatric medicine, although this process evolved gradually over many years and varied from State to State and region to region within States. While the difficulties posed by the split between Commonwealth and State responsibilities had long created problems in dementia care, as identified by Carter in 1981,[17] one unintended impact of this development was the exaggeration of the divided responsibilities between mental health and aged care that affected older people with other mental disorders such as depression and psychoses. Over time, many Commonwealth and State departments for mental health and aged care in whatever administrative structure was in place at the time, tended to 'pass the buck' over who was responsible for policies and services for these individuals with the consequence that they became a neglected group.[18]

In community care, the spouse carer's pension, now known as the carer payment, was introduced in 1983. The first coordinated approach in the provision of community aged care services occurred with the Hawke government's introduction of the Home and Community Care (HACC) Program, a joint Commonwealth–State program, in 1985. There were eleven eligible types of services that included home help, personal care, home maintenance and modification, meal preparation and home delivered food, respite care, transport, paramedical services and home nursing. It targeted individuals who were at risk of premature admission to residential care. People with dementia and their carers were designated as a special needs group. The major providers of services varied from State to State and included a mix of voluntary groups, State services, and local government services. Commonwealth outlays on the HACC program rapidly increased in the late 1980s and through the 1990s.[19]

During the 1980s locally trained geriatricians started to appear but it would be many years until the workforce would reach anywhere near adequate levels. In 1987, not long after geriatric assessment services were announced by the Commonwealth, Roger Warne wrote a 'point of view' in the *Medical Journal of Australia* about the development of geriatric medicine. He opined that assessment services not integrated into the regional geriatric services might not be able to solve the older person's problems particularly if the services did not include a physician in geriatric medicine (geriatrician). At that time there were few geriatric services in Australia that covered the full continuum of care and many were in detached, under-resourced settings. The lack of specialty trained geriatricians meant that many who fulfilled the role were rebadged general physicians or rehabilitation physicians.[20] One exception was the Newcastle service originally developed by Dick Gibson where geriatric medicine training commenced in this period under the leadership of Kevin Grant and Richard Adams, with Leon Flicker being one of the early trainees. While ACAT assessments did not mandate the involvement of a geriatrician, it soon became apparent that multidisciplinary teams could not function adequately without access to a physician with expertise in treating older people,[21] or from a dementia perspective, with expertise in dementia assessment and management which also included psychiatrists and neurologists. The first Australian multidisciplinary memory clinics for dementia assessment appeared in Sydney at Lidcombe Hospital in around 1982, led by Tony Broe and Sid Williams[22] and at Prince Henry Hospital led by Henry Brodaty in 1985,[23] while in Melbourne the Mount Royal Hospital Memory clinic led by David Ames, Leon Flicker and Robert Helme commenced in 1988,[24] and the Caulfield Memory Clinic first opened in 1990.[25]

The other major development during the 1980s was the establishment of Alzheimer Associations in each State based on the models founded in Canada, the UK and the US a few years earlier, with the first branch being in Western Australia followed by NSW in 1982, and subsequently the formation of the national body in 1985 which became a national federation in 1989. The model involved collaboration between health professionals involved in dementia assessment, care, and research with family carers, the main focus of the Associations being on carer support and advocacy.[26,27] Initially known as the Alzheimer's Disease and Related Disorders Society (ADARDS), the national organisation was renamed Alzheimer's Australia in 1999 and then subsequently renamed Dementia Australia in 2017. Each state branch was established with local nuances. For example, in NSW Henry Brodaty wrote to the NSW Association for Mental Health in late 1981 about establishing ADARDS,[28] and subsequently after a very successful public meeting held in May 1982, ADARDS was established as a committee of the NSW Association for Mental Health with the understanding that it would eventually become a separate Society.[29] After a year of formation it had four hundred members.[30] ADARDS in NSW became an autonomous Society in 1989 at which time Henry Brodaty was its President and there were over 1500 members (and by coincidence, John Snowdon was then President of the NSW Association for Mental Health).[31]

The timing of the formation of the Australian Alzheimer's Association was fortuitous as the federal Labor Government used a participative approach to policy and involved the nascent Alzheimer's Association along with the Australian Carers' Association and service providers input to develop its Aged Care Reform Strategy. Thus, from the outset the Alzheimer's Association was an important influence on dementia policy development and was also able to secure some of the HACC funding for support services, respite care, and community education.[32]

The mid-term review of the Aged Care Reform Strategy commenced in 1990. According to Anna Howe, there was high demand for the background paper on *Dementia Care in Australia 1990*.[33] The review recommended that as dementia needs were only going to increase, 'that measures be taken to develop an integrated national action plan for dementia care to advance dementia care within the overall framework of aged care policy'.[34] This translated into the 1992 National Action Plan for Dementia Care (NAPDC), the first in the world, which weaved strands of dementia care throughout the aged care program rather than having a separate dementia program, the rationale being that around fifty per cent of expenses in the aged care program related to dementia. Enhancements in dementia care were based on improving existing services rather than setting up new ones.[35] One long-term impact of this approach was that in the absence of aged care services, few services for dementia assessment and management were to develop, as noted in a NSW survey for the period 2006/7.[36] It would also accentuate the difficulties experienced by persons with young onset dementia who were to later report that services embedded in the aged care system were unsuitable for their needs.[37] But in the context of the lack of historical precedent of any society seriously valuing older people with senility,[38] it was a sensible starting point to facilitate the development of dementia services within the support of an established service framework and was welcomed by the Alzheimer Associations.[39]

The five-year NAPDC covered the seven elements of the Aged Care Program: assessment; services for people with dementia; services for carers; quality of care; community awareness; research; and policy and planning.[40] Funding focused on addressing gaps in programs, improving quality of services through demonstration projects, increased support for carers, research consultancies, and training initiatives. The role of ACATs in dementia assessment was extended by providing resources and a training package to undertake the assessments.[41] The Psychogeriatric Assessment Scales (PAS) developed at the Australian National University by Tony Jorm, Scott Henderson and colleagues in this period had widespread use in ACATs as part of the supplied resources. The PAS, which focused on assessing cognition and depression, were designed to be administered by lay interviewers after training and thus covered two key areas of dementia assessment in a user friendly format.[42] Support was provided by the NAPDC for field testing of the PAS.[43] Forty-one demonstration projects were funded during the first year of the NAPDC, but subsequently larger more targeted funding was provided to groups such as those from Culturally and Linguistically Diverse (CALD) communities. A clearing house was established to disseminate information from the demonstration projects.[44] Overall, however, the demonstration projects lacked coordination and adequate evaluation.

The NAPDC and the first National Mental Health Plan were both released in 1992, with the NAPDC mentioning that the National Mental Health Policy and Plan did not specifically address issues associated with the provision of aged care services, although it did mention the need to strengthen linkages with other health and community services including service integration and workforce training. It also noted that a small percentage of people with dementia required admission for acute or medium to long-term psychiatric care and would thus be directly covered by the National Mental Health Plan.[45]

The 1993 Report of the National Inquiry into the Human Rights of People with Mental Illness by the Human Rights Commission (known as the Burdekin Report after Brian Burdekin the Federal Human Rights Commissioner) had an extensive chapter on older people in Part III that covered people with particular vulnerabilities. The difficulties experienced in getting adequate assessment and care were stressed. While not exclusively focusing on dementia, most of the chapter addressed the challenges faced by people with dementia and their carers. Long-term care in psychiatric hospitals was felt to be inappropriate for most people with dementia. Older people with comorbid mental disorders and dementia were reported to experience discrimination with difficulties in accessing aged care services and approval for residential care due to the ways in which legislative guidelines were interpreted and the reluctance of some service providers to accept such individuals into their care. Poor standards of care in nursing homes, inappropriate facility design, overmedication, inadequacies of the Resident Classification Instrument for funding psychogeriatric issues, and the inability of people with dementia to understand and express their rights as described in the 1990 Charter of Rights and Responsibilities for Nursing Homes were identified as key problems. Burdekin recommended that the solutions included Special Dementia Care Facilities such as Flagstaff Gully in Hobart, Lefroy Hostel in Perth, and the NSW Confused and Disturbed Elderly (CADE) Units which he felt offered a better alternative but that there were significant financial and bureaucratic obstacles to overcome. The lack of psychogeriatric services and the difficulties in attracting staff into the field were mentioned and the desirability of having psychogeriatric services and aged care services under one budget. While not specifically describing the neglect of the human rights of older people as being ageist, Burdekin does mention the prejudices, attitudes, neglect and abuses that they experienced in a manner that is consistent with ageism.[46]

In the 1994–95 Federal budget, $12.4 million was provided over four years in a joint NAPDC and National Mental Health program initiative for six pilot psychogeriatric care and support units, one in each state. The units operated through the ACATs and supplemented State psychogeriatric services by way of providing support to residential aged care facilities in assessment and management of behavioural and psychological problems associated with dementia.[47] The program was evaluated in 2004 and was transformed into the national Dementia Behavioural Management and Advisory Service (DBMAS) in 2005.[48] Research projects were funded under the NAPDC to examine different aspects of challenging behaviour in people with dementia in residential facilities. One project examined care needs and found that sixty-nine per cent of hostel level care for moderate to severe challenging behaviour was provided by mainstream hostels and ninety per cent of nursing home level care for moderate to severe challenging behaviour was provided by mainstream nursing homes. Apart from the replacement of inappropriately designed facilities, the report concluded that more appropriate funding for behavioural care needs and access to better specialist support services was required along with the promotion of special dementia care practices.[49] A second project, on which I was one of the investigators, examined models of care for nursing home residents with dementia complicated by psychosis or depression with the premise being that effective management of these psychological features of dementia would improve behaviour. The randomised controlled trial (RCT) compared three models of care: a psychogeriatric outreach service that provided direct care in the nursing home; a psychogeriatric outreach service that provided a consultative service without direct care; and standard nursing home care. Irrespective of the model of care, each group improved on the outcome measures and it was speculated that the presence of the research team with the indirect support it provided in the nursing homes had a positive impact on care.[50] These projects demonstrated that the care needs of people with dementia and challenging behaviour in residential facilities was high and required extra resources to improve outcomes, although direct care by psychogeriatric services was not likely to be required in most cases.

The mid-term report of the NAPDC was completed in 1996 and was generally positive. It, however, noted that more could be done to increase the capacity of ACATs and GPs in dementia assessment and care, that the central role of carers in all care planning needed to be reinforced, communication between agencies providing care needed to improve, and that the needs of those from ethnic and Aboriginal and Torres Strait Islander backgrounds and those living in rural and remote areas had not been well met.[51] The NAPDC ended a year later in 1997 with its evaluation being completed in February 1999 but not released into the public domain, possibly due to political reasons with the Coalition Howard Government having been recently elected. According to Cecily Hunter and Colleen Doyle, the evaluation was largely positive with the national framework being generally well supported. The capacity of the aged care system to address the needs of people with dementia and their carers was being enhanced, in part through improving quality of care by focusing on training of care providers. The split between State and Commonwealth responsibilities required their active collaboration due to the federal government being responsible for funding of services but not their provision. This meant that there was variability across the States in how federal policy was implemented. Some states, such as NSW and Victoria, were more advanced in their integration of Commonwealth dementia and aged care policies into the delivery of State-run geriatric medical, psychogeriatric and community aged health services in part because they had more dementia and aged care expertise. By the end of the 1990s, the lack of a formal national dementia policy to build on the work of the NAPDC alerted the re-branded Alzheimer's Australia with its new executive director Glenn Rees that a different approach to dementia advocacy that focused on causes in addition to symptoms of dementia would be required in the new millennium.[52]

Under the HACC program, brokerage style services known as 'Community Options Projects' were trialled from the mid-1980s in which 'case coordinators' put together packages of care from different service providers for people with complex needs and these were particularly suited for people with dementia. They proved to be very popular and in 1992 led to the introduction of Community Aged Care Packages (CACP) which were designed as an alternative to hostel care, required an ACAT assessment for eligibility, and were targeted to older people with complex needs. They offered an integrated individualised package of services co-ordinated through one agency to make it easier for the older person and their carer.[53] In 1998 Extended Aged Care at Home (EACH) packages were developed for people with higher dependency needs that would qualify for nursing home care, with the evaluation in 2001 supporting their continuation.[54]

In 1997, the Howard government undertook further aged care reform with a structural reform package as the system was considered incapable of responding effectively and efficiently to the changing needs of older people and the aged care industry. One particular problem was that nursing homes and hostels had different funding models and were operating as distinct service sectors and this system was not thought to be financially sustainable. The 1997 Aged Care Reforms brought nursing homes and hostels together in a unified system as 'aged care facilities' with a single funding tool and a new funding system. This removed barriers to 'ageing in place' thus allowing older people to remain in the one facility as their needs changed. New Residential Care Standards and Accreditation Standards were introduced and an independent Aged Care Standards and Accreditation Agency commenced the accreditation process in 1998. A quality improvement process known as certification was introduced to improve the physical standards of homes.[55]

From a clinical perspective, the major development during the 1990s was the emergence of cognitive enhancing drugs in the cholinesterase inhibitor class that primarily focused on the treatment of Alzheimer's disease. The first drug to be given approval by the Therapeutic Goods Administration (TGA) for release in Australia was tacrine (Cognex) in 1993. Its release was controversial as it had very high rates of adverse effects and was rarely used once the much better tolerated donepezil (Aricept) was released in 1997, followed by rivastigmine (Exelon) in 2000, and galantamine (Reminyl) in 2001.[56] Some of these trials were conducted in Australia with many local leading dementia experts involved as investigators. Pharmaceutical Benefits Scheme (PBS) listing was obtained in 2001 with stringent criteria regarding their prescription which required specialist diagnosis of Alzheimer's disease and monitoring of cognition with the Mini-Mental State Examination (MMSE) for continued prescription,[57] an unpopular process that was not lifted until 2013.[58] Although these drugs, along with memantine (Ebixa) that obtained PBS listing in 2008, have at best modest benefit in the treatment of Alzheimer's disease, their availability signalled to clinicians and the general public that dementia was a medical disorder that could be treated and was not an inevitable part of ageing. Referrals for specialist dementia assessment increased over the decade after PBS listing with 73.7 per cent increase in prescriptions of 'dementia drugs' between 2002/3 and 2009/10.[59] While some people with

Alzheimer's disease and Dementia with Lewy bodies improve markedly, for many people with dementia most benefit was probably best attributed to being linked with dementia services for themselves and their carers.[60] It was indeed fortuitous timing that the arrival of these drugs coincided with the change in direction of dementia advocacy by Alzheimer's Australia as well as the increasing availability of community dementia services.

The growth of community aged care and dementia services over the years following the Aged Care Reforms of the mid-1980s had been largely uncoordinated with numerous demonstration projects, inflexible eligibility criteria, and poor integration with existing services resulting in both service gaps and overlaps, rivalry between Commonwealth and States, and uncoordinated planning of services. In essence by the early 2000s the whole system had become too bureaucratic and confusing for carers, care recipients, and health professionals alike. In August 2002, a coalition of nine professional bodies that included the Alzheimer's Association, Aged and Community Services Australia and the Australian Society for Geriatric Medicine (formerly the Australian Geriatrics Society) released a discussion paper funded by the Myer Foundation on a vision for aged care. The vision involved 'seamless' service delivery with less bureaucracy, fewer assessments, less overlap and better coordination and integration of services provided by health professionals in different settings. The philosophy of care emphasised greater flexibility in service delivery to provide person-centred care with better recognition of the knowledge, skills and capacities of care recipients, rather than just their deficits. An element of this vision that was taken up by the Rudd government in 2010 was a single funding system with only one level of government being responsible for all community care that would incorporate all existing programs and interfaces with general practice and acute hospitals to promote better co-ordinated care.[61] In response to these concerns, the Commonwealth reviewed the community care system in 2004 resulting in reforms that included the adoption of consistent approaches (known as 'common arrangements'). These related to the way services were accessed, the criteria for service eligibility, assessment practices, financial reporting, quality reporting, and information management across the community care programs. A nationally consistent assessment process was developed for the needs of care recipients and the eligibility and needs of carers.[62]

Although in the early 2000s the Howard government did not develop a national dementia policy, in many ways the direction taken under the NAPDC of the mid-90s continued but without a specific dementia strategy. Hunter and Doyle commented that government rhetoric about aged care services in general focused on sustainability of public funding. Alzheimer's Australia sought to influence policy by releasing position papers on dementia as a major health problem in 2001, the economic impact of dementia and quality dementia care in 2003, and dementia terminology in 2004.[63] Access Economics prepared the economic impact report and this was probably the most influential of the Alzheimer's Australia papers, as it estimated that in 2002 dementia costs in Australia were $6.6 billion, $5.6 billion in real costs such as health, community and residential care and indirect costs to carers, with $1 billion in transfer costs such as foregone taxes and carer payments. Over fifty per cent of the real costs were accounted for by residential care. Although these costs represented nearly one per cent of Gross Domestic Product (GDP) in 2002, the report predicted that it may exceed three per cent of GDP by mid-century. Having outlined the economic impact, the report proposed some solutions to be encompassed within a national strategy that included five pillars which were clearly linked with the elements of the previous NAPDC and its evaluation. Early diagnosis and intervention with improved GP access to specialists, possibly through memory clinics, and the dementia drugs was one of the pillars. A second pillar focused on expansion of community support, education and respite services with a person-centred approach for the person with dementia and their carers. Another pillar focused on improving the quality of appropriately financed residential care that was also person-centred. A fourth pillar identified groups with special needs that had not received adequate attention in the NAPDC including those with young onset dementia, people from CALD and Indigenous backgrounds, those residing in rural and remote areas, and people with behavioural and psychological symptoms of dementia (BPSD). The final pillar called for a significant increase in funding research on cause, prevention, and care.[64]

The impact of these reports was eventually seen at the 2004 federal election in which the government largely adopted the title and contents from Alzheimer's Australia's policy documents.[65] After re-election the government included the policy in the 2005 budget and it became known as the Dementia Initiative, focusing on prevention, research, early intervention, improved care and training and was funded for $320.6 million over five years, but was also included in Forward Estimates beyond that. Alzheimer's Australia was allocated the funding to run the National Dementia Support Program (NDSP) which included the National Dementia Helpline, the 'Living with Memory Loss Program' and other early intervention programs as well as counselling, support and education services including for those from CALD and Aboriginal and Torres Strait Islander backgrounds.[66] The 'Living with Memory Loss Program' was a seven-week early intervention course for people with early dementia and their carers that was based on research led by Henry Brodaty at Prince Henry Hospital in Sydney in the late 1980s. The course involved education, skills training and emotional support interventions delivered in a group setting. The evaluations showed reduced carer stress and delayed placement into residential care. Alzheimer's Australia had been running the courses prior to the Dementia Initiative and incorporated them within the NDSP.[67,68]

The Alzheimer's Association was also funded to promote community awareness and the centrepiece of this was the 'Mind your Mind' program. Training was supported at four universities (Dementia Training Study Centres) and for the aged care workforce. Research was supported with research grants and the establishment in 2006 of three Dementia Collaborative Research centres to bring together key national and international ageing and dementia researchers to progress major dementia research areas by translating research into practice. A Minister's Dementia Advisory Group was established and there was funding included for evaluation of the Initiative.[69] A five-year National Framework for Action on Dementia was agreed to by federal, state and territory health ministers at the Australian Health Ministers' Conference in 2006 to provide a structure to bring together strategies from all jurisdictions.[70]

The bulk of the funding of the Dementia Initiative was allocated to two programs that focused on the emerging recognition that it was the challenging behaviour of some people with dementia that required extra resources in the system. Over seventy per cent of the funding was directed to establishing two thousand new Extended Aged Care at Home Dementia (EACHD) Packages, which were designed for people with dementia and associated behavioural and psychological symptoms that were impacting on their ability to live at home. The packages provided the same high level of support provided in EACH packages but with the addition of service approaches and strategies to assist in minimising the effects of the behaviour on the daily life of the person with dementia and their carers. A second component of the initiative, the Dementia Behaviour Management Advisory Services (DBMAS), was established to expand and refocus the existing Psychogeriatric Care Unit Program to assist health and aged care staff in Commonwealth-funded residential and community care services in assessing and managing challenging behaviour in people with dementia.[71] These two programs were well received but would not be enough to counter the mounting stress on services in the Commonwealth aged care program and State geriatric and older people's mental health services to address the needs of these people with dementia and their carers. The transition of long-term residential care from State-run psychiatric hospitals to nursing homes run by a range of public and private organisations, a move generally supported by State mental health authorities and the families of people with dementia, had exposed the extent to which severe challenging behaviour required a skilled workforce and well-designed facilities.[72] This was accentuated by the inadequate nursing numbers that Commonwealth funding for nursing homes allowed with State-run long-term residential care in psychiatric hospitals and nursing homes having extra State funding to bolster nursing numbers, a problem that is ongoing.[73] Severe behaviour disturbance in persons with dementia had been the main precipitant for their admission to nineteenth-century asylums as noted in earlier chapters. This was not a new phenomenon and it was now apparent that the largely untrained aged care workforce in residential care with input from general practitioners was resorting to twentieth-century versions of restraints, both chemical and physical, to manage behaviour. That such approaches to care would eventually result in scandal in the media as had happened numerous times around the country commencing in the nineteenth century was entirely predictable.

By the early 2000s, Australian studies had replicated work from North America and Europe demonstrating the high usage of psychotropic drugs in nursing homes and hostels with more than half the residents being prescribed at least one psychotropic drug and many on multiple psychotropics.[74, 75] One study found despite being prescribed antipsychotic and antidepressant drugs, many residents still had high rates of depression, psychosis and behavioural disturbances that suggested limited effectiveness.[76] It should also be noted that as far back as the 1980s concerns had also been expressed about the high rates of prescription of psychotropic drugs to older Australians residing in the community. In 1987 an analysis of Pharmaceutical Benefits Scheme data conducted by the Royal Australasian College of General Practitioners for the Mental Health Foundation of Australia and the Australian National Association for Mental Health estimated that twenty-nine per cent of people aged 65 years and older attending a GP were using psychotropic drugs, much higher than other age groups.[77] Similar rates were found in a smaller community survey of older people undertaken by John Snowdon in the Sydney suburb of Botany in 1985.[78] Thus while the issue of overuse of psychotropic drugs in older people was concentrated in residential care, it was by no means restricted to that setting.

One of the dilemmas faced by clinicians was that in the mid-1990s the research evidence for managing behavioural disturbances associated with dementia was of low quality for both drug and non-drug treatments. Antipsychotic drugs, such as the older 'typical' antipsychotic haloperidol and the newer atypical antipsychotics such as risperidone and olanzapine, were being used for treating psychosis and behavioural disturbances in dementia with only weak research to support their use. In Australia these drugs had obtained TGA approval for schizophrenia and related psychoses and were being used 'off-label' in dementia. High quality RCTs were conducted in the late 1990s and early 2000s which demonstrated that risperidone in particular had modest efficacy in treating aggression, agitation and psychosis associated with dementia. This was sufficient for this indication to be added to risperidone's PBS indications meaning it was no longer off-label. But the last of the studies that led to the PBS listing, an Australian and New Zealand study led by Henry Brodaty, had a sting in its tail. Unexpectedly it was reported that participants taking risperidone had cerebrovascular adverse events five times greater than the placebo group, although the overall number of adverse events was similar in both groups.[79] As noted in chapter 9, this eventually resulted in warnings about the safety of antipsychotic drugs in dementia. When combined with a large multisite US RCT published in the prestigious *New England Journal of Medicine* in 2006 that found the adverse effects of the atypical antipsychotic drugs (risperidone, olanzapine, quetiapine) offset their benefits, there was clearly limited support for the routine use of these drugs in treating behavioural disturbances in dementia.[80] Use of antipsychotic drugs had to be well targeted, and as recommended in the handbook, *Assessment and Management of People with Behavioural and Psychological Symptoms of Dementia (BPSD),* prepared for NSW Health by the RANZCP Faculty of Psychiatry of Old Age, only after an adequate trial of non-drug treatments.[81] But of course non-drug treatments required a trained workforce to implement them and that was deficient in the aged care workforce.

The extent to which specialist older people's mental health and geriatric services should be managing behavioural disturbances associated with dementia had been troubling policy makers for some time. Studies in community and residential care settings worldwide indicated that nearly all persons with dementia had a significant behavioural issue over the course of their illness.[82] It was obviously not feasible for specialist services to be involved in the ongoing management of virtually every dementia case in Australia, quite a different proposition to just being involved with the diagnostic process as required for prescription of the dementia drugs. Yet there was no clear guidance from research about how many cases needed specialist services involved and this was required to enable accurate service planning. This was resolved in 2003 when Henry Brodaty, Lee-Fay Low and I published a seven-tiered triangular model of service delivery for BPSD in the *Medical Journal of Australia.* The model envisaged prevention as an essential component thus supporting the view that if basic dementia care was being delivered by a trained workforce and family carers in a dementia-friendly environment then challenging behaviour could be minimised. The base tier of the model had people with no dementia obviously implying that preventing dementia was the best way to prevent BPSD. The tiers then went from dementia without BPSD through increasing behavioural severity to the pinnacle of extreme BPSD with the estimated percentage of dementia cases based on cross-sectional epidemiological research (although the numbers in the top tier were based on an estimate by the authors). Each tier was assigned a health workforce that was mainly responsible for management and this clearly showed that it was only around ten per cent of dementia cases that required case-management by a specialist team and/or needed to reside in a dementia-specific facility, while another twenty per cent of cases specialist services would likely be needed to provide consultative advice to primary care or mainstream residential care (See

Figure 3, page 298).[83] This model was quickly adopted by Commonwealth and some State policy makers as the basis upon which to plan services for managing BPSD and supported the emphasis on upskilling the primary care medical and nursing workforce as well as informal family carers, although even at this point there was clearly a lack of benchmarks and a national plan for the management of those with very severe to extreme BPSD that were unmanageable in residential aged care.[84]

After the Rudd government took office in 2007, concerns about how the residential aged care sector was able to manage people with 'psychogeriatric disorders' led to the Minister for Ageing Justine Elliot in 2008 commissioning a departmental report to identify current innovative and appropriate service delivery models. The report involved broad stakeholder consultation and made nine recommendations mainly designed to improve leadership, guidelines, education and training of the aged care and GP workforce. One recommendation was the establishment of an expert reference group comprising old age psychiatrists, nurses and service providers to keep the issue of psychogeriatric issues 'front of mind' for senior level aged care administrators and planners and that would report to the new Australian Ministerial Conference on Ageing.[85]

The Psychogeriatric Expert Reference Group (PERG) was convened in February 2009 and I was appointed as its Chair. It developed a comprehensive 'Framework for service planning and care delivery for people with psychogeriatric disorders' that was endorsed by the Ministerial Conference on Ageing in December 2010.[86] It also had input into the Fourth National Mental Health Plan, the draft of which lacked any priority actions explicitly about older people and there were no major age care examples in the plan to highlight care issues. The PERG recommended to the Mental Health Standing Committee, which had oversight of the Plan, that there needed to be a national framework to address issues between aged care and mental health to define principles and responsibilities.[87] It was this interface involving both Commonwealth and State jurisdictions that often led to older people with mental disorders falling through the gap. The PERG also had input into the Department of Health and Ageing's (DOHA) review of the Aged Care Funding Instrument (ACFI) pointing out that it was not adequately capturing the care needs of those residents with complex medical conditions and behavioural disorders who would previously be managed in hospital environments. The ACFI review conceded that residents with psychogeriatric disorders continued to be difficult to accommodate in the residential care environment and that there would be merit to consider options for increasing support for them.[88] The PERG made submissions to the Productivity Commission that had been commissioned by the Labor Government to inquire into the aged care system and to make recommendations for system redesign and a DOHA sponsored review of subacute care that focused on needs and benchmarking.

By 2012 Julia Gillard was Prime Minister and Mark Butler had replaced Justine Elliot as Minister for Ageing. There were also major changes within DOHA with major staff reshuffles, the retirement of Mary Murnane the Deputy Secretary of DOHA who had been a member of the PERG, and reorganisation of DOHA that impacted on its committee reporting structures. The Ministerial Conference on Ageing was disbanded in 2011 which in effect meant that the PERG was disbanded as it no longer had a reporting line and was largely forgotten. This was emphasised in August 2012 when the Minister for Ageing, Mark Butler convened a Ministerial Round Table discussion on 'Medication and Behaviour Management in Aged Care' due to concerns about the use of antipsychotic drugs. A follow-up meeting was held in Parliament House Canberra on October 9 2012 at the same time that Julia Gillard gave her much discussed 'misogyny' speech in the House.[89] Minister Butler attended and although those in attendance at the Round Table included many who were members of the PERG, Butler and his advisers appeared to have no knowledge of the PERG and its work when it was pointed out to him that his department had previously had an Expert Reference Group that could have addressed the issue. There was no further communication about the PERG and the opportunity to progress this policy work was squandered.

Previously in 2010 the Rudd government announced that the Commonwealth would take full responsibility for aged care including the HACC program as part of the National Health and Hospitals Network Agreement.[90] With the exception of Western Australia, the HACC program was combined with other community programs in 2015 and renamed the Commonwealth Home Support Program with four levels of care. In its continuing advocacy for improving the aged care system for people with dementia, Alzheimer's Australia commissioned Access

Economics to model the changes in supply of aged care services (community aged care packages, operational residential aged care places, HACC clients) for the period 2010 to 2050. The *Caring Places* report was published in 2010 and compared projections based on the parameter used by DOHA on persons aged 70 years and over with that recommended by the National Health and Hospitals Reform Commission which factored in growth of the population aged 85 years and older. When the two models were compared, there was a substantial shortfall in the model used by DOHA suggesting that despite the substantial increases projected, this policy setting would result in an undersupply of aged care services. The *Caring Places* report also commented on the lack of additional funding in the 2010–11 budget to address gaps in dementia specific care, particularly related to early diagnosis, older people's mental health services and the dangers of acute hospital care for people with dementia. It also recommended policies that increased consumer choice and flexibility of services such as consumer directed care and graduated care packages.[91] In addition, there remained the significant challenges of meeting the needs of 'special populations' that included those from CALD and Aboriginal and Torres Strait Island background, those residing in rural and remote Australia, those with intellectual disabilities, and those with young onset dementia who had been the focus of a National Consumer Summit organised by Alzheimer's Australia in February 2009 to identify their priorities related to diagnosis and care.[92]

To assist jurisdictions in effective service planning, DOHA funded KPMG under the Dementia Initiative to prepare a guide on dementia service pathways. The guide was published in 2011 and covered four stages of dementia from awareness of first symptoms through to end-of-life care. It had a very broad overview and perhaps its main contribution was to emphasise that dementia is a chronic progressive disorder that presents with different needs at various stages requiring a continuum of care rather than episodic care. It also provided a self-assessment tool for jurisdictions.[93]

The Productivity Commission handed down its report in 2011 and noted that the aged care system was complex and difficult to navigate with significant waiting times, lack of continuity of care as needs changed, restrictions on consumer choice, and lack of incentives for providers to engage in restorative activities. Amongst its numerous recommendations were consumer directed care including a single gateway to services, reform of the regulatory framework to remove unnecessary regulations, changes to aged care funding mechanisms, measures to enhance quality of care, improved use of technology, and better recognition of the needs of diverse populations.[94] The Government adopted many of the recommendations in its 'Living Longer Living Better' reforms announced in 2012 including adopting a single gateway to services 'My Aged Care'. Dementia services were enhanced by expanding DBMAS into acute and primary care settings and support for more timely diagnosis. A new Dementia Supplement designed to address the needs of those in residential care with more severe behavioural issues not well captured on the ACFI was a new innovation.[95] The other change that occurred in 2012 was the addition of dementia to the existing list of National Health Priorities.

By 2011 over half of residents in aged care facilities had a formal dementia diagnosis as recorded on the ACFI although it was acknowledged that the actual number was likely to be much higher due to undetected cases such as in residents admitted for another serious medical disorder particularly over the age of 85. To illustrate the care challenges posed by these residents, fifty-six per cent were rated as having high level behavioural needs while thirty-nine per cent were given another mental or behavioural disorder diagnosis.[96] Thus it is easy to see why the introduction of the Dementia Supplement worth $16.15 per day in 2013 proved to be very popular. Eligibility was based on residents with a mental or behavioural diagnosis being assessed with the Neuropsychiatric Inventory by an approved clinician with only those obtaining very high scores being eligible for the supplement.[97] Within a year it was clear that the uptake of the supplement was much higher than expected from previous Australian research with marked variability between facilities suggesting that some might be rorting the system. Projections suggested this approach to addressing the needs of residents with severe behavioural disturbances was not sustainable. After a period of consultation, it was decided to replace the Dementia Supplement with a new innovative national approach, the Severe Behaviour Response Team (SBRT) that would interface with DBMAS and focus solely on residents referred to DBMAS who posed a significant risk either to themselves or others. The expectation was that the SBRT would respond within 24–48 hours to assist aged care facilities with very severe to extreme BPSD. The SBRT commenced as a stand-alone program in 2015/16 and as planned was amalgamated with DBMAS in 2016/17 and provided by Dementia Support Australia. Unlike DBMAS that did not necessarily have face-to-face contact with the facility, the SBRT would almost always attend the facility with highly experienced multidisciplinary clinicians. Given that this was a national program, the logistics of achieving the operational guideline expectations related to accessibility meant clinicians were often flying in-flying out to various regional and rural locations.[98]

It was apparent that the SBRT initiative could not resolve the more persistent very severe behavioural issues as represented by tiers 6 and 7 of the seven-tiered model. One approach used worldwide is the Specialist Dementia Care Unit that caters specifically for more severe BPSD, but largely due to the challenges of undertaking high quality evaluation in this setting there is only limited evidence of effectiveness.[99] In 2016 the Australian Government committed to establishing at least one specialist dementia care unit in each of the 31 Primary Health Networks in Australia.[100] During the consultation period prior to setting up the Special Dementia Care Program, a series of scandals in aged care facilities occurred with the principal one being at Oakden in South Australia, a State-run older persons' mental health facility receiving Commonwealth aged care funding, where allegations of overmedication, inadequate feeding, overuse of mechanical restraints and injuries had led to a highly critical external review led by Dr Aaron Groves in 2017 (see chapter 15).[101] Further concerns were aired in 2018 about other aged care facilities in the two-part ABC's Four Corners program *Who Cares?* in which families provided footage filmed with hidden cameras showing abuses and neglect of their relatives.[102] Subsequently a Royal Commission into Aged Care Quality and Safety was established in October 2018 with Richard Tracey and Lynelle Briggs appointed as commissioners.[103]

These scandals increased the imperative to establish the Special Dementia Care Program and the prototype special dementia care unit was set up at 'The Village' in Inglewood, Perth in September 2019 and nine other units were scheduled to open around the country in 2020. A second funding round was scheduled for 2021/22. Their focus was on residents with behavioural disturbances assessed as being within tier 6 of the seven-tiered model with the assessment being carried out by the SBRT using standardised tools. The model of care promoted for the units is a person-centred, restraint free approach to care that has a psychosocial focus with a multidisciplinary team.[104] The Special Care Dementia Program is in its infancy and so it far too early to know whether the combination of these programs to address the management of residents with the more severe behavioural problems associated with dementia will suffice. Further, there is still a gap in that those with the most extreme behavioural disturbances are out of scope for the program without a clear alternative location of care.

My Aged Care, a telephone contact centre and an online portal providing information about and access to Commonwealth aged care services, was introduced in July 2013. There were significant implementation challenges particularly for older people with complex needs, such as those with dementia, and limited access to technology. Navigating the system was difficult even for seasoned service providers. Further changes occurred in 2017 when CACPs and EACH packages were combined into the Home Care Package Program and included consumer directed care. In this reform, the packages were allocated to care recipients rather than care providers and a national priority system was introduced. But delays from approval to receipt of a Home Care Package were already becoming a concern which became apparent in 2017 when a National Prioritisation Queue was established and it was noted in September 2018 that there were over 69,000 people with an approved level package who had yet to be offered a lower level package, while over 57,000 people were on an interim lower level package.[105]

From a geriatric medical perspective, the Australian Society for Geriatric Medicine amalgamated with the New Zealand Society for Geriatric Medicine to form the Australian and New Zealand Society for Geriatric Medicine in 2006. According to the 2016 National Health Workforce Survey, there were 619 geriatricians employed in Australia with an average age of only 48 reflecting the rapid growth in the specialty in the previous decade. There was a maldistribution of the workforce with the Northern Territory and Queensland having well below the national average. Over eighty-seven per cent of geriatricians were located in major cities or centres with large populations. Rural and remote parts of the country remained under-resourced in geriatric medical services.[106] As dementia assessment and management in Australia remains closely linked to aged care services, this gives an indication about where gaps remain. Indeed, in 2006 when 23 memory clinics were identified in Australia, the majority being in Victoria, geriatricians were the most common medical specialty to lead or be part of the clinic.[107]

The interim report of the Aged Care Royal Commission was tabled in October 2019 and pulled no punches about the aged care system which it described as a 'shocking tale of neglect' and identified systemic problems requiring fundamental reform and redesign. Despite numerous reviews over the previous 20 years, it described a system that was difficult to navigate and focused on transactions rather than relationships or care. Older people and their families had little voice while the workforce was under pressure, underappreciated and lacked skills. The regulatory model lacked transparency or incentive to improve. The Commission recommended three areas for immediate action: the provision of more Home Care Packages, the use of the Community Pharmacy Agreement to address overmedication, and to stem the flow of young people with disabilities into aged care.[108]

# Chapter 13

# National Developments in Old Age Psychiatry: 1980-2020

Professor Tom Arie visited Australia regularly over the 1980s to provide advice and support for the development of comprehensive older people's mental health services.[1] In 1984 he visited NSW and Victoria with his influence on service development being most marked in Victoria.[2] Service development was slow and haphazard with different approaches appearing in the key states of Victoria, where services were being embedded within mental health, and NSW where there were moves to include them largely within geriatric services, prompting John Snowdon in a 1987 editorial comment in the *Australian and New Zealand Journal of Psychiatry*, to question the overall direction being taken and the need for service guidelines.[3]

From a professional perspective, the initial moves towards the development of a professional group representing old age psychiatrists within the RANZCP can be traced to informal discussions held at the Australian Society for Psychiatric Research meeting in 1986. With the encouragement of RANZCP President Joan Lawrence, this led to a meeting held at Prince Henry Hospital in Sydney in December 1987 attended by over fifty people including Tom Arie at which a formal motion was passed to form a Section of Psychiatry of Old Age (SPOA) in the RANZCP.[4] Edmond (Ed) Chiu from Melbourne was elected as Chair of the steering committee that included Henry Brodaty, John Snowdon, Sid Williams, Manjula O'Connor, Bob Russell and Ute Rosenbilds in its membership.[5] The application for the formation of SPOA was approved at the RANZCP General Council meeting in May 1988, with Ed Chiu being formally appointed as Chair in October 1988 and Manjula O'Connor was the initial secretary.[6] The first annual meeting of SPOA was held in Adelaide and convened by Ute Rosenbilds on 30 November 1988 in association with the annual meeting of the Australian Society for Psychiatric Research, an association that continued through most of the 1990s. At this meeting SPOA set itself a number of priorities including education and training, research, treatment and service delivery guidelines, strengthening relationships with geriatricians, improving services in rural areas, and involvement in commentary on Government policies as they related to the mental health needs of older people.[7] Visits from prominent British psychogeriatricians were a feature of the late 1980s which apart from Tom Arie included Elaine Murphy, Brice Pitt and Raymond Levy.[8] Their impact and influence on the development of the infant old age psychiatry subspecialty in Australia should not be underestimated with each having authored and edited influential texts.

Ed Chiu was integral to the early development of old age psychiatry as a subspecialty in Australia. Chiu was born in Guangzhou and raised in Hong Kong until the age of 13 when he migrated to Australia in 1952 to live with his sister at Ingham in North Queensland. Educated at the Cardinal Gilroy College operated by the Christian Brothers at Ingham, he then studied medicine at the University of Queensland in Brisbane. Having decided on a career in psychiatry, Chiu moved to Melbourne for his training. He spent his first year at Beechworth Mental Hospital before being transferred to Royal Park Hospital in Melbourne to work with John Cade who became his mentor. Cade had discovered the therapeutic benefit of lithium in bipolar disorder in the 1950s. The other influential mentor was Professor Brian Davies who was the Foundation Cato Chair of Psychiatry at the University of Melbourne. Davies facilitated postgraduate training for Chiu in England where he obtained his Diploma of Psychological Medicine. On return to Australia and Royal Park in the early 1970s, Davies gave him responsibility for Huntington's disease and working with the likes of social worker Betty Teltscher, developed a best practice service delivery model that received international acclaim through his academic publications. This experience in working with families and individuals with a progressive neurodegenerative disorder stood him well for his move into old age psychiatry in the early 1980s, again at the suggestion of Brian Davies who recognised that Herbert Bower needed a successor. Chiu was sent to Nottingham to attend the Arie course and on return to Australia established the psychogeriatric unit at Royal Park hospital with Manjula O'Connor in 1984 and took over from Herbert Bower in providing consultations at Mount Royal Hospital. From the outset Chiu recognised the imperative for old age psychiatry to form a Section within the RANZCP, as had occurred in the UK in the 1970s, to facilitate the development of the subspecialty and older people's mental health services. He was also acutely aware of the lack of old age psychiatry training opportunities in Australia and in February 1989 organised the first Arie course 'down under', a joint program between SPOA and the Office of Psychiatric Services of Victoria, featuring the international speakers Tom Arie, Ken Shulman and Chris Gilleard. The courses continued through the 1990s being the sole provider of old age psychiatry training until formal advanced training in old age psychiatry in the RANZCP Fellowship commenced in 1999. Ed Chiu became a Member of the Order of Australia in 1988 and received the highest RANZCP award, the College Medal of Honour in 2000.[9,10,11]

With the formation of SPOA, old age psychiatry as a subspecialty had the structure and just as importantly the leadership of Ed Chiu as Chair and David Ames, who had taken over from Manjula O'Connor as secretary in June 1990. Ames had returned in the late 1980s from training in the UK under the guidance of Nori Graham and Anthony Mann at the Royal Free Hospital, where he completed a study of depression in local authority homes, to work with Chiu at Royal Park Hospital. After Chiu moved to Mont Park in 1989, Ames took up the senior lecturer position at Royal Park where he was involved in setting up the memory clinic and was promoted to Associate Professor in 1995. He was the secretary of SPOA between 1990 and 1995. After editing the *IPA Bulletin* for many years, Ames became the Editor-in-Chief of the journal *International Psychogeriatrics* in 2003 and during his tenure it had a marked improvement in its quality and impact. In 2007, he became the Director of the National Ageing Research Institute. He has edited numerous books on dementia and old age psychiatric topics. His research has been varied and includes being a principal investigator on the Australian Imaging, Biomarker and Lifestyle Flagship Study of Ageing (AIBL) that is investigating early diagnosis of Alzheimer's Disease. An excellent speaker, in 1995 he was able to combine his passion for opera with a plenary presentation at the Sydney IPA meeting. He was awarded a RANZCP citation in 2017, the Order of Australia (AO) in 2018 and is currently an Emeritus Professor at the University of Melbourne.[12,13]

With the highly successful first Arie Course 'down under' demonstrating their capacity to organise meetings, the next international meeting was convened by Chiu and Ames in Melbourne in November 1990 under the auspices of SPOA and the Geriatric Psychiatry Section of the World Psychiatric Association on the theme of functional psychiatric disorders in old age.[14] It was a well-attended meeting with over 180 registrants and a mix of international and local speakers, but just as importantly it also doubled as the SPOA Annual Meeting and provided another forum for members of SPOA to get together and forge ties from around the country and from New Zealand.[15] The meeting was transformed into a book 'Functional Psychiatric Disorders of the Elderly' edited by Chiu and Ames, the first Australian old age psychiatry text.[16]

One of the requests made to Chiu by then RANZCP President Joan Lawrence at the formation of SPOA was for SPOA to develop 'Guidelines for Psychiatric Services for the Elderly'.[17] A RANZCP Position Statement on 'Psychiatric Services for the Elderly', originally drafted by John Snowdon after he had corresponded with the College Secretariat, was presented at the Section of Social and Cultural Psychiatry meeting at Coffs Harbour in 1986. After feedback and revision it was forwarded by Chiu for the Section of Social and Cultural Psychiatry when he was its secretary and was adopted by General Council in May 1987 before SPOA was formed.[18] Sid Williams, who had recently chaired a Psychogeriatrics Working Party as part of the 1988 Barclay Report on mental health services in NSW, based the guidelines on the recommendations of the Psychogeriatrics Working Party. Apart from providing a description of the principles of care and the structure of a comprehensive psychogeriatric service, the recommendations were quite prescriptive about the number and type of staff, beds and services required.[19] Formal presentation of the guidelines to the General Council of the RANZCP were delayed until October 1992 when a draft revised Position Statement on 'Geriatric Psychiatry Services for the Elderly' that had been prepared by a SPOA sub-committee on psychogeriatric service delivery chaired by John Snowdon were available as a companion document.[20] Meanwhile a joint Position Statement with the Australian Geriatrics Society on 'Relationships between Geriatric and Psychogeriatric Services' had been adopted by General

Council in May 1990 with only minor amendments and no controversy.[21] Thus, the reaction of General Council was surprising but informative of the barriers that remained to the development of older people's mental health services in Australia. Two NSW General Councillors expressed specific concerns. Noel Wilton, who was also the NSW Director of Mental Health, claimed that the Position Statement ran counter to the thrust of the recently released National Mental Health Policy in terms of integration, mainstreaming and equity in psychiatric services. To suggest, however, that having specialised older people's mental health services ran counter to the National Mental Health Policy in terms of integration, mainstreaming and equity was nonsense as these elements were about how mental health services related to general health services and not how mental health services were internally organised to best meet the needs of people. John Ellard objected in principle to age being used as a determinant of where services were to be provided. These attitudes of general adult psychiatry were similar to those encountered in the UK by its own Section in Psychiatry of Old Age of the Royal College of Psychiatrists and involved a mix of ignorance about the needs of older people and misinterpretation of broader policies. Objections to the guidelines with their detailed prescription of staffing and service components were more fundamental and reflected the RANZCP policy of not preparing generic standards for psychiatric services. Nevertheless, both documents were circulated to the College branches for comment.[22] SPOA revised the Position Statement which was finally accepted by General Council in October 1993 and withdrew the service guidelines document to the disappointment of many SPOA members who were aware that the Royal College of Psychiatrists had a different approach and regularly prepared such guidance about standards for psychiatric services which proved useful when developing services. The two Position Statements remain in place with minor revisions.

In the early 1990s, SPOA recognised that there was an imperative to improve both mental health services for older people and the training of psychiatrists in the assessment and management of older people. Being mindful of the approach taken to document 'the state of play' of older people's mental health services in the UK through surveys of psychogeriatricians in order to demonstrate the service gaps that existed, in 1992 John Snowdon led a SPOA supported survey of Australian SPOA members and utilised the same methodology, and the assistance of John Wattis who led the UK surveys, so that comparisons could be made between the countries. The survey found that there were 34 psychiatrists in Australia working full time with older people and the ratio of psychogeriatricians to older people in Australia in 1992 at one psychogeriatrician per 30,000 persons aged 65 years and over was similar to that found in the UK seven years earlier but non-medical staff ratios in Australia were lower than the UK and largely absent in states other than NSW and Victoria, particularly in community settings. There were few comprehensive integrated older people's mental health services. About 480 acute hospital beds (approximately 40 beds per 100,000 older people in the catchment areas covered) and 1060 long-stay beds were identified by respondents but actual numbers were difficult to determine as some older people were admitted to general adult wards depending on demand and there was an ongoing transfer of long-stay beds to nursing homes. Within states there was considerable regional variation and services were largely absent in rural Australia.[23] Clearly most parts of the country were under-prepared to address the needs of older people with mental disorders and developments were occurring in a piecemeal fashion. In 1994, I commented in the *IPA Bulletin* that 'any service enhancement is appreciated, but the absence of a coordinated state and Australian government approach to psychogeriatric service planning continues to result in fragmentary services'.[24]

In May 1992, in my role as the Chair of SPOA's Working Party in Training Issues, I surveyed trainee psychiatrists and training program coordinators about psychogeriatric training within the RANZCP psychiatrist training program. Over 94 per cent of general psychiatry trainees indicated that they required at least three months of training in old age psychiatry within their five-year training program but only 70 per cent of trainees were obtaining that in their basic training. Most trainees who received old age psychiatry training enjoyed the experience and felt it was adequate for their needs. Nearly twenty per cent of training programs had no positions available for old age psychiatry training. As with the older people's mental health services survey, there were significant gaps noted, for example Tasmania and the Australian Capital Territory had neither positions nor potential supervisors in old age psychiatry. Although there was no formal advanced training program in old age psychiatry for those planning to become old age psychiatrists in this period, there were six one-year advanced training positions available during the final year of the RANZCP training program, all located in NSW and Victoria. The survey indicated that there were significant gaps in the training of general psychiatrists to treat older patients as thirty per cent of psychiatrists were not obtaining any specific training in old age psychiatry and that there were few training positions available for those who desired to specialise in old age psychiatry and become old age psychiatrists.[25]

In 1989, Ed Chiu and Scott Henderson were appointed to the Board of the International Psychogeriatric Association (IPA) and through that appointment Chiu secured the 1995 biennial IPA International Congress to be held in Sydney in collaboration with SPOA and underwritten by the RANZCP. In the early 1990s, the previous two IPA Congresses had not been very well organised with financial implications for IPA. The 1991 congress was moved from Jerusalem to Rome at a fairly late stage due to Middle East tensions and this had a negative impact on the Congress arrangements, while the 1993 Congress in Berlin lacked local organisers with the predictable outcome of minimal local interest. Thus there was great pressure on the 1995 Sydney Congress with Chiu as Congress President and Chair of SPOA to deliver a successful meeting in terms of both content and financial outcome. The organising committee comprised NSW SPOA members along with Ed Chiu and David Ames from Victoria, while Henry Brodaty chaired the Scientific Committee.[26]

Henry Brodaty has the distinction of being appointed as Australia's first Professor of Psychogeriatrics at the University of NSW, Sydney in 1990. Brodaty was born in Kirchseeon, Germany after the Second World War in a displaced persons camp before his family moved to Sydney in his childhood as refugees. He studied medicine at the University of Sydney and obtained membership of the Royal Australasian College of Physicians in 1973. After a sojourn in England where he worked in the Academic Department of Psychiatry at the Middlesex Hospital, he returned to Australia to commence psychiatry training in 1974, initially at Rozelle Hospital but from 1975 at Prince Henry/Prince of Wales Hospitals in Sydney, becoming a member of the RANZCP in 1977 and winning the College Medallion as the best candidate in the examinations in the process. His academic credentials were established early in his career as he was awarded the 1980 RANZCP Organon Junior Research Award. Brodaty was the Director of the Psychiatry Unit at Prince Henry Hospital throughout the 1980s and in 1985 established the Memory Disorders Clinic and became the Founding Clinical Director of the Mood Disorders Clinic which was the forerunner of the Black Dog Institute. During this period he helped establish NSW ADARDS in 1982, becoming its inaugural president, and Alzheimer's Australia in 1985, becoming the inaugural vice president before becoming president in 1988 (before ADARDS was federated in 1989) in which role he had input into the 1992 National Action Plan for Dementia Care. It was during the late 1980s that Brodaty conducted his seminal research, the Prince Henry Hospital Carers Program that established his international reputation being awarded second prize in the 1989 IPA research awards and eventually becoming the basis of the 'Living with Memory Loss' program run by Alzheimer's Australia. After his appointment as Professor of Psychogeriatrics, in 1991 he became the foundation Director of the Academic Department of Psychogeriatrics (later renamed the Academic Department for Old Age Psychiatry) and the associated clinical service at Prince Henry Hospital. Over the next thirty years Henry Brodaty cemented his position as the leading Australian academic in old age psychiatry undertaking a broad swathe of research mainly with a dementia focus but covering diverse topics including late life schizophrenia, depression, suicidal behaviour, pharmacotherapy and service delivery. His work in advocacy continued throughout this period at local, state, national, and international levels. He became the Chair of Alzheimer's Disease International in 2002 and President of IPA in 2013. His awards include becoming an Officer of the Order of Australia in 2000, the RANZCP Organon Senior Research Award in 2003, and the IPA 'Distinguished Service to the Field of Psychogeriatrics' award in 2009.[27]

The IPA Congress was a resounding success with an attendance of over 1300 that stretched the Congress Venue, the Wesley Centre, to the limits and thus had a financial windfall for both IPA and SPOA. Attendees reported that it was the best old age mental health meeting that they had ever attended and enjoyed both the diverse academic and social program (including holding the Welcome Reception of the Congress in the foyer of the Sydney Opera House overlooking the harbour) and the relaxed, friendly atmosphere. To achieve this, the SPOA Committees worked intensely with one important innovation of developing a group of mainly non-medical volunteers – nurses, allied health and administrative staff from older people's mental health services in NSW – to assist in the daily Congress organisation doing tasks such as filling the Congress bags, ushering, and manning the registration and information desks.[28,29] SPOA was supportive of nurses and allied health being associate members of the Section but unfortunately in the early 2000s after SPOA became a Faculty, the RANZCP notified the Faculty that it could no longer include nurses and allied health as associate members as that term was used in another context.

This 1995 IPA Congress had a major impact on the development of old age psychiatry in Australia. The intense committee work in the years leading up to the Congress forged strong relationships within SPOA, while the meeting itself brought together many local multidisciplinary clinicians, many of whom were the volunteers at the meeting, who had their first opportunity to experience contact with other colleagues in Australia and from overseas. It is likely no coincidence that the NSW Psychogeriatric Nurses Association was formally convened in 1995 although there had been informal groups in place long before then.[30] The meeting provided encouragement to clinical leaders in the States and Territories where services were less well-developed to pursue service delivery improvement and improvements across the country commenced in the mid to late 1990s. It also was instrumental to Ed Chiu becoming IPA president in 1999.

The IPA Congress also provided incentive to SPOA to pursue its goal of obtaining Faculty status within the RANZCP, with the formal decision to pursue the application being made at the SPOA annual meeting in 1996. There were essentially two criteria that had to be met within the RANZCP constitution for SPOA to become a Faculty. It required the determination that there was a recognised body of knowledge regarding the area of interest and the ability to offer a comprehensive accredited training program related to that body of knowledge, that is, for subspecialty training. At that time, Faculties were entitled to representation on the RANZCP General Council which ensured some input on College policies, an issue that incoming SPOA Chair John Snowdon championed, and this was further motivation for SPOA to seek this transformation. During the IPA meeting, as the new SPOA secretary as well as continuing as the Chair of the SPOA Training Working Party, I forged contacts with key leaders in Canada, the UK and the US who had been involved in pursuing subspecialty status within their countries and continued to correspond and/or meet with Ivan Silver, Ken Le Clair and Joel Sadavoy from Canada, Burton Reifler and Gary

Kennedy from the US, and Rob Jones and John Wattis in the UK to ensure that with input from senior SPOA members, the two-year advanced training program content reflected the standards set in those countries and adapted to the requirements of Australia and New Zealand, the latter because the RANZCP is a binational College. As the Faculty of Child and Adolescent Psychiatry (FCAP) was the only Faculty in the RANZCP at this time, with the encouragement of the RANZCP Fellowships Board that had the responsibility for the oversight of College training, the training program structure and by-laws used by FCAP were adapted to become the basis of a generic structure and by-laws suitable for other subspecialties rather than just old age psychiatry, as Fellowships Board was aware of other Sections that were making similar plans to SPOA. After being satisfied that the curriculum and by-laws were satisfactory, it was approved by Fellowships Board with those who completed the training being awarded the Certificate for Advanced Training in Psychiatry of Old Age and offered membership of FPOA. General Council subsequently approved the formation of FPOA in October 1998 with John Snowdon as the Foundation Chair and the advanced training program commenced in January 1999 in the International Year of Older Persons.[31,32]

John Snowdon was born in England and studied medicine at St Thomas' Hospital in London in the 1960s and his experience in his psychiatry rotation under the tutelage of William Sargant and John Pollitt led him to a career in psychiatry. He came to Australia for two years and first obtained his membership of the Royal Australasian College of Physicians. On returning to England he commenced psychiatry training and it was the rotations in which he worked with old age psychiatrists Felix Post and Raymond Levy at Bethlem Hospital and later neuropsychiatrist Alwyn Lishman that eventually influenced his career direction into old age psychiatry. His first research paper was a case report on hypoparathyroidism based on one of Raymond Levy's patients. After completing his psychiatry training, Snowdon decided to return to Australia and in the late 1970s he met Leslie Kiloh, the Professor of Psychiatry at the University of New South Wales, who recruited him to be the Medical Superintendent at the newly opened Prince of Wales Hospital Psychiatry Unit in Sydney. While working as a general psychiatrist and medical superintendent, he was asked to follow up a complaint about an older patient discharged to a nursing home and upon visiting the facility he was horrified in the conditions he found. At the time no one else was involved in old age psychiatry at Prince of Wales Hospital and so he took on the role. He then became the Director of Community Health in 1983, a newly created position that allowed him to do community old age psychiatry but with some access to admission beds. He tried to establish an old age mental health community nursing team but it was rejected by the community adult mental health nurses. During this period Snowdon became involved with the NSW Association of Mental Health eventually becoming the President in the late 1980s. When the Academic Department of Psychogeriatrics was established at Prince Henry Hospital in 1990 with Henry Brodaty as Director, Snowdon became the Associate Director for a short time before moving to Rozelle Hospital as the Director of Psychogeriatric Services in 1991. He remained there transferring to Concord Hospital with the unit when Rozelle Hospital closed. He became the Chair of the Section of Psychiatry of Old Age in 1995 and subsequently became the first Chair of the Faculty of Psychiatry of Old Age in 1999 with Graeme Halliday as secretary. Snowdon's research has tended to have a clinical focus including nursing home psychiatry, squalor syndrome, late life mood disorders, suicide and older people's mental health service delivery. He has received numerous awards including a RANZCP College Citation, an FPOA Citation for special service to old age psychiatry and is a Member of the Order of Australia.[33]

The advanced training program required a significant amount of input from senior FPOA members in the early years as each RANZCP training program across Australia and New Zealand that wanted to offer advanced training in psychiatry of old age had to be accredited, a process involving site visits by external FPOA reviewers. This was a fruitful process as it allowed the local services to use the external site visitor reports to assist them in service development. If accreditation standards were not being met regarding psychiatry of old age training due to service deficiencies then it was a way of convincing administrators about the need for service enhancements. After a decade of operation, 81 trainees had been awarded their Certificates including those from New Zealand and by mid-2021 this had increased to 225, 185 of whom were based in Australia.[34]

The first decade of FPOA witnessed continued growth and by 2008 there were 191 members in Australia with a further twenty nine in New Zealand.[35] By April 2021 this had increased to 286 accredited Australian members, that is, those who had fulfilled the requirements to be recognised as an old age psychiatrist, with a further 317 non-accredited members who had an interest in old age psychiatry, a category of membership introduced in 2014.[36] Annual scientific meetings usually held in late spring and which circulated between the Australian states and New Zealand remained the main vehicle for professional and social contact and a forum for including the advanced trainees at an early stage of their career. This was facilitated from 2001 by adding a subsidised advanced training weekend with presentations by international and national luminaries who had attended the FPOA scientific meeting. The FPOA newsletter, which had humble beginnings in 1995 as a means of communicating with SPOA membership about issues related to the IPA conference, which was very professionally edited and produced by Richard Bonwick over the first decade of Faculty and later by Helen McGowan, was the main source of regular communication for members. As intended, FPOA contributed to policy issues both within the College and externally over the next decade. Within the College, John Snowdon (Chair 1999–2001) ensured that FPOA funds within the College that had been earned at the 1995 IPA meeting remained with FPOA, while Pam Melding (Chair 2001–2005) managed to obtain some administrative support within the binational College headquarters in Melbourne for FPOA affairs. Some of the external policy submissions included to the 2005 Senate Select Committee on Mental Health and the 2007 Review of Subsidies and Services in Australian Government Funded Community Aged Care Programs while Daniel O'Connor was Chair (2005–2007. While I was Chair (2007–2009) election statements on the neglect of mental health in older people were sent to the major political parties at the 2007 Federal election (and perhaps prompted the commissioning of the report by the Minister for Ageing that led to the establishment of the Psychogeriatric Expert Reference Group). A submission to the Productivity Commission was prepared while Gerard Byrne was Chair (2009–2011). A Position statement on the use of antipsychotic drugs in people with dementia was issued in 2006 and has subsequently been regularly updated. During the decade FPOA gave citations to Ed Chiu (2002), John Snowdon (2002), Neville Hills (2005) and to me (2004) for contributions to FPOA and old age mental health in Australia.[37] Later initiatives by FPOA include the establishment of an Older Persons Mental Health Network to accommodate multidisciplinary communication and collaboration and the production by the

NSW branch of a Handbook on the management of BPSD in 2013,[38] and a 2015 Position Statement on the use of antidepressants to treat depression in dementia.[39]

Involvement with IPA conferences continued with FPOA running successful IPA meetings at Lorne in 2001, Rotorua in 2005 and Cairns in 2012. Apart from running these IPA meetings, Australian membership of IPA remained high after the 1995 Sydney Congress compared with other countries. Many Australians have had a significant input into the organisation with two becoming President (Ed Chiu and Henry Brodaty), Daniel O'Connor was secretary, John Snowdon, Gerard Byrne, Wendy Moyle, Nancy Pachana, Carmelle Peisah, Diego De Leo and I were Board members, David Ames edited the IPA Bulletin before editing the IPA scientific journal *International Psychogeriatrics* before handing over the latter role to Nicola Lautenschlager, and Henry Brodaty and I each edited editions of the *IPA Complete Guide to BPSD*.[40]

One of the important features of FPOA has been the large number of members with international academic standing. Apart from Ed Chiu, Henry Brodaty and John Snowdon, others that have full professorial appointments include David Ames, Gerard Byrne, Osvaldo Almeida, Daniel O'Connor, Carmelle Peisah, Nicola Lautenschlager and me. The research has covered a broad range of topics including prevention of dementia and depression, early dementia diagnosis, dementia management, depression, anxiety, suicide, mental health services, ethics, medico-legal issues and numerous clinical trials. There has been considerable collaboration between the researchers. Many books have been written and edited and various teaching activities across Australia and overseas have been provided.

In October 2008, FPOA members were surveyed as there were still concerns that there was an insufficient number of old age psychiatrists for the ageing population. The survey sought to identify barriers to practice. Most respondents had a public appointment, with just over a third working in private practice where lack of a multidisciplinary team and poor remuneration were cited as barriers. But the most pleasing finding was that 88 per cent reported that they were satisfied with their work, the main reasons cited being the work with older people, the intellectual challenge and working in a multidisciplinary team.[41] The challenge of treating older people in private practice was reflected in analyses of specialist psychiatric consultations in the community from Medicare reimbursement data from 2001–2006 where the per capita consultation rates dropped steeply over the age of 65, with the rates of those aged 65–74 being about a third of younger adults, while for those aged 85 years and over it was less than a tenth of younger adults with only home visits being more common. Such a steep drop in specialist consultations suggests that older people were not accessing private psychiatrists at levels consistent with the known epidemiology of mental disorders in late life. Geriatricians were possibly acting as de facto old age psychiatrists particularly in light of their involvement in dementia care and the finding that in persons over the age of 75, hospital care for mental disorders was more likely to be in a general hospital rather than a mental health setting.[42]

It was unlikely that public mental health services were picking up the slack. A survey of publicly funded older people's mental health services was undertaken by Daniel O'Connor and Pam Melding for FPOA in 2003. The Australian survey results showed marked variability between the states and territories on various components of service delivery. Victoria was the state best served by comprehensive services, while NSW and Queensland performed relatively poorly. Estimates of the number of community clients in these public older people's mental health services would not have compensated for the low numbers observed in private practice.[43] This variability was further noted in the 2005 National Mental Health Report that listed per capita expenditure in general adult and older adult mental health for each State and Territory, with Victoria, the State with the highest expenditure, spending more than double that reported in NSW, Queensland and the Territories. In part, this reflected the different approach used in Victoria where there was a strict 65 and over age cut-off for funded services thus requiring a greater service reach.[44] The 2007 National Mental Health Report charted bed changes across the States and Territories between 1994 and 2005 with around 38 per cent reduction in older persons' beds in that period across the country due to closure of long-stay beds. There was a lack of acute beds for older people in Tasmania and the Territories and very few per capita in Queensland.[45]

Opportunities to provide some national guidance about developing older people's mental health services have been missed. Between 2005 and 2008 the National Mental Health Benchmarking Project included older people's mental health services demonstrated marked variability between services but did not result in substantive national change.[46] The 2009 Fourth National Mental Health Plan lacked any priority items related to older people and a 'blueprint' for mental health reform issued by the Independent Mental Health Reform Group in 2011 largely ignored older people.[47] Although the Government response to the Productivity Commission's 'Caring for older Australians' 2011 report had some specific items related to dementia care as noted in the previous chapter, there was nothing specifically related to old age mental health. The 2017 Fifth National Mental Health and Suicide Prevention Plan also lacked priority items related to older people who receive only a few brief mentions.[48] The inadequate consideration of older people in these plans was likely fuelled by findings in the 1997 and 2007 National Mental Health Surveys that reported low rates of anxiety and depression in older adults.[49,50] The accuracy of these surveys has been questioned and subsequent studies identified an age-related bias in the survey methodology that resulted in an underestimate of mental disorders in older people.[51,52,53] But it seems that mental health policy is still driven in part by these data.

A 2015 national survey to map the provision of services for severe persistent behavioural symptoms of dementia by state-funded older people's mental health services showed marked variability between jurisdictions in the availability of older people's mental health services per population of people aged 65 years and over, with South Australia and NSW having the lowest and Tasmania the highest. Compared with the 2003 survey, the provision of services to rural and regional areas had improved in all states bar South Australia and Western Australia. The number of acute old age mental health beds was particularly low in Queensland and NSW which as a consequence were more likely to use other types of admission beds for severe behavioural symptoms that could not be managed in situ. There was no nationally accepted pathway of care for those with dementia and severe behavioural symptoms requiring hospital admission.[54]

Psychological services for older people were slow in development despite there being a number of Australian psychologists with an international profile. In 1991, the year neuropsychologist Wayne Reid from Sydney won the International Psychogeriatric Association research prize for his work on the evolution of dementia in people with Parkinson's disease,[55] a survey of Australian Psychological Society (APS) membership revealed that only one per cent had a primary interest in working with older people.[56] An APS Ageing Special Interest Group had been established under the leadership of Colleen Doyle in the 1980s yet by 2008 the proportion of Australian psychologists that spent the majority of their time with older people had only risen to six per cent, a figure comparable with international studies.[57] Predictors of working with older people included clinical exposure and age-related course content in training programs.[58] Barriers to improving the situation in the training of Australian psychologists include a dearth of experienced supervisors, the optional nature of old age placements, and a content focus on assessment and diagnosis rather than therapy of older people.[59] Australian guidelines for the training of psychologists about older people and the provisions of old age psychology services were published in 2006.[60] Nancy Pachana in Queensland has been one of the leaders in the training of psychologists, research on anxiety, and involvement with IPA. Clinical psychology services for older people remain quite low. In 2018/19, the lowest population-based rates of Medicare-subsidised clinical and other psychology services in adults was to those aged 65 years and over; this was only about a third of services provided to adults aged 18–44.[61] One barrier to accessing these psychology services was for residents of aged care facilities who until 2019 were unable to receive Medicare-subsidised clinical psychology services other than those related to dementia. It is too early to know whether the new Psychological Treatment Services initiative which is organised through Primary Health Networks will overcome this deficiency.[62]

There are some signs that at a national level there is emerging awareness that there are significant mental health needs of older people beyond those related to dementia as witnessed by concerns related to residents of aged care facilities becoming depressed during the COVID pandemic lockdowns and the acknowledgement that men over the age of 85 have the highest suicide rates in Australia. A National Mental Health Service Planning Framework, based on a model developed in NSW, includes older people which has been a challenge but includes clear targets for increasing mental health resources for older people.[63] Whether or not this leads to a coordinated national strategy and improved older people's mental health services remains to be seen.

## Chapter 14

# The Development of Older People's Mental Health Services in Victoria and NSW 1980-2020

One of the consequences of the States and Territories having the responsibility for running public mental health services is the lack of uniformity in service development as was noted in the previous chapter that reported on the national surveys. At times this reflects the different demographic imperatives that the jurisdictions faced, such as with the Northern Territory that until more recent years had relatively few older people. Other factors, however, often influenced the level of priority that the States had in developing their specialised older people's mental health services and the form that they took. This became readily apparent after 1980 and in this chapter the contrasting older people's mental health service development in the two States that had made some progress before 1980, Victoria and NSW, is provided.

### Victoria

In the early 1980s there was a need to reinvigorate old age psychiatry in Victoria. Herbert Bower had semi-retired and it was the realisation of this gap that led Professor Brian Davies to encourage Ed Chiu to move in to old age psychiatry in 1982 and attend the 'Arie Course' at Nottingham. On his return Chiu, together with Manjula O'Connor, established the Psychogeriatric Unit at Royal Park Hospital in 1984.[1]

Meanwhile Arthur Harrison continued his work at Larundel Hospital, a State psychiatric hospital located at Bundoora, an outer suburb of Melbourne, where he ran a comprehensive service for the Outer Eastern and Country

Region that had a population of 550,000. From the mid-1980s Larundel also provided a service for those with functional mental disorders in the Southern Region that had previously been admitted to the Willsmere Hospital, although the organic cases continued to be admitted to Willsmere. The service included an acute ward, two long-stay wards, a small multidisciplinary community team, and provided a liaison service and outpatient clinic at Maroondah Hospital, the nearest general hospital in the catchment area. In reporting on one hundred consecutive admissions from 1985–1986, Harrison and colleagues noted the diagnostic complexity of the cases, the significant medical comorbidity with nearly half of the admissions having significant previously undiagnosed physical illnesses, the importance of having acute and long-term beds, the need to have a community team to assess patients before admission and follow-up after discharge, and that with proper assessment and management the majority of admissions (75 per cent in this study) were discharged to the community. The use of a '65 years and over' age cut-off for the service was justified in part to avoid the beds being filled by younger intractable cases. The study also highlighted the challenges of providing an older people's mental health service in a mental hospital rather than a general hospital. With seven patients requiring transfer to a general hospital, Harrison and colleagues recommended that clearer definition of the responsibilities of public older people's mental health and geriatric services was required.[2]

Another early development in Victoria was the establishment of the Older Veteran's Psychiatry Program at Austin Repatriation Medical Centre in 1986 to provide psychiatric care to ageing Second World War veterans and war widows across the state. Much of the service work was delivered through a day hospital with specific programs for affective disorders, anxiety disorders, organic disorders, chronic psychoses and for post-traumatic stress disorder. The service also had a strong educational focus across the state. Richard Bonwick was a consultant in the service for over twenty years.[3]

In 1987, a general practitioner from St Kilda, Dr R.J. O'Bryan, wrote a viewpoint article in the *Australian Journal on Ageing* poignantly describing the complex challenges faced by his older patients with various types of often chronic mental disorders, from diverse cultural backgrounds, many of whom had also led bohemian lifestyles. He also mentioned the numerous types of formal and informal services that assisted them to remain in the community.[4] This contributed to the widespread recognition that mental health service provision to older people required change to meet emerging needs and to improve coordination, which led to the release of a policy and program statement *Psychiatric services for older people in Victoria* by the Office of Psychiatric Services in May 1988. Largely based on the model of care espoused by Tom Arie, the issues identified that needed to be addressed included that resources were concentrated into providing long-term residential care, poor identification of geriatric psychiatry (the term used in the report) beds within the general psychiatry program, geriatric psychiatry beds not being associated with assessment programs, limited day patient and rehabilitation programs, varied and ad hoc community outreach services, and lack of a specific program in community health centres. Some of the facilities in use were noted to be unsuitable or inadequate with Willsmere Hospital being specifically mentioned and its closure in December 1989 foreshadowed, decommissioning having already commenced in 1987. Other facilities, such as general psychiatry wards, were admitting older people but were inappropriate facilities for their needs. Resources were over-committed to large psychiatric hospitals rather than into community outpatient and residential services. The need for more trained and experienced staff was highlighted.[5]

The policy statement had the objective of developing 'a specific geriatric psychiatry service integrated within the overall health care system for older people'.[6] To achieve this, it was proposed to expand community-based assessment, develop inpatient geriatric psychiatry assessment and treatment services, provide inpatient and outpatient rehabilitation programs, expand home and community support services, provide long-stay residential facilities, ensure an adequate supply of specialist professional expertise, and increase community awareness about mental disorders in older people and the services available. Priorities that were determined would be funded out of the Willsmere Replacement Program and included the establishment of new community psychogeriatric assessment teams in four regions, new acute inpatient units at the Peter James Centre Burwood, Heatherton Hospital, Dax House at Geelong, as well as the recently opened unit at Royal Park, four psychogeriatric nursing homes and cluster homes in the Willsmere precinct, nursing homes for the Mornington Peninsula and Geelong, respite beds, home and community care services, and Chairs of Psychogeriatric

Medicine at Victorian universities. A multidisciplinary Expert Panel in Geriatric Psychiatry was established to advise the Director of the Office of Psychiatric Services.[7]

Most of the priority list was completed with the exception of establishing an acute inpatient unit at Geelong which has yet to occur. As planned, replacement services were set up before Willsmere closed with the Janet H Bowen Day Centre established by Herbert Bower being replaced by the Wildara Day Centre that long-stay patients from Willsmere were also able to attend. For those older long-stay patients with specific needs unable to be met in mainstream facilities (usually related to behavioural disturbance), smaller cluster homes which became known as psychogeriatric nursing homes and three psychogeriatric hostels were established in community locations such as Flemington, St Albans, Bentleigh and Noble Park. Extensive staff training was funded.[8] Academic posts were established with Ed Chiu moving to Mont Park in the North Eastern Metropolitan Psychiatric Service (NEMPS) as Associate Professor at the University of Melbourne in 1989,[9] and New Zealand-born Daniel O'Connor, who had been working in England doing seminal research with Sir Martin Roth on dementia in the community in Cambridge, being appointed as the Professor of Psychogeriatrics at Monash University in 1990. This position was based in the re-purposed Heatherton Hospital, a former tuberculosis sanatorium that was re-named as the Kingston Centre, and included being Director of the Psychogeriatric Service with a community team, acute and long-stay wards, many of the staff being formerly from Willsmere. Daniel O'Connor later became the third Chair of FPOA and was instrumental in organising surveys of older people's mental health service development across the country. His research has focused on management of BPSD with various innovative approaches including aromatherapy and Montessori methods as well as the diagnosis and management of late life depression in primary care.[10] One of the new Community Aged Psychiatry teams funded from the Willsmere Replacement Program and commencing in 1991 was on the Mornington Peninsula with Michael Duke leading the multidisciplinary team that undertook a broad range of educational, advocacy and liaison activities in addition to assessment and management.[11] The positive impact of the Willsmere Replacement Program on the development of older people's mental health services was reflected in the national survey undertaken in

1992 that found Victoria led the way on most of the multidisciplinary staffing parameters reported.[12]

Further developments occurred in the early to mid-1990s under the 'Building Better Cities Program', a joint Commonwealth and State initiative, in which the Victorian Government included the closure of Larundel Hospital in 1998 and the deinstitutionalisation of many long-stay patients into smaller community facilities including psychogeriatric nursing homes.[13] Funds from this initiative also contributed to the establishment of an acute ward at the Caulfield General Medical centre with Kathy Hall as Director. Hall identified four factors that contributed to Caulfield's readiness for the development: an established consultation liaison psychiatry service, an established memory clinic, a psychiatrist director of medical services, and the Caulfield chief executive officer having a long history of psychiatric experience.[14] This was developed alongside geriatric medicine and rehabilitation services as part of the 1995 Victorian overhaul of the governance of health in which seven health networks were established and Aged Persons Mental Health (APMH) services (the term adopted in Victoria from this point) were co-located with geriatric medicine and extended care centres.[15] In 1996 the Victorian Department of Health and Community Services, as part of its overall reform of mental health service delivery, released a framework for APMH service delivery and in 1997 published generic briefs for 20-bed psychogeriatric admission and assessment units and 30-bed psychogeriatric nursing homes including those proposed for Bundoora Extended Care Centre and Eastern Metropolitan Region nursing homes at Hawthorn, Richmond, and Mooroolbark.[16,17,18] Victoria led the way in closure of stand-alone psychiatric hospitals, NEMPS achieving this in 1995 with APMH moving into St George's Hospital, Bundoora Extended Care Centre and Caulfield Hospital.[19] By mid-1998 all had either been closed or were in the process of closure, a process completed by 2004.[20] In the late 1990s concerns were raised about the funding of APMH services compared with Adult Mental Health Services. The Victorian branch of FPOA, led by Kathy Hall and Anne Hassett, in collaboration with the Victorian Hospitals Association produced an issues paper that argued for funding parity which was achieved in the 2000–2001 Victorian budget.[21]

An initiative that distinguished Victoria from the other States and Territories developed out of the Victorian Government's 1997 Ministerial Taskforce on

Dementia Services that was set up after lobbying from the Victorian Alzheimer's Association.[22] The Taskforce, led by Ed Chiu, recommended the establishment of a State Network of Specialist Cognitive Dementia and Memory Services (CDAMS) based in aged care services with strong links to all services relevant to the management of dementia with one service located in each of the State's health regions. These built on the independently developed memory clinics that were already in existence in some hospitals. While largely based within a geriatric medical framework, the co-location of APMH services facilitated the input of old age psychiatrists in the assessment and management of dementia. The State Network with funding linked to clinical indicators that enabled uniformity in assessment and management across the State was innovative.[23] Victoria remains the only state that has a coordinated network of memory clinics covering urban and regional areas.

The 2003 national survey of older people's mental health services found that Victoria was the only state to provide specialist multidisciplinary aged psychiatry teams with community, acute inpatient, and residential care components in all of its major cities. Victoria also recorded the highest bed numbers and number of older people managed by the community teams. Clearly Victoria led the way in older people's mental health service development.[24] This was reflected in another initiative, the Intensive Community Team (ICT) that was piloted in the Aged Persons Mental Health Program in Eastern Health from late 2003 as an alternative to developing the costly infrastructure required for acute inpatient services in a region where the ratio of older people to available bed numbers was high. The pilot was a success in terms of symptom improvement, although symptom severity of those managed by the ICT was less than those admitted to hospital. Carers rated the service highly and from an economic perspective, an ICT admission cost 60 per cent less than a hospital admission.[25] The successful pilot resulted in the expansion of the ICT program over the next five years to other catchment areas, including Barwon, Dandenong, Gippsland and Bendigo, where there was an excess of older people to beds available.[26]

Ed Chiu retired from his post at St Georges Hospital in December 2004, remaining active in an honorary capacity, with David Ames taking over as the Professor/Director of the Academic Unit for Psychiatry of Old Age in 2005 where he remained until September 2007 when he became Director of the National

Ageing Research Institute. Subsequently Nicola Lautenschlager moved from Western Australia in July 2008 to become the Professor/Director at St Georges Hospital.[27]

Guidelines for Victorian mental health services were released in 2005. These confirmed that there was a strict age cut off between adult mental health services (18–64 years) and APMH services (65 years and over). The target population for APMH services included people with long-standing mental illness, people who developed functional illnesses such as depression or psychoses later in their lives, and people with psychiatric or severe behavioural difficulties associated with organic disorders such as dementia. The three service components specified were aged persons' community mental health teams, acute inpatient services and aged persons' mental health residential care.[28]

Although the majority of older people's mental health services are in the public sector, the Melbourne Clinic is an exception with the 25-bed Herbert Bower Unit having a focus on affective disorders in older people, mean age of admissions circa 2011 being 75 years. Richard Bonwick was the director of the unit in this period and noted that the unit had a full multidisciplinary team including trainee psychiatrists, day programs, an ECT service and an outreach service. Many of the admissions came from outside Melbourne where there was poor access to inpatient APMH services.[29]

The 2015 national survey of older people's mental health services showed that Victoria had fourteen APMH services, which was above the national average of services, and had the second highest number of acute beds per population of persons aged 65 years and over. Victorian APMH services reported the greatest capacity to provide daily community visits to older people with severe disorders. However, only one APMH service had access to non-acute beds.[30] When compared with the previous survey twelve years earlier, there had been a reduction in services relative to the population of older people from 2.5 to 1.5 per 100,000 people aged 65 years and over and acute bed numbers had declined from 34.5 to 24.6 per 100,000 people aged 65 years and over.[31]

In February 2019 the Victorian Government called a Royal Commission into the Victorian Mental Health System with an interim report released in November 2019 and the final report in February 2021. The Royal Commission largely focused on youth and young adult mental health as it interpreted the issues of prevention and early intervention that were central to the terms of reference mainly from that perspective. Only one of the sixty-five recommendations related specifically to older people (Recommendation 22) and that was a relatively generic one that largely reiterated the need for parity with adult services and suggested a similar service description as in the 2005 guidelines.[32] There were few submissions about older people though one issued raised in the submissions by the Commissioner for Senior Victorians and COTA Victoria related to the barriers and appropriateness of having a strict age cut-off at 65 years between adult and APMH services. The transition for some older people between services was seen to be problematic.[33,34] With some evidence that APMH services in Victoria are less well-resourced circa 2020 than fifteen years earlier and a Royal Commission that largely ignored the needs of older people, service development appears to have stalled. To add to this, the Older Veteran's Psychiatry Program at Austin Repatriation Hospital closed in June 2021.

## NSW

In the early 1980s, NSW older people's mental health services were largely based in the State Psychiatric Hospitals with only some of these services, notably those at Parramatta under the leadership of Miriam Merlin, providing a comprehensive service to their local area, and at Rozelle Hospital (formerly Callan Park), the Rozelle Outreach Service for the Elderly (ROSE) team provided an assessment and management service. Sid Williams was the main voice that attempted to influence service planning and when the *Inquiry into Health Services for the Psychiatrically Ill and Developmentally Disabled*, chaired by David Richmond from the Public Service Board was commenced in 1982, Williams largely crafted the RANZCP submission related to psychogeriatric services based on the 1977 submission that Miriam Merlin had made to the Mental Health Service Planning and Review Committee. The issues identified included lack of staff training and experience, lack of status of geriatric psychiatry, problems in placing older people with psychiatric illness, lack of adequate community and inpatient facilities for the assessment and management of older people, and poor community awareness of older people's mental health issues. The submission proposed a comprehensive service structure for psychogeriatric services.[35]

Sid Williams had a prominent role in raising public and health professional awareness of dementia and old age mental health, particularly in the 1980s, facilitating education for health professionals, students and carers. Williams worked as a medical officer at the Psychiatric Research Institute (PRI), the forerunner of the Neuropsychiatric Institute, at Callan Park Hospital before undertaking formal psychiatry training in the early 1970s. After completing training, he took up a position at PRI, became the Director after a few years, and then moved to Lidcombe Hospital to work with Tony Broe in the mid-1970s. In the late 1970s he became more focused on old age psychiatry. With others he developed the first Australian carer-oriented, multidisciplinary outpatient dementia clinic at Lidcombe Hospital, older people's mental health services at Lidcombe, Bankstown-Lidcombe and Braeside Hospitals, and a multidisciplinary psychiatry of old age course at the NSW Institute of Psychiatry. He chaired the Psychogeriatrics Working Party for the 1988 Barclay Report. Formerly Associate Professor at the University of Sydney, in later years he provided services to rural and regional NSW and outer south-west Sydney.[36] He was awarded a RANZCP College Citation in 2017.

The *Richmond Report*, released in March 1983, was a major turning point in the organisation of mental health services in NSW. It led to the separation of developmental disability services from mental health services and further deinstitutionalisation of people with chronic serious mental illness into community settings, along with the planned closure of psychiatric hospitals.[37] By 1984, Aftercare was frustrated as it realised that the Richmond Implementation funding was inadequate and utilised a highly flawed process that was partly due to the healthcare system struggling to catch up with decades of increasing population in the western suburbs of Sydney.[38] The failure to adequately fund community-based alternatives to institutional care across the age range resulted in bed reductions across the state without the means to support those with chronic serious mental illness in the community. It led to disruption of mental health services in NSW with serious bed shortages across the age range that particularly impacted on services from the mid-1990s.

Part 4 of the Report was titled *Services for the Confused and Disturbed Elderly and the Future Role of State Nursing Homes* and at the outset noted the inappropriateness of the label 'psychogeriatric' that was felt to add stigma and increase the likelihood of inappropriate care. It recommended that its use be discontinued.[39] Perhaps the key recommendation that influenced older people's mental health service planning in NSW for the next 20 years was that the 'primary focus of services for the disturbed and confused elderly be based on a multi-disciplinary community oriented geriatric assessment service' that should be 'provided in an integrated manner through linkages to appropriate area or regional acute health services (*including psychiatric services*)'(italics added)[40] and 'that assessment should be based on a geriatric service, with the availability of psychiatric consultation as required'.[41] Clearly this was recommending that older people's mental health services should be located within an aged care service structure. It went on to recommend that all older admissions to psychiatric hospitals should be contingent on a joint assessment with the geriatric assessment service. As Richmond commented, 'because of the complex inter-action between organic and psychiatric factors in elderly disturbed patients the only rational approach is one based on joint responsibility of geriatric and psychiatric personnel'.[42] It is important to realise that these recommendations pre-dated the Commonwealth Aged Care Reform Strategy by around four years, although reference was made to the Macleay Report that had been released in 1982 that had also referred to geriatric assessment services. Most of these recommendations had a dementia focus and were largely about ensuring appropriate admissions to long-term care that was felt should not be primarily in a State psychiatric facility. Importantly, the Report stated that funding of the geriatric assessment service should be a Commonwealth responsibility. Functional psychiatric disorders such as depression were dealt with in one sentence of the 31-page section on older people and simply stated that after the joint assessment process, they should receive the same services as other adults but without explaining how that could occur. The State nursing homes Garrawarra Hospital, Allandale Hospital and Strickland House were recommended to be attached to local general hospitals with the view to be rationalised and the services decentralised into smaller community accommodation, day hospitals and other services. The nursing home component of Lidcombe Hospital was recommended to be integrated into the Lidcombe Hospital services.[43] Despite Lidcombe Hospital being the only general hospital in the state to have a functioning older people's mental health service, it lay outside the mental health system and did not have a recognised catchment area. The *Richmond Report* failed to address this issue and also failed to address the lack of community older people's mental health services beyond noting that staff from long-stay ward closures could be redeployed to geriatric assessment services.[44]

The impact of the *Richmond Report*, particularly as it related to dementia, was augmented by a series of judicial interpretations of the *1958 Mental Health Act* by Justice Powell. The first decision in November 1982 involved a case in the Protective Division (*RAP v AEP*) in which the son of a woman with 'senile dementia by reason of arteriosclerotic degeneration' sought to have the appointment of a committee of three persons including himself to manage the estate of his mother. In 1982, there was no guardianship legislation in NSW and so the Mental Health Act (MHA) was the only legal process available to families wishing to manage the financial affairs of an incompetent relative. Justice Powell ruled that for the Act to apply, it had to be demonstrated that the mother was a 'mentally ill person'. He noted that the *1958 MHA* made an intentional distinction between a person with mental illness and a person with mental infirmity from disease or age, and ruled that dementia fell into the second category and thus the MHA could not be applied. A second case in 1986 (*CCR v PS*) involved a patient with Alzheimer's disease who had been admitted to Rozelle Hospital under the *1958 MHA* but an appeal by the Mental Health Advocacy Service was upheld by Justice Powell who ruled that CCR was not a 'mentally ill person' and had to be discharged. In his judgement Powell made a significant distinction between a person with dementia and comorbid symptoms of mental illness such as hallucinations and delusions who could be deemed a 'mentally ill person' from a person with dementia without those additional symptoms who could not be regarded as a 'mentally ill person'. He also noted that medical practitioners might find such distinctions as ridiculous and lacking in psychiatric sense, but while sympathising with that viewpoint, he regarded his duty to be to uphold the law. Other conditions including Down syndrome, anorexia nervosa and alcohol dependence were also deemed in other Powell decisions to not be mental illnesses.[45]

A third issue that contributed to uncertainty was the failure of the NSW government to proclaim the new *1983 MHA* due to concerns about the definition of mental illness that had been exposed by the Powell judicial interpretations.

Although it was eventually proclaimed in 1986, the definition of mental illness was not clarified until the *1990 MHA* which based the definition on symptoms such as delusions, hallucinations and severe mood disturbance or irrational behaviour suggestive of these symptoms.[46] Thus, as previously indicated by Justice Powell, persons with dementia could be admitted as a 'mentally ill person' under the *1990 MHA* if they had those symptoms. However, the combination of the *Richmond Report* and the Justice Powell decisions meant that from the mid-1980s onwards, medical superintendents of psychiatric hospitals became increasingly wary about admitting people with dementia under the MHA. In 1995, I noted in correspondence with Noel Wilton the NSW Director of Mental Health that medical superintendents in NSW were still making incorrect interpretations of the MHA regarding dementia citing the Powell decisions without recognising that a person with dementia could also legally be mentally ill.[47] The shortage of mental health beds across the State was impacting on the system by this time and was likely to be contributing to the decision-making of the medical superintendents.

In implementing the *Richmond Report*, it quickly became apparent that a large proportion of the patients needing to be deinstitutionalised into local community facilities were older patients and that there were inadequate and insufficient alternative facilities available. The imperative to find such community placements had been amplified by the Powell decisions about dementia. Richard Fleming, working with John Bowles, designed small residential units that accommodated sixteen patients in two wings using cutting edge design principles that utilised the structured physical environment to minimise the impact of confusion on daily living. Fleming trained as a clinical psychologist in London and occupied the positions of Head of Psychology, Kenmore Hospital and Regional Coordinator of Mental Health Services in the South East Region of NSW between 1979 and 1992. He was the Founding Director of HammondCare's Dementia Centre in 1995 where he remained until 2010. Subsequently he was appointed as a Professorial Fellow at the University of Wollongong in 2010 where he was the Executive Director of the Dementia Training Study Centre and Dementia Training Australia. Since 2019 he has been Honorary Professorial Fellow at the University of Wollongong specialising in environmental design for people living with dementia.[48]

The Confused and Disturbed Elderly (CADE) Units, the title acquired from the *Richmond Report,* became the solution that the NSW Government desired. The pilot unit, Pepper Tree Lodge, was built at Queanbeyan and opened in June 1987, populated largely from Kenmore Hospital and although most had dementia,[49] four of the residents had alcohol-related dementia,[50] a situation that geriatrician Terry O'Neill felt was unrelated to the real world accommodation needs of people with dementia.[51] The NSW Government initially planned to build twenty seven CADE Units but only nine were constructed between 1989 and 1991, and these in a rather rushed haphazard and uncoordinated process by the Richmond Implementation Team in terms of location, management and connection with aged care and older people's mental health services.[52] Indeed Sid Williams, in correspondence with Health Minister Peter Anderson in December 1986, expressed the frustration and concern of many in old age mental health that the CADE unit program was being poorly implemented and that there was an urgent need to develop community older people's mental health services.[53]

In the Hunter region, in the early to mid-1980s Ross Chambers managed four long-stay wards, one called Boronia at James Fletcher Hospital (Watt Street) and three at Morisset Hospital. Stephen Ticehurst, who trained at Lidcombe Hospital with Sid Williams in 1984, moved back to Newcastle and after completing his advanced training in old age psychiatry in 1987 (and attending the Arie course in Nottingham), he became the Director of the older people's mental health service in 1988. While the Boronia ward was largely a long-stay dementia ward with many of the patients there because local nursing homes were unable to cope with 'wanderers', the wards at Morisset had a range of poorly assessed or unassessed patients that had accumulated for long-term care. According to Ticehurst,

> 'we spent some time finding out the diagnoses and needs of the patients and moving them around. We ended up with one ward of people who had been there with non-dementing illnesses most of their lives, one with ambulant dementing patients and a smaller one with bed bound patients in the old "Medical Ward".'[54]

With the Powell rulings on dementia, some wards were degazetted. Gradually the Morisset patients were discharged or transferred with funds freed up to support a community team and a State-government run nursing home ward. Eventually, the older people's mental health service at James Fletcher Hospital that had focused on dementia care was given responsibility for all patients aged 65 years and over when it relocated to the Mater Hospital in 2009 but without additional resources. At this point, admissions were controlled by the Psychiatric Emergency Care Centre rather than the older people's mental health service that resulted in people with dementia less likely to be admitted.[55]

The legacy of the *Richmond Report* and the way it was implemented was long lasting in NSW. It stymied development of comprehensive older people's mental health services within mental health programs. During the second half of the 1980s, the few enhancements were largely through the Commonwealth Aged Care Reform Strategy. An example of this was in the St George District of southern Sydney where from late 1985 I was employed at St George Hospital as a staff specialist general psychiatrist but with a focus on older people. In 1985 there were no dementia assessment services and I collaborated with Andrew Cole, who had just been appointed as the Director of the Community Rehabilitation and Geriatric Service (CRAGS) based at St George Hospital, to establish a new community-based dementia assessment and management service utilising the nurses, social workers and psychologists from CRAGS. As with all dementia assessment, some of the referrals had other mental disorders, particularly depression, and with these cases community mental health nurses became involved. Within 18 months of developing the service, community enhancements from the Aged Care Reform Strategy started to flow, and the work already accomplished by the collaborative community dementia program facilitated developments based in CRAGS and so extra staff for the new Geriatric Assessment Team and new dementia day care centres were funded. Eventually in 1989, funding for a new specialist old age psychiatrist was obtained which allowed me to move full time into old age psychiatry in a position funded by the aged care program but also positioned within psychiatry. Similar service development occurred at Royal North Shore Hospital where the Psychogeriatric Unit with Bob Russell as team leader was established within the Rehabilitation and Geriatrics department but with joint appointments in psychiatry.[56]

The major positive development in NSW in the 1980s was the commencement of the Psychiatry of Old Age year-long course in 1987 at the NSW Institute of

Psychiatry under the leadership of Sid Williams. It featured lectures (in a two-week block), workshops, and seminars provided by key experts on a broad range of topics and placements as observers into services. Intentionally designed to attract multidisciplinary participants, it was particularly popular for psychogeriatric nurses and allied health and became one of the main sources of postgraduate old age mental health training in NSW along with the quarterly SPOA NSW half day seminars.[57] For nurses in this era, this was the main source of specific old age mental health education available as there were no postgraduate old age mental health nursing courses, although the NSW College of Nursing had a geriatrics course.[58]

In 1987, the direction that NSW was taking with older people's mental health services being part of aged care services rather than mental health services contributed to John Snowdon raising concerns in an opinion piece in the *Australian and New Zealand Journal of Psychiatry*.[59] A change of government which saw the Greiner Liberal/National Party Coalition take power in 1988 resulted in a Ministerial Review of NSW mental health services under the leadership of Bill Barclay, in particular the Richmond implementation process. A Psychogeriatrics Working Party convened by Sid Williams, and including Richard Fleming, John Snowdon and geriatrician Michael Price, completed a report for the Minister that recommended that the NSW Health Department 'provide comprehensive geriatric psychiatry services by 1992' based on the principles and minimum standards outlined in the report. The detailed recommendations left the model of service organisation to be determined by local area or regional authorities, noting that some might opt for the 'Health Care of the Elderly' approach (the term used by Tom Arie) which would be similar to the direction NSW had been taking. The level of detail and specifications about staff, hospital and community services was daunting and to a large extent based on UK experiences.[60] Given the limited older people's mental health service development in NSW in 1988, the Warrina team based at Cumberland Hospital (formerly Parramatta Hospital), now under the leadership of Dr C.S. Balaraman who had succeeded Miriam Merlin, remained the only comprehensive older people's mental health service in NSW,[61] the recommendations were clearly not feasible and were largely aspirational. But in outlining the complexity of the needs of older people with mental disorders and the broad range of services required to meet those needs, the report for the first time in NSW gave a clear message about the serious gaps that existed.

One issue that the report failed to clearly identify and that had long lasting ramifications for adult and older people's mental health services of all ages was the relationship between the new Area Health Services that were first established in 1988 and the Schedule 5 psychiatric hospitals that were initially placed outside of the Area Health Service structure. This meant that resources tied up in the large psychiatric hospitals were not necessarily connected with the local regions that they served, particularly since many of the Area Health Services had no psychiatric hospitals within their geographical catchment. One specific issue that needed to be addressed but did not occur was how to rationalise and redeploy resources based in the psychiatric hospitals to geographical areas that they served. Later when the psychiatric hospitals were put under the administration of the Area Health Services in which they were located, the failure to have addressed this issue properly left some Area Health Services resource rich and others resource poor particularly as it related to rehabilitation and long-term residential care facilities across the age range. A good example in old age mental health occurred in South West Sydney Area Health Service that used to be covered by Cumberland Hospital but the resources from Cumberland were solely deployed to Western Sydney and Wentworth Area health services.[62]

Despite the Psychogeriatric Working Party report, not much changed with the Strategic Plan for NSW Mental Health Services 1990–1995 having inadequate plans for old age mental health.[63] The only major development of note was the establishment with State funding from the closure of Strickland House of the Academic Department for Psychogeriatrics including the resources for a ten-bed ward at the Prince Henry site of the Prince Henry/Prince of Wales Hospitals with Henry Brodaty as Professor/Director and until early 1992, John Snowdon as his deputy until he moved to Rozelle Hospital. I moved from St George Hospital to Prince Henry Hospital to replace John Snowdon in April 1992. The ward was co-located with the Neuropsychiatric Institute led by Perminder Sachdev. Although only funded for an inpatient service, it quickly established an outreach service particularly into residential care.[64] After the unit moved to Prince of Wales Hospital in 1999 there was a long period where there was limited access to beds in the adult ward while the new ward was being refurbished and two inpatient nurses were redeployed to the community within an integrated team structure. After the refurbishment was completed, bed numbers were reduced to six allowing the nurses to be permanently redeployed as they were still being funded through the inpatient budget. A new 32-bed psychogeriatric ward was built at Kenmore in around 1990 replacing old wards. Most were long-stay patients with a diverse array of disorders including alcohol-related brain damage, Huntington's disease and chronic psychoses.[65]

In the early 1990s Gavin Andrews was a contributor to the debate, as in his work on health services research and the future of Australian psychiatry he suggested that geriatricians would primarily manage most older psychotic, confused and disturbed older patients and somewhat flippantly suggested, in an exchange of correspondence with John Snowdon in the *Australian and New Zealand Journal of Psychiatry*, that 'about one psychogeriatrician per million should suffice if geriatricians are going to treat the elderly'.[66] Snowdon was understandably sceptical about Andrews' viewpoint, noting in particular the large number of older residents in nursing homes with chronic serious mental disorders that were not receiving any specialist care.[67] In an effort to estimate the number of acute mental health beds required for older people, Snowdon retrospectively examined all mental health admissions aged 65 years and over from the Eastern Suburbs of Sydney, who resided in the Prince Henry/Prince of Wales Hospital catchment areas in the period 1977–1987. From these data he estimated that 22 acute beds were needed for a population of 32,000 people aged 65 years and over but warned that caution was required in drawing conclusions from the data due to varying management practices and availability of alternative options.[68] It is interesting to note that in the thirty years since this publication, the Eastern Suburbs catchment area covered by the older people's mental health service has operated throughout with less than 50 per cent of these bed estimates.

The regular planning meetings for the 1995 Sydney IPA Congress were held in conjunction with the quarterly SPOA half day seminars that rotated around various Sydney locations. It brought together multidisciplinary clinicians and academics and helped establish a sense of camaraderie during a period in which NSW appeared otherwise directionless in old age mental health planning. As noted in chapter 13, the Sydney IPA Congress was a resounding success. The extent to which the meeting came to the attention of the new Labor Government with Premier Bob Carr that had been elected in March 1995 is unclear, but it is noteworthy that in 1996 it established two Ministerial Task Forces. The first, chaired by Beverley Raphael who was the Director of the NSW Centre for Mental Health, examined the problem of inappropriate prescribing of psychotropic drugs in nursing homes after extensive media coverage occurred following a study published by John Snowdon from nursing homes in Central Sydney. Although the Taskforce came up with a series of educational, research, practice, resource, and legislative recommendations, the Commonwealth announced its intention of reforming residential aged care a few months after the Taskforce was formed and requested that recommendations be modified or withdrawn as it was unclear what role the States would have in ongoing regulations.[69]

The second Taskforce was on the Mental Health Care of Older People and was co-chaired by Henry Brodaty and Beverley Raphael. It undertook a thorough examination of the issue and came up with a comprehensive report and recommendations. The NSW Government response in its 1999, 'Caring for Older People's Mental Health', was a disappointment that was eloquently summarised by the NSW FPOA Chair, Bob Russell, as being a 'damp squib'.[70] The response was full of generalities about health promotion, prevention and education, ignoring any recommendations concerning service models and resources.[71] Bob Russell also noted that perhaps as a 'consolation prize', the NSW Centre for Mental Health allocated $150,000 to NSW FPOA 'for the purpose of advancing old age psychiatry' but with an eye to a needs assessment of ACATs throughout the State regarding access to psychiatric advice and expertise.[72] This funding was used to survey aged care services, adult mental health services and older people's mental health services in 2001 about their perceptions of mental health service delivery to older people in NSW. Only 59 per cent of aged care services and adult mental health services felt that their local mental health services for older people were adequate with resource (such as old age psychiatrists and other staff, acute and long-stay beds) and budget limitations portrayed as the main reasons for inadequacy. The marked variability of service structures, settings and activities of older people's mental health services across NSW was noted. Inexperience in old age mental health and lack of staff training hindered aged care services and adult mental health service efforts to fill the gap.[73] These findings were reflected in the 2003 national survey of older people's mental health services with NSW slipping in service development from 1992 and having particularly low staff numbers.[74]

The closure of the Lidcombe Hospital site in 1995 in readiness for the site to become the Olympic Media Village for the Sydney 2000 Olympic Games resulted in the amalgamation of the hospital facilities with Bankstown Hospital to become Bankstown-Lidcombe Hospital with the acute older persons' mental health unit being co-located with the acute geriatrics ward. It was administered through geriatric medicine but with old age psychiatrists managing the patients, the only such ward with this service arrangement in NSW. An evaluation undertaken in the mid-2000s showed favourable results compared with other State services on various routinely collected outcome measures and length of stay.[75] In 2020, the service arrangement was altered by the Local Health District with the ward being put fully under geriatric medicine management with old age mental health only providing consultations.

In 2002, concerns about the lack of adequate resources in NSW residential aged care facilities to manage severe and persistent behavioural disturbances related to dementia, led to a joint NSW Centre for Mental Health and FPOA project chaired by John Snowdon to examine options including special care dementia units to best address the issue. The project found that there were insufficient older people's mental health services in NSW and that residential aged care facilities in NSW did not have the resources to address the issue in a systematic and reliable way.[76] Detailed reference was made to the then recently published seven-tiered model of service delivery as an approach to guide service delivery planning.[77] In 2004, Kate Jackson was appointed as the Principal Policy Officer for Older Persons Mental Health, the first such position in NSW, and in 2006 Rod McKay was appointed as Clinical Advisor. The Older Persons Mental Health Policy Unit was subsequently established in December 2007, with Kate Jackson as Director, based at Orange.[78] Under Jackson's leadership the NSW Service Plan for Specialist Mental Health Services for Older People (SMHSOP) for the decade 2005 to 2015 was produced. This included a detailed implementation plan which focused on community mental health service developments for the first five years with over $63 million enhancement funding for the period. Within the plan and influenced by the earlier report, Behavioural Assessment and Intervention Services (BASIS) were established as the components of community SMHSOP teams that would outreach into residential aged care and other community settings to manage severe and persistent challenging behaviour. The second new initiative was the establishment of two Special Care Dementia Units within residential aged care facilities to be operated in partnership with NSW Area Health Services and the local SMHSOP teams, a model influenced by the Psychogeriatric Nursing Homes in Victoria that had combined Commonwealth and State funding. A third initiative involved the service redesign of the long-stay CADE units into what was termed the short to medium-term T-BASIS model of care. The overall service plan with its range of strategies was striking for both the detail and linkage of staged service developments across the comprehensive array of service components to research evidence, benchmarks, performance indicators and resources. One key feature that stood it in contrast to Victoria was that it did not have a rigid age cut-off at 65 to delineate from adult mental health services, as it recognised that some older individuals were appropriately managed in adult services and should not be forced to change service based on chronological age. This reflected a combination of long standing practice and resource availability. The NSW SMHSOP Service Plan certainly led the way nationally with regard to the comprehensive detail it provided along with a clear pathway for staged service development. It also introduced SMHSOP as a new acronym for older people's mental health services in NSW.[79]

The reason for the major turnaround in attitudes towards older people's mental health service development in NSW probably reflects a conjunction of events. Certainly having Kate Jackson as the older persons' mental health policy officer helped, a position supported by Beverley Raphael the director of the Centre for Mental Health and other senior staff within the Centre such as Robyn Murray, but the political situation is also likely to have played a part.[80] When the plan was developed, Morris Iemma was Minister for Health before becoming NSW Premier in August 2005 and he had already demonstrated his willingness to provide extra funding to train psychiatrists through the Institute of Medical Education and Training.[81] In a National Press Club address in June 2006 Iemma spoke about his commitment to a mental health reform, 'I want to be remembered as the Premier who brought hope to some of the most marginalized and disadvantaged people in our community'.[82] This involved a five year $939 million package of mental health reforms and thus the SMHSOP service plan was able to attract funding, although it should still be noted that the amount was less than seven per cent of the total mental health enhancements.[83]

Within months of the BASIS service being established, the Commonwealth's Dementia Behaviour Management and Advisory Services (DBMAS) were announced. DBMAS was similar in concept to BASIS but with a few differences related to scope and function, for example DBMAS services were limited to individuals receiving Commonwealth funding in residential or community care but BASIS services had a broader remit. NSW Health won the tender for running DBMAS in NSW and so BASIS and DBMAS were essentially rolled together to be implemented across the State.[84] The pilot psychogeriatric care and support unit funded under the joint National Action Plan for Dementia Care and National Mental Health Program had been established at Wollongong in the mid-1990s and this became the coordinating unit for DBMAS and BASIS in NSW until the second round of DBMAS tenders at which time the HammondCare group won the tender and took over DBMAS in NSW in 2013.

Guided by the National Framework for Action on Dementia 2006–2010, NSW developed a three year Dementia Action Plan followed on by a five-year (2010–2015) Dementia Services Framework that was produced by the NSW Dementia Policy Team led by Henry Brodaty with Anne Cumming and Troy Spiers supported by an Expert Advisory Group.[85] This was a very detailed framework but it was not given additional resources for implementation, possibly another victim of the NSW Electoral cycle as there was a change of government in 2011. Some parts were implemented such as the appointment of Dementia Clinical Nurse Consultants at major hospitals.

A survey in 2006/2007 reported that there were fourteen SMHSOP services in NSW which were mostly located in major cities, with only three in inner regional areas and none in outer regional and remote areas. Of 120 hospitals that did not have any aged care or SMHSOP beds, only 11 had a visiting old age psychiatrist while 21 had non-medical SMHSOP team member visits, few of which were to rural locations. Only six SMHSOP services were based in major general hospitals, three were in subacute/non-acute hospitals, while despite the closures of psychiatric hospitals in NSW, five SMHSOP services were still based in stand-alone psychiatric hospitals (for example Rozelle Hospital closed in 2008 and the SMHSOP service moved to Concord Hospital). It is noteworthy that for the same time period that witnessed the start-up of BASIS/DBMAS services in NSW, less than half of SMHSOP services reported that they were doing initial assessments of referrals for dementia-related behavioural disturbances in residential aged care facilities.[86] Clearly this survey near the commencement of the SMHSOP service plan (2005–2015) justified the focus on developing community services as the priority for the initial five years.

By the early 2000s the uncoordinated development of CADE Units meant that some were managed by aged care services, some by mental health, and others by both. The degree of clinical and administrative input also varied and thus it had become a fragmented system as predicted by Sid Williams in 1986. A review of the CADE Units found that two of the CADE Units were already utilising a T-BASIS model of care effectively but the effectiveness of the other units was less obvious and recommended that the remaining units follow the same model with strong input and clinical governance from Aged Care and SMHSOP services but within the SMHSOP program.[87] One of the CADE Units, Yathong Lodge at Wagga Wagga that had been identified as the 'model unit', had transitioned from the CADE long-stay model into a short-to-medium stay assessment and treatment model in 2004 with the assistance of Commonwealth Aged Care Innovative Pool Program funding that enabled an increase in the care level to allow the unit to provide services for patients with more severe behaviour disturbance and fund a small community outreach team. It was found to be a cost effective model of care compared with acute hospital admission.[88]

The T-BASIS model of care linking specialist community mental health teams with short to medium term residential assessment and management was implemented in 2006. The initial T-BASIS evaluation in 2008/9 in the remaining five units found that substantive progress had been made in the transition to the new model of care. The outreach teams were regarded as a critical component, particularly as four of the T-BASIS units were located in rural and regional locations with limited access to SMHSOP teams. A higher level of medical, nursing and allied health staffing was recommended in part due to the clinical complexity of cases. Staff training remained an issue requiring further attention and there was early evidence of drift from the goals of the program in some units. Future expansion of the program was envisaged but to date this has not occurred.[89] To develop consistency across the T-BASIS units, a network was established that allowed use of benchmarking data at regular meetings.

The Mental Health Aged Care Partnership Initiative (MHACPI) was a pilot of two purpose-designed special care dementia units within residential aged care facilities operated by not-for-profit organisations (HammondCare and CatholicCare) aimed at people living with severe dementia but with input from the local SMHSOP services. The MHACPI units were staffed by a multidisciplinary team skilled and experienced in behavioural interventions. The intent was for the units to be transition units. The initial evaluation of the MHACPI program undertaken in 2009 was generally positive, especially regarding the well-designed service agreement and model of care, but overall was limited in being able to assess various issues such as resident outcomes due to the small number of patients.[90] The program was expanded with an additional three units (with a fourth planned) under another project, the Pathways to Community Living Initiative, which aims to transfer long-stay psychiatric hospital patients with chronic serious mental illness into smaller community facilities. Around one hundred of these patients were originally admitted under the age of 65 and were now over the age of 65. These have been complemented by two specialist mental health residential aged care facilities for those unable to be transitioned.[91]

The mid-term evaluation of the SMHSOP Service plan was largely complimentary but noted that 'although improving over time, access to SMHSOP is well below the level indicated by estimated need. Rates of access per head of population are also much lower compared with most other Australian states and territories', and this was particularly apparent in priority groups such as Aboriginal and Torres Strait Islander, culturally and linguistically diverse, and rural populations.[92] The evaluation foresaw that the next phase of implementation would be critical to the future of the program. It noted that adult mental health services provide about one-third of the total community contacts and around sixteen per cent of the overnight acute episodes for the SMHSOP target group, with a further fifty-two per cent provided by other admitted units.[93] Indeed, even by 2015 the low number of acute beds in NSW was starkly apparent in the national survey in which the only state to fare worse was Queensland.[94] This was despite new inpatient units being established at Wollongong in 2008 and at St George Hospital in 2013, the latter technically a subacute unit but largely operating as an acute unit. However, the Older Persons Mental Health program did produce a good practice model of care for acute inpatient units in 2012.[95] In 2017 there were sixteen acute inpatient units in NSW providing specialist mental health care, some providing a mix of acute and subacute care. Two units were under development, one in Western Sydney LHD and the other on the Mid North Coast.[96]

The Older Persons Mental Health Policy unit instigated a number of initiatives in the second half of the service plan many that were being introduced in adult mental health services including a focus on the mental health needs of older Aboriginal and Torres Strait Islanders, alcohol and other drug misuse in older people, early intervention and prevention of mental disorders and suicide, recovery-orientation as applied to older people, and the physical health of older mental health patients.[97] An acute inpatient model of care was developed under the leadership of John Dobrohotoff in 2016 and built on an earlier systematic review of acute inpatient unit facility design undertaken with Robert Llewellyn-Jones.[98,99] One pleasing feature has been the evidence that there has been a considerable improvement in the number of services in rural health districts between 2005 and 2018 with community teams increasing from three to twenty six and acute inpatient units increasing from two to five. There was also evidence of increased access to services.[100] The service plan was updated through to 2027 with a continued focus on community initiatives including partnerships with other organisations with a Community Model of Care being published in 2020.[101] A focus on non-acute inpatient models and services programs was also planned along with extra attention to various priority groups. The acronym SMHSOP also disappeared as services were now called Older People's Mental Health Services.[102]

While the overall strategy and service plan in NSW remains impressive, much will depend on the level of resources allocated to the Older People's Mental Health Program to determine if developments for older people adequately meet their needs.

# Chapter 15

# The Development of Older People's Mental Health Services in Other States and Territories 1980-2020

Unlike Victoria and NSW, the other States and Territories entered the 1980s with very little service development for older people beyond long-stay psychiatric wards in their mental hospitals. Acute inpatient care was largely co-located with general adult psychiatry while community care was limited and mainly provided by adult mental health. In the early 1980s, Western Australia and South Australia were the next states to show signs of recognising the need to develop comprehensive services for older people.

### Western Australia

It was the combination of fortuitous circumstances rather than evidence of service planning that gave Western Australia the opportunity to develop a contemporary older people's mental health service system. The decision taken in 1979 to close Swanbourne Hospital due to its poor conditions and use funds from the sale of the land to provide capital for new services included those for older people, as Swanbourne had a large long-stay elderly population. This provided a greenfield opportunity to develop older people's mental health services.[1]

Into this situation came Neville Hills who had been appointed Deputy Psychiatrist Superintendent at Swanbourne in 1979 after previously working in forensic psychiatry for nearly a decade. When Peter Reed, who had commenced steps towards a British model of old age mental health assessment and care, retired later in 1979, Neville Hills became the Superintendent and devoted himself to old age psychiatry for the rest of his career. Hills had an interesting background. Born and educated in Western Australia (WA), he completed undergraduate medicine in Adelaide although his final year was based back in Perth. He initially worked at Claremont Hospital from 1964 as a medical officer but in that era there was no psychiatry training program in WA, and so he decided to move to England with his family where he worked at St John's Hospital Aylesbury, obtained the Diploma of Psychological Medicine (DPM) in 1967 and subsequently worked for two years as a forensic psychiatrist at Rampton Special Hospital. He returned to Western Australia and took up a psychiatrist position at Shenton Park Day Hospital.[2] In this period he was a Captain Medical Officer in the Citizen Military Force where he learned the concept of having small regimental aid posts close to the action that could triage as required. He later felt that these principles could apply to medical planning in community psychiatry with outpatient clinics being small accessible contact places that could leapfrog over existing hospitals. In espousing these principles in an examination for Major's rank, he failed as the accepted wisdom of the time was for medical strategy based on desert warfare which Hills felt was outdated in the Vietnam War era. It was this willingness to challenge the accepted way of doing things based on evidence that showed a better approach irrespective of whether it put him at odds with authorities that characterised Hills approach throughout his career. In 1970, Hills moved to the WA Department of Corrections as a forensic psychiatrist where he spent five years but found himself in conflict with government over his views on parole and probation which Hills saw as contributing to incarceration rather than relieving it especially for Aboriginal people who had little chance of working the system in their favour. Due to this conflict, Hills returned to England for a second stint at Rampton Hospital being unaware there was an investigation into institutional abuses underway. He returned to Australia being thankful that his earlier conflict with government did not prevent his appointment to Swanbourne Hospital.[3]

Hills was keen for any new developments to reflect the cutting edge of service delivery models in old age mental health. He returned to the UK and Europe for six weeks in 1981 to examine developments in old age psychiatry to help inform the direction policy should take in replacing Swanbourne Hospital. He met Tom Arie in Nottingham and visited other facilities in England, Scotland, Germany, and the Netherlands. No single model or architectural blueprint for design emerged as ideal, although the principles, such as working closely with geriatric medicine and simpler referral pathways, and the range of services became clearer. He visited newly opened NHS psychogeriatric units at Edinburgh and Stockton but was unimpressed with the standardisation of design and warehousing approach. What most impressed him was not in the NHS but within Social Services. Woodside House in Birmingham was initiated by the eminent geriatrician Bernard Isaacs and many of its features were incorporated into WA facilities including the Lefroy Hostel built in Perth by Anglican Homes in 1986. This included having more staff working in the evenings to deal with sundowning, single room accommodation with décor and fittings typical of a private home in a normal village street, exercise areas, well-trained staff and activities.[4]

Replacement facilities for Swanbourne Hospital were based on the 1982 Campbell-Miller Report largely prepared by architect and health planner Bob Miller from a private firm of architects/developers, Campbell and Associates, who established current and projected service utilisation patterns for older people's mental health services across the State and consulted with staff and patients. Arguably the report contains the first clear Statewide strategy for older people's mental health services in WA with recommendations including that: all older admissions with mental disorders be subject to specialist review in order to establish admission policies; specialist psychogeriatric services based on acute psychogeriatric admission wards be located in general hospitals in association with geriatric medicine and general psychiatry with 90 beds provided per 100,000 population; four 24-bed Psychogeriatric (acute) Assessment Units be established in teaching hospitals in Metropolitan Perth by 1991; the needs of patients eligible for home care should be met; patients with young onset dementia be cared for with the dementia group; eight psychiatrists (two per team) would be needed by 1986 and ten by 1991; and facilities for continuing care of existing older Swanbourne patients, Psychogeriatric Extended Care Units, should be organised in units of 24 and 48 beds each with day places and located according to geographical distribution of older people.[5]

Only one of the 24-bed Psychogeriatric Assessment Units was built at Bentley Hospital alongside a 24-bed geriatric medical unit and this was eventually taken over by geriatric medicine in 1992 after the departure of the unit psychiatrist. Six Psychogeriatric Extended Care Units, known as Lodges (Selby, Bentley,

Osborne, Swan, Armadale, and Moss Street), were opened as planned and in 1985 210 patients were transferred from Swanbourne over a six-month period. These Lodges became the core of comprehensive older people's mental health service delivery in WA having day hospitals and housing the community teams covering metropolitan Perth with agreements about rural and regional areas, and eventually taking on an acute inpatient assessment role, filling the gap left by the absence of purpose built acute assessment units, and being gazetted under the Mental Health Act.[6]

A third element was a hostel type community housing project for those who were considered capable of residing in conventional housing but only with staff support. Eight three-bedroom homes in Eden Hill cluster housing project in a normal suburban area were purchased in 1982. After a successful start in which the facility transitioned numerous long-term Swanbourne patients who had been pre-assessed by former Swanbourne staff into community living and began to accept community referrals, problems developed with an industrial dispute regarding relationships with community health that were accentuated by the unexpected 1987 amalgamation of State Mental Health Services into the Health Department. The amalgamation changed the governance structure in which Neville Hills, as the Psychiatrist Superintendent from Swanbourne had also been the Statewide coordinator of older people's mental health services, was now replaced by Health Department business managers. Pre-admission assessments and community follow-ups were halted, new referrals dried up and staff morale declined. It was soon closed and labelled as being a failure.[7] In retrospect, it was an initiative ahead of its time.

The change in governance after 1987 resulted in a loss of services funded by the Swanbourne hospital closure and a reduction in bed numbers over the next seven years. The gains made in the 1980s that put WA at the forefront of older people's mental health service developments were not entirely lost but had certainly had some pull back, in part due to the weak economic climate in WA at the time. There was also a change from a Statewide service model to a regional one, a move that involved Neville Hills position being lost and led to his redundancy. In the mid-1990s Hills noted that there were only three old age psychiatrists in WA at a time when ten were required,[8] a deficiency also found in the 1992 national survey.[9]

The next significant change in WA came in the late 1990s with the arrival of Osvaldo Almeida and Leon Flicker in 1998 to take up Chairs in Geriatric Psychiatry and Geriatric Medicine respectively at the University of Western Australia (although Osvaldo Almeida's formal appointment as Chair in Geriatric Psychiatry occurred in 2001). Together they forged an impressive portfolio of research in late life mental disorders that has had an international impact. But just as importantly they provided the foundation for high quality training in the broad field of geriatrics and the encouragement for psychiatry trainees to commence sub-specialty training in psychiatry of old age when that commenced in 1999.[10] By 2004 there were eleven psychiatry trainees in WA enrolled in the psychiatry of old age advanced training program and the sites used for training had expanded into the teaching hospitals and outer areas of Perth.[11]

After a period without Statewide leadership following Neville Hills' redundancy, the position of Lead Psychogeriatrician was established in July 2000, in part to ensure that resources earmarked for older people's mental health were not siphoned off, with Alan Wood taking up the post and developing a service plan.[12] But by 2001 in the context of funding cuts across mental health, the position was initially reduced in hours and resources thus impeding its effectiveness, before being abolished in 2003.[13,14] In 2003, WA was faring quite well when compared with other states and territories in the national survey. By this time the Lodges had completed their transition from subacute to acute care units and this was reflected in the survey with WA having the highest number of per capita acute beds in the country, with the trade-off being that it now had the lowest number of subacute beds. The number of old age psychiatrists and allied health staff were also the highest per capita in the country and only Victorian services were managing a higher number of community patients.[15] High Dependency Units were established in some residential aged care facilities for severe behavioural disturbance in dementia (tiers 5 and 6 in the seven-tiered model) and were prototypes for the Commonwealth Special Dementia Care Units, the pilot of which also occurred in WA with a partnership between the Northern Metropolitan Health Service and the Brightwater Care Group and support of the Mental Health Commission.[16]

In the early 2000s a regional model of memory clinics aligned with departments of geriatric medicine was established, not as extensive as in Victoria, as they were mainly located around Perth and funding was less secure.[17] A Statewide model of dementia care was established in 2011 at which time identified gaps included lack of systematic screening of cognition with culturally appropriate tools, inadequate training of mainstream clinicians in the management of challenging behaviour, variable and limited access to dementia specialists in emergency departments, a broad need for culture change in the health system, inadequate community supports for carers and lack of policy about the management of dementia with comorbid delirium, mental disorders or behavioural issues. The model of care envisaged an integrated array of complex care services that would be introduced on a continuum based on the needs of the person with dementia or their carer. The model commenced with health promotion and dementia prevention, and contained reference to primary and specialist health care, community and residential services through to end of life care.[18]

There have been no substantive resource enhancements for older people's mental health services in WA for some years and this is reflected in the 2015 survey that showed lower per capita acute bed numbers than in 2003.[19] According to Helen McGowan, the co-lead of the Older Adult Mental Health Sub-network that was established in 2014, there has been a trial of intensive 'hospital-in-the-home' approaches in the Northern Metropolitan Health Service which has reduced length of stay in the acute wards but funding to expand the service has not been forthcoming.[20] The Older Adult Mental Health Sub-network of the Mental Health Network, which is not a decision-making body but reports to the Department of Health and the Mental Health Commission, held its inaugural open meeting in August 2016. The sub-network has broad multidisciplinary representation from consumers, carers, community organisations, health services, agencies, and the Mental Health Commission. Key issues identified at the inaugural meeting included suboptimal integration and coordination of services, need to engage families in care planning, inadequate staff training, lack of services for young onset dementia and lack of appropriate accommodation options for older people with mental health problems.[21]

The WA Mental Health Commission released the *Western Australian Mental Health, Alcohol and Other Drug Services Plan 2015–2025* in 2015 and an updated version in 2018 that included revised weightings for older people as 2025 population projections increased from 14.9 per cent to 17.6 per cent of the WA population. In the draft plan, it is proposed that the number of acute old age mental health assessment beds be reduced from 144 in 2017 to 84 in 2025, being counter-balanced by an increase in high intensity 'Hospital in the Home' places from eight in 2017 to 52 in 2025 and the establishment of 122 new subacute/non-acute beds. Such a reconfiguration and enhancement of services will be the first substantive change since the turn of the century, but it remains in draft form and leaves doubt about how much will occur.[22] The Northern Metropolitan Older Adult Mental Health Service developed an approved model of care in 2014 but attempts to make this a Statewide model have not succeeded so far.[23] There has been a lack of overarching governance in WA regarding older persons' mental health and the absence of a policy officer in the field has perhaps contributed to the lack of progress. Rural WA has almost no services with only one community rural team in the south west, the other rural adult teams provide limited services to older people but have no formal links with metropolitan services. There have also been difficulties in recruiting to vacant positions.[24]

## South Australia

In the early 1980s there was cause for some optimism about the future of older people's mental health services in South Australia (SA). Downey Grove, a newly built 128-bed long-stay complex with four wards had been opened in March 1979 at Glenside Hospital near the assessment ward at Downey House and this was joined in November 1982 with a similar modern psychogeriatric unit at Hillcrest Hospital that replaced substandard accommodation.[25] Thus by 1985, Hillcrest had a 30-bed assessment unit (Howard House), four long-stay wards with 93 beds and was the base for two community teams that covered the eastern and north eastern suburbs of Adelaide.[26] This burst of development was not maintained and little changed for the next two decades. Services were centralised at a State level and largely hospital-based with only limited community outreach. In the 1992 national survey, South Australia had eight psychiatrists working in old age psychiatry, six in the public sector, with only NSW and Victoria having more, but numbers of allied health and community nurses were comparatively low.[27]

With the closure of Hillcrest Hospital in 1992 and devolvement of services to other settings, the older people's mental health services, the 30 bed assessment ward at Howard House, and the long-stay wards in what was known as the Oakden complex remained.[28] By 1997, a third of the long-stay beds on psychiatric hospital sites had been reclassified as State nursing home beds.[29] In 1998 it was decided to seek Commonwealth accreditation for two of the Oakden complex wards (Makk and McLeay) which meant that they transitioned from State funding to the lower Commonwealth funding with its subsequent impact on staffing with the use of less skilled personal care assistants.[30]

In the late 1990s, the organisation of 'Services to the Elderly' in SA became regionalised with each of the three metropolitan services linked to a teaching hospital – Eastern Region to Royal Adelaide Hospital, Southern Region to Flinders Medical Centre, and the North Western Region to the Queen Elizabeth Hospital. There were plans to establish psychogeriatric units in the teaching general hospitals including Daw Park Repatriation Hospital in the south.[31] Little changed in the 2000s and this is reflected in the 2003 national survey in which SA had only two older people's mental health services that covered the whole state, the lowest per capita in the country, with neither being based in a general hospital. In terms of bed numbers, staffing and community patients, SA ranked in the middle of the States.[32]

It took a decade from the time that the first proposals to develop acute old age mental health wards in general hospitals to the State Government eventually agreeing to funded recommendations in 2007 for 70 acute beds and a further decade until the work was completed.[33] As part of the redevelopment of the Lyell McEwin Hospital, a 20-bed old age mental health unit was included which replaced the 26 acute beds at Howard House and this opened in 2010. Subsequently another 20-bed acute ward replacing the 24-bed acute ward at Glenside Hospital was opened at the Queen Elizabeth Hospital in 2013.[34] A third 30-bed acute unit, originally based in ward 18 of the Daw Park Repatriation Hospital, was opened at the newly expanded Flinders Medical Centre in 2017.[35]

The 2007 report from the Social Inclusion Board titled *Stepping Up: A Social Inclusion Action Plan for Mental Health Reform 2007–2012* upon which the acute inpatient service recommendations were based, also included a recommendation about the remaining long-stay wards that combined a need for SA to have 'a clear plan of action for the future management of long-term residential aged care that is consistent with good practice and contemporary policy' with a focus on early intervention for older people in the community as well as the essential need to develop partnerships with the Commonwealth and aged care providers.[36] A draft comprehensive Statewide service plan and model of service for the Older Persons Mental Health Service in South Australia was developed after the *Stepping-up Report* that included replacement of the Oakden facility, but this was never endorsed by the Department of Health.[37] There is evidence, however, that the broad thrust of the *Stepping-up Report* recommendation linking long-term residential beds with community mental health services was being followed, as by early 2011 approximately 40 extended care beds had been closed with funds earmarked to increase workers in the community teams,[38] with ongoing evidence of progressive extended care ward closures and plans to transfer further beds to non-government organisations.[39] But in 2012 budgetary problems in SA resulted in the funds that had been released by bed closures not being allocated to the community teams.[40] There was also no evidence that in closing the extended care beds that there were adequate resources left to manage those with the most severe degree of behavioural disturbance (tiers 6 and 7 in the seven-tiered model) and in reality the Oakden facility was the only one in the State with that potential.[41] Overall, these events were very unsettling to staff in the older people's mental health service. Despite these concerns, when SA was benchmarked against the other States in the 2015 national survey it was around the average on most parameters of staffing and bed numbers.[42] In this period there was lack of an overall plan and a general disinterest of older people's mental health services, both in the health networks and politically. Morale in older people's mental health services was low. According to Duncan Mackellar, the attempt by the Central Adelaide health network to integrate older people's mental health services into a 'lifespan mental health service' in 2015 brought old age psychiatrists together with the support of the new Chief Psychiatrist, Aaron Groves.[43]

In 2016 allegations emerged of staff physically abusing patients at the Oakden facility. This led to the CEO of the Northern Adelaide Local Health Network to request that South Australia's Chief Psychiatrist, Aaron Groves, undertake a review focusing on five broad areas of clinical care: the model of care; staffing model; quality and safety of care; culture; and restrictive practices. At the same time the CEO made immediate staff enhancements. The *Oakden Report* found that there were considerable problems and this attracted media attention particularly with the ABC throughout 2017 and, as noted in Chapter 12, became the forerunner to the Aged Care Royal Commission. When the Oakden review looked back over the history of the Oakden facility, there was clear evidence of concerns regarding the quality of care that dated back to 1999, the year after it transitioned to Commonwealth funding. Between 2001 and 2007 Oakden only received one- or two-year periods of Commonwealth accreditation, less than what was usual, due to concerns about care issues. In December 2007, the facility failed 25 of the Commonwealth's 44 care standards and sanctions were applied. In 2010, after an external review, Oakden was returned to State mental health funding but retained Commonwealth funding for the Makk and McLeay wards, and subsequently passed the 44 accreditation standards. By this time, one of the long-stay wards had closed and Howard House had moved, leaving Oakden as a relatively isolated facility.[44]

The *Oakden Report* made recommendations related to the five areas of clinical care in its terms of reference. Regarding the model of care, the *Oakden Report* found that was no endorsed model in operation and the one being used was largely inconsistent with best practice nationally and internationally. It recommended in considerable detail the need to establish a specialised contemporary model of care and made specific reference to the NSW service plan. It also noted in detail that the design and condition of the Oakden facility was inappropriate for the management of residents with severe behavioural problems and recommended that it be replaced with a purpose built facility. The staffing model was deficient in terms of staff numbers that were hard to ascertain, the level of skills and training of the nurses, and inadequate numbers of allied health and medical staff. The recommendations were very detailed and prescriptive about what the staffing model should be, indeed reminiscent of the FPOA guidelines rejected by the RANZCP in the 1990s due to being too prescriptive. In terms of the quality and safety of care, the Report found that there was a failure of clinical governance where warning signs such as injuries, falls, medication errors, use of restraints, poor documentation and failed accreditation were not acted on. There was poor clinical leadership, lack of accountability, lack of training and no processes to improve care quality. The Report recommended the need to establish a new clinical governance system and gave a detailed list of what it should encompass noting that it would take three to five years to make a difference. The culture of Oakden was found to be 'characterised by poor morale, disrespect and bickering, secrecy, an inwardly looking approach, control, a sense of entitlement and indifference', although there was also a sub-culture of those who cared.[45] Here the recommendations were that there was a need to have a change of senior leadership and other new staff to drive change to a culture of dignity, respect, care and kindness. With regards to restrictive practices, there was evidence that these were being used excessively and outside of the relevant legislative framework by staff who did not have the sufficient level of training. Lack of leadership was also noted. The recommendation was to develop an immediate Action Plan based on trauma informed principles developed by the National Centre for Trauma-informed Care and to comply with relevant policy directives and guidelines.[46]

The considerable media interest garnered by the *Oakden Report* and the community and political reaction meant that the South Australian government needed to make a significant response. It established a Response Oversight Committee chaired by Tom Stubbs that had broad representation from consumer, carer, community, government and professional groups. Six working parties were charged with examining the five areas of clinical care featured in the Report plus one to examine the physical design of the new facility. The work of the committee and working groups was reported in June 2018. One of its recommendations was the establishment of a 24-bed Statewide Neurobehavioural Unit. The other recommendations were broad ranging and included in-reach services to residential aged care facilities modelled after the Rapid Access Service that had been piloted in Southern Adelaide in the previous decade. Indeed, the response went well beyond Oakden and building on the *Oakden Report* outlined a service strategy for Older Persons Mental Health Services in South Australia, an approach accepted by the State Government.[47] This was important as the impact of Oakden permeated throughout older people's mental health services in South Australia as it is a relatively small close knit community. Staff were traumatised and were ashamed of what happened. The crisis provided an opportunity for transformational cultural change that is well underway.[48]

While it is too early to determine how much of this will lead to further positive developments in SA, a new 18-bed neurobehavioural unit was opened in 2021 at the Repat General Hospital at Daws Park, albeit that it was not purpose built but one that had significant renovation and refurbishment.

## Queensland

There was little development of older people's mental health services in Queensland during the 1980s. Joan Ridley, who had trained at Newcastle-upon-Tyne where she was influenced by Sir Martin Roth, had been appointed as medical superintendent of the Baillie Henderson Hospital, Toowoomba in April 1977 at which time, despite housing around 2000 patients many of whom were elderly, there was no psychogeriatric ward. She is credited with establishing the first older people's mental health service in Queensland in the late 1970s to early 1980s by setting up an acute assessment ward at Baillie Henderson Hospital to accompany the long-stay ward and an outpatient clinic and multidisciplinary community liaison service located in an old colonial house in Royal Street, Toowoomba (known colloquially as 'Royal Street') that was run by Dr John McIntyre from 1982. McIntyre's background was in liaison psychiatry and when he eventually went into private practice, Bill Rowntree took over as the Director of the older people's mental health service. Joan Ridley later moved to the Northern Territory in 1986 to become the Director of the Territory's psychiatric services.[49,50,51]

Psychiatric hospital populations gradually decreased over the 1980s in Queensland by around 43 per cent between 1980/81 and 1991/92, a process that was a bit slower than in most other States. Although the main growth in nursing homes during the 1980s was in private and non-profit nursing home, State government and semi-government nursing home populations also increased by over thirteen per cent, a change that was also in contrast to the direction being taken in other States.[52] This increase in the State government funded nursing home population is likely to be due to the transfer of chronic mental health patients from psychiatric hospitals. When Gerard Byrne provided a visiting psychiatrist consultative service in the early 1990s to the Eventide Nursing Home at Brighton, which evolved out of the Sandgate asylum that originally housed former Dunwich asylum residents, he was surprised to discover than many of the residents that he was asked to see were former psychiatric hospital patients with chronic serious mental illnesses such as schizophrenia, bipolar disorder and psychoses related to epilepsy and other organic brain syndromes.[53] The focus on institutional care is reflected in the 1992 national survey that found Queensland to have no community nurses in the three identified services and very few allied health staff, although the number of psychiatrists, while lower than required, was more reasonable, albeit some such as Don Grant were either neuropsychiatrists or general psychiatrists with an interest in older people.[54]

The first modern older persons' mental health unit in a general hospital in Brisbane occurred by chance. In April 1990 there were devastating floods in the outback town of Charleville which required the whole town to be evacuated. Some of the nursing home residents from the State government's Waroona Multipurpose Centre were relocated to Grevillea ward in the geriatrics department at Princess Alexandra Hospital. Subsequently it was decided to keep Grevillea ward as an older persons' mental health unit within the geriatrics service. Interestingly this harkened back to a proposed development at Princess Alexandra Hospital suggested by Basil Stafford in the early 1960s. Dr Michael Leong became the Director of the unit, while Paul Varghese was the Director of the geriatrics service. Together they established a memory clinic.[55]

In 1995, the new mental health wards at the Royal Brisbane and Women's Hospital were opened and Gerard Byrne was appointed as the Director of Geriatric Psychiatry (later renamed the Older Persons' Mental Health Service). New Zealand born, Gerard Byrne is an old age psychiatrist and the Mayne Professor of Psychiatry, Faculty of Medicine, University of Queensland. Byrne migrated to Australia with his family as a child. He studied medicine at the University of NSW, moving to Brisbane in his second post-graduate year to work at Prince Charles Hospital having rotations in the Winston Noble neuropsychiatric unit before he undertook psychiatry training. He then completed a doctorate on bereavement in older men under the supervision of Beverley Raphael. He is a past Chair of the Faculty of Psychiatry of Old Age and a past Board Member of the International Psychogeriatric Association.

With the assistance of a Commonwealth grant, the older people's mental health service was launched in 1996 which included a small community outreach team, outpatient clinics and 12 beds within the adult mental health unit. At the time there were no community older people's mental health services in Queensland with resources largely locked in to long-stay wards.[56] In 1994, I provided a week-long consultancy to the ACAT based at Nambour on the Sunshine Coast where the absence of any resources or interest in older people within the mental health service was striking.

Queensland released its first service plan for *Mental Health Services for Older People* in 1996 as a component of the ten-year Queensland Mental Health Plan. The plan outlined a comprehensive service structure including community, acute inpatient, and extended inpatient services. Population based bed numbers were supplied with the aim for 45 acute beds and three extended inpatients per 100,000 population, these to be co-located with geriatric services while remaining part of the mental health program. The number of acute beds was consistent with the 40 per 100,000 identified in the 1992 survey but the key difference to the then existing services in Queensland was the very low number of extended inpatient beds. Consistent with the overall Queensland Mental Health Plan, long-stay psychiatric facilities at Wolston Park Hospital at Wacol, Baillie Henderson Hospital at Toowoomba, and Mosman Hall Hospital at Charters Towers were to be phased out with resources reallocated to improving access through community (including outreach to residential aged care) and acute inpatient services. Similar to NSW, there was no rigid age cut-off at 65, older people whose needs could be met appropriately by adult mental health services could be managed by those services with age-related comorbidity being the key criterion for older people's mental health to be regarded as the more appropriate service. While detailed staffing profiles were provided, the broad number of community clinical staff for older people was one per 10,000 population aged 65 years and over. These staff were seen to be part of the overall community mental health teams rather than separate services with the exception of services where there was sufficient population to establish a discrete Psychogeriatric Assessment and Treatment (PAT) service. The usual range of linkages to aged care services, general practitioners, carers, mental health organisations and disability support services was envisaged and required strengthening.[57]

The effects of having a plan quickly became apparent with a lot of local interest being generated. In 1997, Michael Leong summarised the services available in Queensland noting that five hospitals now had acute inpatient beds (Princess Alexandra Hospital, Royal Brisbane Hospital, Wolston Park Hospital, Prince Charles Hospital and Baillie Henderson Hospital at Toowoomba), four had community outreach teams, three had extended care/long-term care beds, and each had psychiatry trainees allocated to their services. More than 25 psychiatrists in Queensland were expressing an interest in old age psychiatry.[58]

Despite this initial enthusiasm, developments in Queensland were slow but according to a report from David Lie the Chair of FPOA in Queensland, by 2001 the number of community teams had increased from one in the mid-1990s to eight and the downsizing of the stand-alone psychiatric hospitals led to the opening of a number of extended inpatient units in regional centres. The number of full time old age psychiatrists in Queensland had increased to five in 2001 but workforce shortages were a concern across all of the disciplines particularly in regional areas.[59] In 2001, Gerard Byrne became Head of the Discipline of Psychiatry at the University of Queensland and provided a solid academic base for the further development of old age psychiatry research and training, in particular, he was responsible for the oversight of the advanced training program in old age psychiatry in Queensland and later became the Chair of the binational Committee for Advanced Training in Psychiatry of Old Age.[60]

The 2003 national survey showed that further gradual developments were occurring in Queensland as there were now thirteen community teams, albeit most having less than ten full time staff equivalents, which was understandable as Queensland had a large regional population with only Tasmania being less centralised of the Australian States. The larger regional developments were based at Ipswich, Toowoomba (where Eddie Tan was based from 1999) and on the Gold Coast. However, in other ways Queensland still lagged having the lowest number of old age psychiatrists per capita and with only NSW having less acute and non-acute psychiatric bed numbers and Tasmania having less allied health staff.[61] David Lie, who had taken over from Michael Leong as the Director of the Aged Care Mental Health Services at Princess Alexandra Hospital in 2001, provided a snapshot of the service in 2003. Although the acute inpatient ward with 16 beds remained co-located with the geriatrics ward, the service was formally a part of the Division of Mental Health. A consultation-liaison service was provided to the geriatrics wards. The community old age mental health team was co-located with the adult community team. There were no day hospital, respite, or continuing care beds.[62]

In 2004 Queensland Health released a strategy for mental health services for older people within a broader aged care strategy. There were five key action areas to be developed: assessment; access; service delivery; carers; and partnerships. Strategies identified for assessment included the development of comprehensive assessment protocols and processes, while telehealth was suggested as an important strategy to improve access along with clinical care pathways. Indeed Queensland was the national leader in telehealth in part due to its degree of decentralisation. Recommended strategies to improve service delivery included the development of evidence based service models and data systems to better monitor older people with mental illness. The involvement of carers in individual and overall service planning was proposed and recommended strategies around carer needs included education and support. The development of formalised partnerships, inclusion of key stakeholders in policy and supporting Commonwealth initiatives related to shared care were recommended.[63]

The 2007–2017 Queensland Plan for Mental Health included a major enhancement to older people's community mental health services with the allocation of over $18 million to fund 46 clinicians, a much larger enhancement than for the adult services and one that according to David Lie was a greater than 50 per cent increase. This was the only specific enhancement to old age mental health in the comprehensive plan although some of the other hospital and community enhancements might well have benefitted older people too.[64] A submission put together by a working party of interested clinicians to assist the Queensland Director of Mental Health, Aaron Groves, in order to inform the State plan obviously worked as it provided evidence of the low funding of older people's mental health services in Queensland based on data in the 2005 National Mental Health Report and put at the top of the list funding of community older people's mental health services.[65] The lack of focus on acute beds for older people in the Queensland Plan for Mental Health was reflected in the 2015 national survey that placed Queensland at the bottom of the States for acute beds for older people at only 6.6 per 100,000 aged 65 years and over, although the community services were at least comparable to other States and had the highest proportion of services located outside the capital city.[66] It has been a complete turnaround in the imbalance of services shifting from having an almost total institutional focus in the mid-1990s to having a reasonable community service provision with inadequate acute inpatient services to back that up, although a new 10-bed ward for the management of severe behavioural disturbances in dementia was subsequently opened at Princess Alexandra Hospital in the geriatric service.[67] There has also been some re-branding of subacute beds located on the Gold Coast and at Ipswich without any bed gains or noticeable change in function, while the opening of the Sunshine Coast University Hospital has seen the consolidation of scattered bed access at Nambour Hospital into a 12-bed unit. There are plans to provide five beds in the new purpose built mental health unit in Cairns due to open in 2022.[68]

## Tasmania

David Kay remained at the helm of the Tasmanian Mental Health Commission for eight years until his return to Newcastle-upon-Tyne in the UK in 1984. During his tenure he brought greater integration of clinical and research activity,[69] collaborating with Scott Henderson and others to produce epidemiological studies based in Hobart of the mental disorders in older people who lived alone and those residing in nursing homes and the long-stay wards of Royal Derwent and St John's Park Hospitals.[70,71] Upon Kay's departure John Tooth became the Chair of the Tasmanian Mental Health Services Commission, a position he held until 1990. Tooth became aware of the inadequacies of the institutional care being provided for people with dementia in mental health facilities. While Chair of the Tasmanian Mental Health Services Commission, Tooth developed plans to transform large old-fashioned psychiatric wards into smaller community-oriented residential facilities. In particular, there was a need to develop facilities that could accommodate persons with dementia and severe behavioural problems in a humane manner and in homelike surroundings.[72]

This, of course, was consistent with the desire to shift the balance of mental health services from an institutional to a community focus by ensuring direct transfers of residents and ward closures such as that which occurred with the opening of a community facility in Hobart in 1987. In 1989 the Mental Health Commission was integrated into the Department of Health Services, a move consistent with the national trend to mainstream mental health.[73] John Tooth continued working on the smaller community-oriented residential concepts as President of the Tasmanian Branch of the Alzheimer's Association. The Alzheimer's Association had for some time been concerned about the types of residential care available for persons with dementia and so this proved to be a very fruitful partnership of like minds. In 1991 the 36-bed ADARDS nursing home was opened in Hobart with John Tooth as the honorary consultant old age psychiatrist. The ADARDS nursing home set a world standard for residential dementia care by providing an environment designed to minimize the effects of dementia by creating a comforting atmosphere reminiscent of the person's home while at the same time being safe. From the mid-1990s, Japanese aged care workers began to visit the ADARDS nursing home and in September 2000 Tooth was invited to address the two major aged care associations of Japan after the Japanese Diet had passed a bill making it illegal to use physical restraints in dementia units. Other visits followed with an increase in the number of Japanese doctors, nurses and care workers visiting the ADARDS Nursing Home and attending the 3-day training courses that Tooth ran. At the request of his Japanese students, Tooth wrote a book on dementia management that was published in Japanese in 2002. The dementia residential care guidelines established by John Tooth at ADARDS were to a large extent adopted by the Japanese Department of Health. John Tooth received an Order of Australia Medal in 2001, was the Tasmanian recipient of Australian of the Year in 2007 and received a RANZCP College Citation in 2008.[74]

Few nursing homes are featured in the international gerontology journals but ADARDS nursing home had an article written about it by the eminent residential aged care and dementia researcher Jiska Cohen-Mansfield in the leading journal *The Gerontologist* in 2006. She was particularly impressed by the flexible management practices which perhaps contributed to the low staff turnover and high staff morale as well as fewer issues with disturbed behaviour in the residents and greater satisfaction of family carers.[75] It also featured in the 2020 World Alzheimer Report on design for dementia facilities as one of the ten ground-breaking paradigm-shifting designs for its homelike features and lively garden.[76]

Unfortunately, problems were on the horizon. The ADARDS nursing home was Commonwealth funded and when the new Aged Care Funding Instrument (ACFI) was introduced in 2007 it resulted in a significant reduction in its funding, in large part due to its small size. Tooth had long been aware of this potential risk and believed that he had secured a promise of State top-up funding in this eventuality from Ray Groom in 1989 when he was Minister for Health. However, when he turned to the State government for top-up funding it was declined in 2008. The situation became quite acrimonious and led to the forced sale of the facility to Presbyterian Homes of Launceston in September 2008. Tooth long believed that the standards of care established at ADARDS diminished from this point on largely through the discarding of the flexible management practices in place such as allowing residents to get up at times that suited them and have breakfast when they wanted, which was allegedly replaced by a rigid routine of when residents had to get up, wash and have breakfast. In a submission to the Senate Enquiry on the care and management of younger and older Australians living with dementia and BPSD in 2013, Tooth alleged that Tasmanian Department of Health and Human Services and the Commonwealth Department of Health and Ageing had met secretly over the issue of top-up funding. Through Freedom of Information legislation he obtained minutes of the meetings. Tooth's interpretation was that the bureaucracies intentionally denied ADARDs such funds and aimed to force its closure or change of ownership.[77] In contrast the State government believed that it had taken a facilitating role with the Commonwealth to ensure the long-term viability of the facility and that the quality of care had not suffered.[78] Whatever the case may be, the style of State top-up funding that had by this time become established in Victoria and was being trialled in NSW was not offered in Tasmania.

In the early 1990s the innovation witnessed at the ADARDS nursing home was not matched with other service developments in Tasmania. In the 1992 national survey Tasmania was the only state to report that it had no comprehensive older people's mental health services, although there was a full time old age psychiatrist.[79] It was not until 2000 that the first older people's mental health centre was established, the Roy Fagan Centre at Kalang, Hobart, a Statewide facility that had 40 beds, twenty for dementia, ten long-term beds and ten acute beds along with a day centre and hub for a community team with Dr Laurence Herst as its inaugural director.[80] By late 2000, Herst was reporting on the challenges of placing the last 70 patients from the Royal Derwent Hospital, thirty of whom were elderly. Many of the difficulties related to staff resistance and industrial action occurred presumably to prevent the imminent closure of the hospital.[81] Telepsychiatry commenced in 2001 improving access for patients in remote parts of the state such as King Island.[82] Martin Morrissey joined Herst in 2002 as the second old age psychiatrist. By 2003 the improved service configuration in Tasmania was reflected in the national survey where overall bed numbers were relatively high though acute bed numbers were still relatively low as were allied health staff in the community.[83]

There has been little further service development since this period. Fortunately, the number of old age psychiatrists in Tasmania has increased to five with four locally trained. The Roy Fagan Centre now has two ten-bed acute units, one managed by old age mental health and the other by the geriatrics service with close relationships between the services.[84] On the 2015 national survey Tasmania was at around the average number of per capita bed numbers.[85] The service based in Hobart has taken on an increasing role in the assessment and management of various neuropsychiatric disorders and young onset dementia, particularly those relating to the well-known high incidence of Huntington's disease in Tasmania. There is a maldistribution of services across the state's three health regions with the north and north-west of the State having difficulty in attracting psychiatrists in part due to management issues in the health service and thus in the most part locums are used.[86] Despite this maldistribution and the fact that Tasmania has the most ageing population in Australia, there is no State older people's mental health plan. The State mental health plan for 2020–2025 barely mentions older people.[87] In contrast, the Primary Health Network recognised that older people should be a priority population for suicide prevention and obtained Commonwealth funding in the national suicide prevention program and were the only site in the program to target the older population.[88] In the absence of a strategic plan for older people's mental health there seems little likelihood of new developments in the short term.

### Australian Capital Territory

Prior to 1999 there were no specific older people's mental health services in the Australian Capital Territory (ACT). Keith Fleming had been the geriatrician in the ACT since the early 1980s and was the main clinician oversighting dementia care.[89] Older people with mental disorders were managed within general adult mental health services, by private practitioners, or went interstate. Yet the Australian National University through the Social Policy Research Unit established by Scott Henderson in 1974 with later collaborators that included Tony Jorm and Helen Christensen were international leaders in epidemiological research into dementia and depression in late life. There was disconnect between research and clinical practice in the ACT.

In 1999, Judy Raymond, who had completed most of her psychiatry training in the ACT but had spent a year in Newcastle completing advanced training in old age psychiatry with Stephen Ticehurst, at her instigation was appointed to a part-time old age psychiatrist position and with the appointment of Helen Kirkwood, a nurse experienced in old age mental health, the nucleus of the older people's mental health service was formed.[90] In their account of the early days of the service, the challenges that had to be met included a lack of direction from ACT Health about service development, lack of administrative support and infrastructure, and the burden of budget management without the appropriate business management support. With only two team members, the initial service model was a consultation-liaison style and involved collaboration and partnerships with a wide range of stakeholders including GPs, residential aged care facilities, case managers in the adult mental health service, ACAT, geriatric medicine, Carers ACT and the Alzheimer's Association. A collaborative shared care model of service delivery based upon the GP evolved and eventually a GP was employed as a member of the multidisciplinary team, a first in Australia, although this innovation did not last. The team gradually developed over the first five years and in December 2002, after a service review by Ed Chiu, the establishment of the multidisciplinary Research Centre for the Neurosciences of Ageing funded through ACT Health brought an academic component and Jeff Looi into the service.[91] This position has evolved due to university and health service changes but continues to bring a strong academic representation to the service with Jeff Looi becoming the Head of the Academic Unit of Psychiatry and Addiction medicine at ANU in 2016 as well as oversighting advanced training in old age psychiatry.[92] Keith Fleming fostered two beds on the geriatrics ward for old age mental health admissions as in this period it was difficult to admit older people to the adult mental health ward where ageist attitudes were encountered.[93]

The 2003 national survey reported that the ACT had now grown to have more than ten staff, was seeing more community patients per capita than most states, and that it had acute beds for older people but the latter referred to the use of beds in the adult mental health ward rather than a specific unit.[94] A 20-bed subacute psychogeriatric unit opened at the Calvary Hospital at Bruce in

February 2007 with initial utilisation limited by staffing constraints and only fifteen of the beds have ever been commissioned for the older people's mental health service.[95] There was no single factor responsible for the development of the unit but likely a combination of lobbying by Judy Raymond, carers and consumers and perhaps the cost savings from the closure of Hennessy House, a unit for those with chronic mental disorders that included ten older patients.[96] Although described as a subacute unit, few patients are too behaviourally disturbed to require management in the acute adult mental health unit. One drawback has been the lack of geriatric medicine services at Calvary Hospital. There are no long-stay psychiatric beds in the ACT and the only unit for severe behavioural disturbance in dementia is the new Commonwealth-funded Special Dementia Care Unit.

Innovative programs since 2010 include the development of a community older persons' intensive treatment service that has had success in preventing or delaying admissions and a physical health monitoring team that interacts with GPs. There have also been changes in the governance of the service. Originally an integrated community and inpatient service, since around 2016 it has been aligned with adult mental health service governance and now has separate community and inpatient services reporting to generic mental health line managers in a 'lifespan' approach to mental health management and thus has lost its integration.[97] In addition the ACT Mental Health and Suicide Prevention Plan for 2019–2024 lacks specific detail for older people.[98] Whether a lifespan approach to mental health management can benefit older people when it has not succeeded elsewhere remains to be seen.

## Northern Territory

With a small and younger population than the rest of Australia, it is perhaps understandable that the Northern Territory (NT) has lagged in service development for older people. The first geriatrician was Dr S. Mahajani who was funded through the HACC program in the 1990s. The initial service development was the Territory Older Persons Support Service (TOPSS) that was established in 1999 by Frontier Services Aged Care in Darwin and from February 2000 had a dementia focus with Judy Ratajec as the sole staff member. It evolved to having outreach workers in Katherine (Mary Ingrames) and Alice Springs and extra staff in Darwin alongside Judy Ratajec by 2005, with services of visiting old age psychiatrists (Ray Chenoweth and Bob Penhall both from 2000 until around 2004) and then Jill Pettigrew. With the introduction of the DBMAS in 2007, this replaced TOPSS but was still run by Frontier Services with Judy Ratajec as the program manager and Jill Pettigrew the old age psychiatrist until 2010 after which Philip Morris visited quarterly from 2011 to 2013. Initially the team operated from Darwin, Katherine, and Alice Springs and grew to include a music therapist, holistic therapist as well as behaviour advisors but later reduced to Darwin and Alice Springs offices, with face-to-face regular outreach service across the entire NT. During this period it created culturally appropriate dementia behavioural educational resources for the Top End, the Kimberley region of Western Australia and North Queensland in conjunction with Alzheimer's Australia. It serviced the Kimberley region for Western Australia DBMAS and joint trips with the Western Australia team through to 2014. Mary Ingrames took over as program manager in 2012. In 2014 Australian Regional and Remote Community services took over all Frontier services aged care business across the NT. Then in 2016 HammondCare won the national contract to provide DBMAS services Australia wide via Dementia Support Australia (DSA). There is an office in Darwin with local behaviour advisors but since change to a national service there has been variable ability to provide dementia behaviour support in the NT, although more recently more linkages and staff to increase this service. Of note, the person must have a dementia diagnosis to be referred. Steve MacFarlane, the old age psychiatrist overseeing DSA, visits as required.[99,100,101]

The community based multidisciplinary NT Psychogeriatric service is part of Aged Care Services in Darwin and Alice Springs and started in 2010. They took all community referrals for psychogeriatric support/chronic disease aged related criteria. It has always been separate from DBMAS and is not an acute service. There have long been difficulties in obtaining acute mental health services for older people with access via the general adult Mental Health Access Team. Geriatrician Michael Lowe provides clinical oversight while Samantha Loi, old age psychiatrist from Victoria, provides monthly video-link clinical support. There are no specific older persons' mental health beds in the Northern Territory with all acute admissions being to the adult mental health ward at Darwin.[102]

# Chapter 16

# Services for Aboriginal and Torres Strait Islander Peoples after the Second World War

Aboriginal and Torres Strait Islander peoples first became eligible for pensions in 1942 if they were not subject to a State law 'relating to the control of Aboriginal natives' or if they lived in a state where they could not be exempt from such laws. It was not until 1962 that the Aboriginal and Torres Strait Islander peoples had the right to vote, and it was only in 1966 that nomadic Aboriginal Australians became eligible for the age pension. In 1967, a national referendum recognised them as 'people of their own country', and included them in the national census, the first time being in 1971. Thus it is only in the last 50 years that reasonable demographic information about Aboriginal and Torres Strait islander peoples became available. In 1992 the High Court of Australia declared that the legal concept of terra nullius ('land belonging to no-one') was invalid as applied to Australia.[1,2] In 2007, the Rudd Government issued a formal apology to Aboriginal and Torres Strait Islander peoples that focused on the stolen generation (those forcibly removed from their families) and its impact. Despite these advances, there is a lack of reconciliation and numerous unresolved issues remain that impact on the health and well-being of Aboriginal and Torres Strait Islander people. These include: land rights; the lack of a treaty that acknowledges in some way the rights of Aboriginal and Torres Strait Islander people and the wrongs that occurred; Aboriginal and Torres Strait Islander control over their affairs; self-determination; and the lack of consensus about whether or not there should be any compensation such as by financial reparation or by extending some positive discrimination to Aboriginal and Torres Strait Islander people in various contexts.[3]

Since the turn of the century, there has been a focus on the shorter life expectancy of Aboriginal and Torres Strait Islander peoples than the general population, which has resulted in the *Closing the Gap* initiative of 2008.[4] The difference in life expectancy has shrunk since 2008. In 2018 it was estimated that Aboriginal and Torres Strait Islander males live 71.6 years, 8.6 years less than other Australians, females live 75.6 years, 7.8 years less; a decade earlier the differences had been 11 years less for males and 10 years for females.[5] However, in recent years the gap has not been shrinking due to a similar increase in life expectancy in other Australians and the *2020 Closing the Gap Report* noted that progress on the life expectancy target was not on track.[6] Importantly the differences in life expectancy between Aboriginal and Torres Strait Islanders and other Australians decreases with age,[7] many of the reasons for lower life expectancy occur in early and mid-life and continue to impact on Aboriginal and Torres Strait Islanders who survive into old age.[8] As a consequence of shorter life expectancy, the Commonwealth uses the age of 50 for Aboriginal and Torres Strait Islander peoples for planning and eligibility for aged care services. The explanation for the differences in life expectancy involves a complex mix of socioeconomic (poverty, low education, unemployment), behavioural (tobacco, alcohol, exercise and diet), psychological (life stressors), biomedical (high blood pressure, obesity) and environmental factors (discrimination, racism, removal from family, remoteness of residency).[9] Most of the poor health is accounted for by chronic disease and injuries.[10] The impact of this is that older Aboriginal and Torres Strait Islander people are more likely to need assistance with self-care, mobility or communication tasks than other Australians.[11] The Aboriginal and Torres Strait Islander population, however, is ageing rapidly. While only five per cent of the Aboriginal and Torres Strait Islander population was aged 65 years and over in 2016 (compared with 16 per cent of the general population), this had increased from just three per cent in 2006.[12] Over the next 30 years, it is projected that there will be a 200 per cent increase in those aged 60–64 years and 800 per cent increase in those aged 85 years and over.[13]

There was little investigation of mental and cognitive disorders in Aboriginal and Torres Strait Islander populations until the 1960s. John Cawte, using a lifespan ethnopsychiatric approach, undertook a series of investigations in Central Australia. In the early 1960s, Cawte realised that with the rapid acculturation of Australian Aboriginal peoples, there was a need to obtain a better understanding of traditional explanations of mental illness in Aboriginal and Torres Strait Islander cultures before modern explanations replaced them. He undertook a field trip to a region in the Northern Territory located between the Hart Range and Lake Nash near the Queensland border where the Eastern Aranda people, a subgroup of the Yowera people, lived. There had been reports of a high incidence of mental instability in the region. Cawte devised a pragmatic classification of mental disorders for Aboriginal and Torres Strait islander mental illnesses – organic disorders (such as epilepsy, head injury, neurosyphilis), disorders predominantly associated with traditional beliefs (such as sorcery, evil beings), and disorders predominantly associated with assimilation stresses and cultural transitions. He did not abandon modern psychiatric diagnoses which were used as well in his series of case vignettes, one of which was of a 60-year-old man, 'Bushranger', whose illness dated from the previous year when one night, while camped alone by a bore, he had visual hallucinations in which a mob of animals, devils or Kurdaitcha (an Aranda term for a party of men appointed by the council of elders to avenge a tribal misdeed by assassination) were coming to get him. He fled to another bore where an older couple were camped and then all three fled. Subsequently he was unable to be reassured and had remained unsettled, appearing older, inactive, and unlikely to camp alone again. While Cawte's modern diagnosis of 'hysteria' is questionable, the psychological reaction described with likely depressed mood and its severe impact on function is illustrative of a severe mental disorder.[14]

In a second study, in collaboration with Malcolm Kidson, Cawte examined the lineage of mental disorders in the Walbiri people who lived nearly three hundred kilometres north-west of Alice Springs in the Northern Territory. Here the three living index cases were each in their 60s and from a psychiatric perspective, the first was a man with a paranoid psychosis that developed mid-life and who had a tendency to fly into rages, the second a near-blind woman with a cantankerous nature, and the third a man with a lifelong truculent personality prone to getting into fights. None had evidence of a cognitive disorder but each exhibited aggressive behaviour regarded by their community as being abnormal.[15]

Cases of dementia did not feature in either of these studies and so traditional views about dementia were not canvassed. Aboriginal society is nominally regarded as gerontocratic, in that the elders hold paramount authority but age alone is not the criterion for becoming an elder. The Aboriginal person must have something to offer and this is the major criterion.[16] According to A.P. Elkin, those who are too old to take an active, sensible part in daily life are regarded as 'close-up dead'.[17] Here Elkin was referring to traditional settings and it would presumably include some older Aboriginal people with dementia. There does not appear to be a specific word in Aboriginal languages for dementia but in her overview of dementia in Aboriginal Australian communities, Penelope Pollitt noted that terms such as 'childlike' and 'tiredness' were often used with mild to moderate cognitive impairment in old age, while behavioural change associated with more severe dementia might be regarded as 'madness' or 'gone off his head'. One challenge noted by Pollitt in the mid-1990s was to get Aboriginal communities to recognise dementia as a 'sickness' rather than a 'madness', in part due to the stigma attached to 'madness'.[18] Older Aboriginal people who were unable to care for themselves were looked after by their community,[19] with the exception of the desert peoples who in bad seasons might be forced to leave older people behind to starve or die of thirst.[20]

The first population-based mental health study that included a reasonable number of older Aboriginal participants was published by Malcolm Kidson in 1965. He undertook a survey of the mental disorders in 650 Walbiri people residing at Yuendumu in the Northern Territory, of whom 80 (12.3 per cent) were aged 60 years and over, a high proportion due to older people being more likely to reside in a settlement. Rates of mental disorder increased with age but overall rates (5.4 per cent) were quite low. Of the seven cases of mental disorder in those aged 60 years and over (8.7 per cent), three had definite evidence of dementia, most likely felt to be senile dementia, and while another two were blind with abnormal behaviour that might have represented early dementia too. The last two cases were of a paranoid psychosis and a personality disorder. Across the age range, in this largely traditional setting, there was no evidence of suicidal behaviour. Bearing in mind the later research that found high rates of dementia, only 3.8 per cent of those aged 60 years and over could be regarded as having definite evidence of dementia and there were no cases under the age of 60. However, the survey methodology that relied heavily on observed behaviour as reported by Aboriginal informants is likely to have underestimated dementia prevalence.[21]

A markedly different picture of the lifestyles encountered in fringe-dwelling Aboriginal communities was painted by NSW rural general practitioner Dr R.E. Coolican in a medical student lecture reproduced in John Cawte's book *Medicine is the Law* in the early 1970s. Coolican vividly described the high rates of alcohol abuse, poverty, gambling, poor nutrition, poor physical and mental health, and premature ageing in an Aboriginal fringe-dwelling community in the far west of NSW. He also mentioned the poor neonatal health with increased neonatal mortality and the suicides and accidental deaths in those intoxicated with alcohol.[22] Alcohol was then implicated as a significant cause of dementia in Aboriginal and Torres Strait Islander populations in two studies. A neuropathological study of Wernicke's encephalopathy by Clive Harper in Western Australia in 1983 found that Aboriginal people had five times higher rates than other people.[23] Wernicke's encephalopathy is the acute phase of the Wernicke-Korsakoff Syndrome, a form of dementia that is due to thiamine deficiency often caused by alcohol abuse in the context of poor nutrition. It often overlaps with alcohol-related dementia so much so that they are frequently described together as 'alcohol-related brain damage'.[24] The age distribution of the cases in Harper's study was consistent with other studies of alcohol-related brain damage with nearly 80 per cent of cases aged under 70.[25] The second was a population-based study that focused on dementia prevalence in an Aboriginal and Torres Strait Islander community and was undertaken in six small towns in Northern Queensland in the early 1990s. It utilised a modified version of the Psychogeriatric Assessment Scales as well as recorded diagnoses in hospital records. There were 133 people aged 65 years and over, representing three per cent of the total population. The prevalence of confirmed and suspected cases of dementia was 20 per cent with half of the cases previously diagnosed, the rest being identified in the survey. Alcohol-related dementia was the main cause identified in the study.[26]

These studies contributed to the misperception that alcohol abuse was one of the main causes of dementia in Aboriginal and Torres Strait Islander populations and for around fifteen years this was featured in various publications including the *Dementia Learning Resource for Aboriginal and Torres Strait Islander Communities* published by the Commonwealth in 2007. In that publication it was stated that 90 per cent of cases of dementia in Aboriginal and Torres Strait Islander populations were preventable as they were due to alcohol, vascular disease or head trauma (some presumably due to a combination of these factors).[27] Subsequent better quality research has not supported this contention about the role of alcohol as a cause of dementia in Aboriginal and Torres Strait Islander populations, but this does not mean that alcohol abuse should be entirely excluded as either contributing to cognitive impairment or more generally to late life mental disorders. Alcohol-related harms are experienced disproportionately in Aboriginal and Torres Strait Islander populations across the age range but peak between the ages of 45 and 59, remaining high in males over the age of 60.[28] The distribution of these harms across Australia varies considerably by geographic location, peaking in the Central and Northern parts of the country.[29]

One of the challenges that was identified in early dementia work was the lack of a culturally appropriate cognitive assessment tool that could be used in rural and remote populations with high levels of illiteracy and non-English speaking older populations. There are large numbers of Aboriginal and Torres Strait Islanders who speak little English. For example, in remote and very remote parts of Australia in 2009–10, an Indigenous language was the preferred language of 19 per cent of dementia residents in residential aged care facilities.[30] This was addressed with the development of the Kimberley Indigenous Cognitive Assessment (KICA) tool which was work initially undertaken with the support of the Kimberley ACAT who seconded Kate Smith, an occupational therapist to work with geriatrician Dina LoGiudice who was on sabbatical there.[31,32] Using the KICA, supplemented with a specialist medical examination by a geriatrician or old age psychiatrist, a study of 363 Aboriginal Australians aged 45 years and over residing in the remote Kimberley region of north west Western Australia reported a dementia prevalence of 12.4 per cent with a further eight per cent having 'cognitive impairment not dementia'. For those aged 65 years and over, dementia prevalence was 26.8 per cent. This dementia prevalence represented a rate 5.2 times that estimated in the general Australian population of the same age range. Importantly the higher dementia prevalence was most apparent in those aged 45–69 where it was 26 times that in the general population. Of the 45 cases of dementia identified in the study, only two were attributed to alcohol.[33] Factors that were found to be associated with dementia were older age, male sex and lack of a formal education. After adjusting for age, sex and education, factors associated with dementia included current smoking, previous stroke, epilepsy, head injury and poor mobility, incontinence and falls.[34] At five-year follow-up, dementia incidence was comparably higher than other populations and the longitudinal risk factors for cognitive decline similar to those found in the original study.[35]

Around 75 per cent of Aboriginal and Torres Strait Islander people live in urban and regional Australia and are predominantly English-speaking and thus these findings from the remote Kimberley region needed to be replicated in these settings. Tony Broe led the Koori Growing Old Well Study (KGOWS), of which I am one of the investigators, that investigated dementia prevalence in 336 Aboriginal and Torres Strait Islander people aged 60 years and over at five sites, two in Sydney and three on the mid-north coast of NSW. Tony Broe has been a leader in geriatric medical research and service provision for over fifty years. He graduated in social sciences and medicine from the University of Sydney. He trained in general medicine, geriatric medicine and neurology in Sydney, the University of Glasgow and the Mayo Clinic. He was head of the University Clinical School and Neuroscience at Lidcombe Hospital (1975 to 1985); Professor of Geriatric Medicine at Concord Hospital and University of Sydney (1985 to 1999); and at Prince of Wales Hospital, Neurosciences Research Australia, and University of NSW (1999 to 2021). He set up health services in neurosciences, aged care, community health and Aboriginal health. He is a Member of the Order of Australia.[36]

The Koori Growing Old Well Study reported an age-standardised dementia prevalence of 21 per cent with an estimated prevalence of Mild Cognitive Impairment of 17.7 per cent, with notably high rates in those who were aged in their 60s. Most cases of dementia were due to Alzheimer's disease, vascular dementia or mixed dementia with no cases of alcohol-related dementia, although alcohol was determined to be a factor in some cases of mixed dementia.[37] Factors associated with dementia were similar to those found in the KICA study and included age, unskilled work, stroke and head injury with the addition of childhood trauma that had not been measured in the KICA study.[38] In KGOWS, a lifespan approach was taken to investigating the possible modifiable risk factors for dementia and this included a standardised measure of childhood trauma that was found to be associated with events such as separation from family, poor childhood health and frequent relocations as well as late life outcomes that included Alzheimer's disease, depression, anxiety and suicidal behaviour but not alcohol abuse.[39] Importantly, from the practical perspective of how best to assess cognitive functioning in the urban-dwelling English-speaking Aboriginal and Torres Strait Islander population who are likely to access mainstream services, the Mini Mental State Examination was found to be culturally acceptable and to perform marginally better than a modified KICA and the Rowland Universal Dementia Assessment Scale.[40]

A third study from the Northern Territory used a different approach by examining routinely collected dataset sets from hospital admissions, aged care and primary care services, and death certification to determine dementia prevalence. Similar to the KICA and KGOWS research, the study found that the prevalence of dementia in the Aboriginal and Torres Strait Islander population was nearly three times higher than in the general population and was occurring at a younger age.[41] A fourth study in the Torres Strait islands and Cape York also found high rates of dementia and cognitive impairment.[42]

Mental disorders in older Aboriginal and Torres Strait Islander populations have been examined in three studies. A survey of nearly two thousand Aboriginal and Torres Strait Islander people from NSW aged 45 years and over (mean age 58 years) found that 23 per cent reported a past history of depression compared with thirteen per cent in the general population. There was also a higher prevalence of psychological distress and lifetime anxiety in the Aboriginal and Torres Strait Islander population.[43] The KICA study reported on the prevalence of depression in 250 participants aged 45 years and over (mean age 61 years) and found that 7.7 per cent were currently depressed with higher rates in women. Depression was associated with having heart problems. A culturally appropriate depression scale, the KICA-Dep, was devised for the study.[44] Only KGOWS had all participants aged 60 years and over and reported the highest rates of mental disorder with a third of participants having a history of lifetime depression, 30 per cent lifetime anxiety disorder and 19 per cent lifetime suicidal behaviour. Similarly, there were high rates of current loneliness (48%), dissatisfaction with life (30%), current depression (18%) and current suicidal ideation (11%). Suicidal ideation was strongly associated with current depression. Other factors associated with depression were living in a regional (as opposed to urban) location, sleep disturbances, a history of childhood trauma, perceived racism, low resilience, loneliness, life dissatisfaction, anxiety disorder, cardiac disease and lung disease. These factors indicate contributions to late life depression from across the life course and from a range of biopsychosocial issues.[45] Suicide rates in the Aboriginal and Torres Strait Islander population is approximately double that in the general population but this is not the case in the Aboriginal and Torres Strait islander population aged 65 years and over where the rates are lower than in the general population.[46] Historically, suicide in the Aboriginal and Torres Strait Islander population was quite rare and it is unclear whether the birth cohort that first showed higher suicide rates as adolescents and young adults in the early 1990s will persist with high suicide rates into old age.[47] This will become clearer in the next twenty years.

Overall these studies consistently show that Aboriginal and Torres Strait Islander peoples have much higher rates of dementia and late life depression than other Australians and that a variety of preventable health and psychosocial factors across the lifespan are likely to be contributing to this. Furthermore, dementia is occurring at a younger age than in other Australians. Programs to address dementia prevention across the lifespan are currently being trialled.

Mental health and dementia service provision to older Aboriginal and Torres Strait Islander peoples is influenced by broader health service provision. The 1989 National Aboriginal Health Strategy is regarded as the landmark document in Aboriginal health policy probably in large part due to the comprehensive and inclusive consultative process behind it. Consequently, it was widely owned by the Aboriginal and Torres Strait Islander population as it enunciated their health aspirations and goals within a rights-based framework. It is a holistic approach that focuses on spiritual, cultural, social and emotional well-being in addition to physical health. An evaluation of the strategy in 1994 found that the strategy was never effectively implemented due to a range of reasons that included underfunding, lack of partnerships with Aboriginal and Torres Strait Islander communities, lack of accountability, lack of political will from various governments, and the failure to include non-health portfolios in the strategy.[48] Although the National Aboriginal Health Strategy addressed the low life expectancy of Aboriginal and Torres Strait Islander peoples, it did not focus on ageing or age-related disorders. The Aboriginal and Torres Strait Islander Aged Care Strategy was developed in 1994 after broad community and service provider consultation about the provision of aged care services. The 1996 mid-term evaluation of the 1992 National Action Plan for Dementia Care reported that the needs of the Aboriginal and Torres Strait Islander population and those living in rural and remote areas were not being met.[49] The Aboriginal and Torres Strait Islander Aged Care Strategy addressed issues of service access by establishing the Aboriginal and Torres Strait Islander Flexible Services for rural and remote communities. This provided a mix of community and residential services, many in remote areas where no aged care services were previously available. These are now funded by the Aboriginal and Torres Strait Islander Flexible Aged Care Program, which in small rural and remote locations, are usually part of multi-purpose services that bring together health and aged care services under one management structure, being a more feasible care and treatment model.[50] These services complement rather than replace services available through mainstream services.

Little changed over the following decade. The 2003 Access Economics Report on the economic impact of dementia included meeting the special needs of the Aboriginal and Torres Strait Islander population within one of its strategic pillars.[51] When the Alzheimer's Association was funded to run the National Dementia Support Program, the Aboriginal and Torres Strait Islander population was included as a specific focus.[52] Despite the high rates of dementia and the Aboriginal and Torres Strait Islander Flexible Aged Care Program, a 2011 report by the Australian Institute of Health and Welfare found that relatively few Aboriginal and Torres Strait Islander people accessed Commonwealth support programs, particularly those who resided in remote areas. For example, only one per cent of EACH-D package recipients were identified as Aboriginal and Torres Strait Islanders with no identified clients under the age of 65. While the Aboriginal and Torres Strait Islander population has proportionally higher utilisation of residential aged care services than other Australians under the age of 65, the reverse is true for those over age 65. Overall total usage rates of residential aged care are lower in Aboriginal and Torres Strait Islander populations.[53] Low access of Aboriginal and Torres Strait Islander peoples to specialist mental health services for older people was also found in a 2011 evaluation of the NSW Service Plan.[54]

In 2017, the Commonwealth released its Aged Care Diversity Framework from which, out of the national consultation process to develop Aboriginal and Torres Strait Islander Action Plans, arose the National Advisory Group for Aboriginal and Torres Strait Islander Aged Care.[55] These were regarded by Aboriginal and Torres Strait Islander people as the first time effective recognition had been given to the specific needs of Aboriginal and Torres Strait Islander people in the national reform agenda for Australia's aged care system.[56] These action plans, one for consumers and the other for aged care providers, were released in 2019. They outlined six outcomes that would improve care including making informed choices, improved accessibility and support, flexible proactive care, respectful and inclusive culturally competent services, meeting the needs of the most vulnerable, and partnership approaches to service planning and implementation.[57,58]

There are multiple reasons for low access of Aboriginal and Torres Strait Islander peoples to formal services but perhaps most fundamental of all is the lack of trust in mainstream services stemming from such diverse factors such as European colonisation, government policies that led to the forced removal of children until around fifty years ago, and a long history of poor outcomes of interventions that were often instigated with good intent.[59] Historically, mainstream services have tended to lack cultural competency and respect for Aboriginal and Torres Strait Islander peoples, such as failing to recognise sensitive issues, grief and loss that results in the lack of acceptance of the services. In its submission to the Aged Care Royal Commission in 2019, the National Advisory Group for Aboriginal and Torres Strait Islander Aged Care outlined some of the barriers in the Aged Care System that reduced access for Aboriginal and Torres Strait Islander peoples. At the top of the list was the My Aged Care (MAC) system that is heavily reliant on computer literacy, internet access, phone access and internet navigation skills. While the MAC system has adversely affected many older Australians, it is particularly difficult for those living in remote communities. Furthermore, the lack of culturally appropriate navigation coupled with the previously mentioned mistrust of mainstream services has led to avoidance of the system. Fear of institutionalisation especially in an aged care system that lacks culturally appropriate aged care services providing trauma-informed care was another issue identified. The lack of mandatory cultural safety training for assessors of aged care packages and services was noted along with the lack of contextualisation of the training that was available. The concept of person-centred care as practiced in Australia was noted to be incompatible with Aboriginal and Torres Strait Islander understandings of health and well-being, although there was potential for modification to fit in with family/community/kinship models of care. The lack of Aboriginal and Torres Strait Islander people working in aged care was a hindrance and the importance of Aboriginal controlled care emphasised. The importance of flexible and adequate funding particularly for those in rural and remote areas was seen as another key issue.[60]

Coupled with these broad issues related to service delivery are those specific to dementia and mental health. Misconceptions about dementia are common among Aboriginal and Torres Strait Islander peoples and as noted earlier one of these relates to regarding dementia as a 'madness' rather than 'sickness'.[61] Due to the role of Elders in using their memories to pass on cultural knowledge to younger generations, entire communities can be affected by dementia. Furthermore, communities may also become distressed if cultural taboos and norms are broken by a person with dementia.[62] Thus service delivery needs to take these facets into account.

There is synergy between the recommended approaches to improving aged care and mental health care for Aboriginal and Torres Strait Islander peoples. Aboriginal and Torres Strait Islander peoples have a different construct of mental and physical health and prefer the term 'social and emotional well-being' that brings with it a more holistic approach that incorporates a network of relationships between individuals, family, kin, and community. It also includes connections with land, culture, spirituality, and ancestry along with their effects on the person that can change over the life course. Importantly these understanding vary between cultural groups and individuals. Seven domains of social and emotional well-being are recognised with connections to body, mind and emotions, family and kinship, community, culture, country, and spirituality and ancestors. A National Strategic Framework for Aboriginal and Torres Strait Islander Peoples' Mental Health and Social Well-being was developed to assist in the delivery of services consistent with the Fifth National Mental Health Plan. It is based on nine principles that include a holistic approach, self-determination, culturally competent services, trauma-informed care, a human rights approach, recognising the impacts of racism, stigma and social disadvantage, the centrality of family and kinship, understanding that there are numerous Aboriginal and Torres Strait

Islander cultural groups, and recognising the strengths of Aboriginal and Torres Strait Islander communities. The Framework signalled a new approach for mental health programs in the care of Aboriginal and Torres Strait Islander peoples that is based on Aboriginal and Torres Strait Islander leadership and partnership, social determinants of mental health, addressing racism, person-centred care as adapted for Aboriginal and Torres Strait Islander peoples, a focus on children and young people, integrated approaches, trauma-informed care, culturally appropriate, affordable and clinically appropriate care. As with the Fifth National Mental Health Plan, there is little that is specific for older people although important areas mentioned include the role of Elders in promoting community wellness and in the lives of children, while the only aspect of ill-health mentioned was to assist older members of the Stolen Generations outside of institutional contexts to avoid re-activation of trauma from childhood institutionalisation.[63]

For mainstream services that have attempted to improve service delivery for Aboriginal and Torres Strait Islander communities, the importance of having Aboriginal Health Workers, developing partnerships with the local communities and Aboriginal Health Services, pathways to care, and cultural competence staff training has been emphasised. Another successful approach was the development of an Aboriginal Mental Health First Aid for Elders Program at Orange in NSW by an Aboriginal Mental Health clinical leader. This program was consistent with the National Strategic Framework's vision for the role of Elders.[64]

It appears that services to older Aboriginal and Torres Strait Islanders with mental disorders and dementia and their carers is on the cusp of significant change and improvement with much of the policy guidance in place and now the difficult translation into practice is under way.

# Chapter 17

# The Impact of the Ageing Culturally and Linguistically Diverse Population on Service Development

By the 1980s, the number of older people born overseas was increasing and in 2016 this reached thirty-three per cent of those aged 65 years and over, while twenty per cent of people aged 65 years and over were born in a non-English speaking country. The most common non-English languages spoken at home being Italian and Greek, which represented the two main non-English speaking countries that were the source of post-war migration in the 1959s and 60s. Easing of the White Australia Policy in the 1970s led to a surge in Asian migration, particularly from Vietnam and Hong Kong, so that by 2016 Chinese languages were the third largest non-English language spoken at home by older Australians.[1] From the perspective of mental health and dementia assessment and services, this evolution of Australia into a culturally and linguistically diverse society added further complexity to the field and the need for specific services including health interpreters and ethno-specific aged care.[2, 3]

The Culturally and Linguistically Diverse (CALD) population is heterogeneous with considerable diversity in terms of cultural background, life experiences, education, socioeconomic status, English literacy, and the circumstances and timing of migration to Australia. Specific issues that impact on mental health include the post-traumatic stress experienced by older refugees, such as by Holocaust survivors, and increased isolation and loneliness as contemporaries die, particularly for the non-English speaker. These factors impact on late life mental health and cognitive disorders in multiple ways including the risk of illness, recognition of key symptoms, access to services, availability of interventions, and impact on carers. Furthermore, over time different ethnic groups have ageing populations. For example, while in the late 1900s and early 2000s European groups from Italy, Greece, Germany, and the Netherlands were the main ageing CALD populations, in more recent years ageing Asian populations from China, Vietnam, India, and the Philippines have become more prevalent. These changes impact upon service planning and development and will also vary from one part of Australia to another; indeed, even different local areas within major cities such as Sydney and Melbourne vary. Although CALD community leaders and mainstream service providers have long been aware of the challenges that these issues bring to mental health and dementia service delivery, ethno-specific and multicultural services and research has been relatively limited. In addition, most of the CALD research and service development has focused on dementia rather than old age mental health, which has received little attention despite evidence of unmet need.[4]

A 1992 report from South Western Sydney, *A Double Jeopardy*, highlighted that CALD communities had low access and utilisation of dementia services due to lack of information, language barriers, cultural factors, community concern, and the cultural appropriateness of services.[5] Under the 1992 National Action Plan for Dementia Care (NAPDC) some of the initial small demonstration projects were targeted towards CALD communities and were mainly education focused but overall there was limited attention to CALD issues. For example, the South Australian branch of the Alzheimer's Association produced radio scripts on dementia for ethnic communities. The mid-plan report of the NAPDC noted that there was a need for culturally appropriate assessment tools.[6]

Service evaluations from Melbourne published in 2001 indicated that CALD presentations to a memory clinic had more severe cognitive impairment and were more likely to have psychiatric disorders.[7] Concerns that CALD issues were not being adequately addressed led to the formal establishment of the National Cross Cultural Dementia Network in 2003. It provides advocacy and advice to Dementia Australia, Commonwealth and other governments, and organisations regarding CALD dementia issues. Its membership is multidisciplinary and represents a diverse range of cultures and ethnicities with organisational representation from Dementia Australia, ACATs, Partners in Culturally Appropriate Care, and migrant resource centres. It has been a strong advocate for the development of culturally appropriate assessment, research, resource development and training.[8]

The 2003 Access Economics report, prepared for Alzheimer's Australia on the economic impact of dementia, again reflected that CALD communities were one of the special needs groups that had not received adequate attention in national dementia policy and programs.[9] One of the challenges that was identified by an expert group in 2008 was the lack of research on dementia incidence and prevalence in CALD populations.[10] The Access Economics *Keeping Dementia Front of Mind* report from 2009 provided dementia incidence and prevalence estimates for 2010 and projections to 2050. In 2010 it was estimated that there were over 35 thousand CALD persons with dementia which was nearly 14 per cent of those with dementia. Projected increases in the CALD population through to 2050 were less than for the general population due to population demographics.[11]

The 2009 Survey of Disability, Ageing and Carers was reanalysed for the 2012 Dementia in Australia report, which found that a third of persons with dementia residing in the community were from countries where English was not the main language compared with less than 20 per cent in residential aged care facilities. Most of the non-English speaking CALD dementia population in residential aged care facilities at this time were in major cities.[12] Initial analysis of Aged Care Funding Instrument (ACFI) data in 2011 revealed that Victoria had the highest numbers of residents with dementia for whom English was not the preferred language. Across the country, Italian, Greek, Polish, German, and Cantonese were the top five preferred languages. The proportion of residents with dementia born in Italy and Greece was lower than in the general community, while the proportion born in Poland was higher than in the general community. It is unclear whether the relatively high numbers of Polish residents with dementia reflects underlying differences in dementia prevalence or availability of community supports.[13]

There are a number of issues that have to be kept in mind when interpreting data from surveys and service utilisation. Dementia and mental health literacy is low in ethnic minorities with some variability between ethnic groups. One study that examined Italian, Greek and Chinese Australians found that first-generation migrants had less understanding of dementia and more negative attitudes towards dementia than third generation descendants. The first-generation migrants were more likely to believe that dementia was a part of normal ageing. Level of acculturation was associated with dementia literacy. It was noted that the term used for dementia in Chinese literally translates to 'old person crazy/ stupid/retarded disease' and thus introduced stigma.[14] An earlier report from the Cultural and Indigenous Research Centre Australia that did a small qualitative study of the understanding of dementia in Italian, Chinese and Vietnamese people in Sydney found more similarities than differences, although the Italians were more likely to talk of shame, the Chinese were more fatalistic about life's path, and the Vietnamese were more comfortable with talking about the future.[15] Another project in 2008 from Victoria that studied twelve ethnic groups found a broad lack of knowledge about dementia but perceptions about dementia, and what it was, varied between the ethnic groups.[16] This low dementia literacy acts as a barrier to dementia assessment and the view that memory impairment being part of normal ageing and not requiring medical attention is reminiscent of the nineteenth century understandings encountered in earlier chapters.

Diagnosis can be challenging, particularly where there are only mild symptoms, even in those from a non-English speaking background who are fluent in English such as participants in the prospective longitudinal Sydney Memory and Ageing Study. The study found that the prevalence of Mild Cognitive Impairment (MCI) was two to three times higher in those from a non-English speaking background than those from an English-speaking background due to performance on objective neuropsychological tests, although the incidence of MCI, incidence of dementia, and incidence of conversion of MCI to dementia did not differ. This demonstrates the challenges that clinicians face in early diagnosis in CALD populations due to the risk of 'over-diagnosis' of cognitive impairment.[17] The challenges of cognitive assessment in CALD communities led to the development of the Rowland Universal Dementia Assessment Scale (RUDAS) that operates as an equivalent of scales such as the Mini Mental State Examination (MMSE) and the Montreal Cognitive Assessment (MoCA) for cognitive screening in multicultural populations. It minimises the number of items that rely on education and acculturation. Since the initial publication in 2006, the RUDAS has become well-accepted in CALD communities, which has helped remove one barrier to dementia assessment. Being a screening tool, however, it does not overcome the challenge of accurate early dementia diagnosis requiring a more detailed assessment.[18] Other approaches have been to use translated versions of the MMSE or MoCA but one limitation here is that the translations have usually been undertaken in other countries and not for CALD populations in Australia.

Overcoming the cultural and language barriers to accurate dementia assessment in CALD populations remains a challenge to mainstream services. An assessment by an adequately trained clinician who speaks the person's language and is from the same cultural background would be ideal, and although a few mainstream services have that capacity, this is where bilingual general practitioners fill an essential role, so long as they are adequately trained in dementia assessment. Cultural competency training for all staff and employment of bilingual clinicians who speak the main languages of the ethnic groups in the local catchment area have become approaches well accepted in mainstream services. But an area where there has been less attention is work with interpreters. In some parts of Australian capital cities, up to a third of new assessments might be with a person who speaks no or limited English. Interpreters are required for the assessment. Many clinicians turn to family members to translate, and while this might be essential in an emergency, in routine mental health or dementia assessment this is poor practice that increases the likelihood of inaccurate assessments and may impact on confidentiality. The training of interpreters on how to translate cognitive assessments and of clinicians on how to work with interpreters has not been a priority.[19] Research is lacking into the training of interpreters and clinicians and how interpreters are best used by services.[20] Yet, research into use of interpreters has not been deemed a priority for CALD dementia research by the National Institute of Dementia Research.[21]

In the 2005 Dementia Initiative, Alzheimer's Australia was allocated the funding to run the National Dementia Support Program (NDSP) which included counselling, support and education services for those from CALD backgrounds.[22] There are some misconceptions about the extent to which extended families provide care for family members with dementia. The Victorian consultation with twelve ethnic communities in 2008 found that while there was consensus that family members are expected to provide care, the reality was that for many families other commitments with work and children and weaker family ties due to migration prevented this from happening.[23]

In 2011, the Productivity Commission Inquiry on *Caring for Older Australians* recommended that aged care services should cater for greater diversity.[24] As part of the Australian Government's response, the *Living Longer, Living Better Aged Care Reform Package* of 2012, a CALD Ageing and Aged Care Strategy was developed following extensive community consultation and released in December 2012. There were five broad principles in the strategy – capacity building, quality, access and equity, empowerment, and inclusion. One of the action areas identified in the CALD strategy was to develop initiatives in dementia assessment and early diagnosis services. Following a 2015 analysis of Dementia Programs which found a wide divergence in the quality of training programs, the National Dementia Training Program that commenced in 2016 includes addressing the needs of CALD consumers as a key performance indicator. While continued funding was provided for a number of initiatives including the National Cross Cultural Dementia Network and other support and educational activities provided by Alzheimer's Australia, there were no new initiatives to improve early diagnosis. Another area identified in the 2015 analysis of Dementia Programs requiring attention related to the need to address CALD issues in behavioural assessments provided by DBMAS and the Severe Behaviour Response Teams. Other dementia projects that addressed behavioural issues were also funded along with some locally focused projects which had a dementia or mental health focus. Partners in Culturally Appropriate Care (PICAC), a program funded by the Australian Government at a state level since 1997 to help older people from a CALD background to understand and access the aged care system, had a large role in the strategy including improving CALD access to My Aged Care and facilitating the provision of cultural competency training for the aged care workforce.[25] Alzheimer's Australia South Australia developed the Cultura smartphone app to assist with the provision of appropriate dementia care for people of CALD and Aboriginal and Torres Strait Islander backgrounds. There are 21 nationalities or cultures featured in the app that enables aged care workers to identify the cultural needs of the person for whom they are caring.[26]

There are three broad types of service models that provide community and residential dementia care. The first type is ethno-specific dementia services that provide care for one language group. These are usually run by ethnic community groups such as the Australian Greek Welfare Society or CoAsIt for the Italian community. This model works best when there is a large local community of the language group. The second type is the multicultural model that provides care to numerous language groups and might be best suited to areas where there are diverse migrant populations. The third type, mainstream services, often have greater dementia capacity but may enhance their cultural competency through training and partnerships with ethnic community groups.[27] These are not competing models of care but rather complementary models that depend on the needs and size of the various ethnic communities.[28] Whatever type of service model used, the importance of personalised support to dementia carers was demonstrated in a randomised controlled trial in Adelaide that involved ten ethnic groups and in which the carers receiving the personalised support reported a greater sense of competence.[29]

For many families from CALD background, placement into residential aged care is delayed until the person has more advanced dementia and the family is no longer coping.[30] Ethno-specific residential aged care facilities are preferred by many families who express greater satisfaction with care due to the facilities being more able to meet the residents' language and cultural needs, social and leisure activities, and food preferences than mainstream facilities. Bilingual staff and support for families at the time of admission were key factors in family satisfaction that could be adopted in mainstream facilities.[31] There is also evidence that residents with dementia in ethno-specific facilities are more likely to communicate with each other than those in mainstream facilities, although staff-resident communication may not differ. In addition, residents in ethno-specific facilities had a lower rate of antipsychotic drug prescription.[32] Another study reported that ethno-specific facilities were more likely to have activity programs, use interpreters and have other services for their non-English speaking residents than mainstream homes.[33]

Mainstream facilities remain the only option for many from small ethnic groups and those from larger groups who are unable to access ethno-specific care. The challenge that this presents to mainstream facilities in cities such as Melbourne and Sydney was captured in a Victorian survey of 220 aged care facilities in 2015 that found just over two-thirds had at least one non-English speaking resident and that overall there were 55 non-English languages spoken in the facilities. On average, each facility had between nine and ten non-English languages spoken by their residents with one facility having 22. In 16 per cent of cases, the resident was the sole speaker of the non-English language in the facility. Overall around three quarters of facilities had at least one non-English speaking staff member. When compared with ethno-specific facilities, mainstream facilities had fewer staff that spoke non-English languages.[34] Communication is a key issue in dementia care and this is accentuated in CALD populations as there is a tendency for languages acquired later in life to be affected and for the person to return to the language of their upbringing. There is a shortage of adequately trained bilingual staff in the aged care program and this was identified in the 2017 review of the CALD Ageing and Age Care Strategy. Other issues identified in the review included a disconnect between organisational and individual views of the effectiveness of the strategy with organisations much more positive than individuals, a need to address 'diversity within diversity', and further work to improve equity of access and cultural competence in organisations.[35]

Old age mental health service delivery to the CALD population in Australia has received limited attention despite evidence that they have a high risk of mental disorders, particularly depression, related to social isolation, loneliness and chronic ill health.[36] There is some evidence that where older migrants do not integrate into mainstream society their risk of depression is higher.[37] Similar to dementia services, poor access to old age mental health services has been a concern. The factors associated with poor access are not dissimilar to those relevant to dementia services, although stigma perhaps has a larger role.[38] An investigation of admissions to an acute psychogeriatric unit in Melbourne in 1996 found that admissions from a non-English speaking background were more likely to be married males admitted involuntarily, were less likely to receive an affective disorder diagnosis and more likely a dementia diagnosis than those from the general population. For most ethnic groups, the proportion of admissions was similar to that in the catchment area, except for an under-representation of Vietnamese and over-representation of 'other European' that essentially included a large number of smaller European ethnic groups, perhaps suggesting a potential role of social isolation in the admissions.[39] Subsequently in 2002, access to the community aged psychiatry arm of the same service was noted to vary between ethnic groups, with low access found in Asian and non-European communities. Overall just over 40 per cent of referrals to the service over a one year period were from a non-English-speaking background with around 80 per cent of these needing an interpreter. Those from a non-English speaking background had low levels of education and previous employment in unskilled occupations. Clinical details and outcomes did not vary significantly between groups.[40]

The NSW Specialist Mental Health Services for Older People (SMHSOP) service plan for 2005–2015 identified the CALD population as a priority group. The NSW Transcultural Mental Health Centre undertook a three year project to build and inform capacity within SMHSOP services. Recommendations from the project included use of culturally relevant assessment tools, interpreters and bicultural/bilingual mental health clinical specialists and to develop more partnerships with organisations that work with older people from CALD backgrounds.[41] In the mid-term evaluation of the plan after the three year project, the proportion of older service contacts from CALD background had doubled and there had been a 174 per cent increase in unique CALD contacts by NSW mental health services.[42] The factors responsible for the increase are not clear but making the CALD population a priority group and having some practical ways to improve quality and safety of mental health care were likely contributors. Going forward, developing partnerships with bilingual GPs in the Primary Health Networks might improve access. Training of staff on working with interpreters and to attain cultural competency for the main ethnic and cultural groups in the local region is essential.

In 2019, the Australian Government incorporated CALD, Aboriginal and Torres Strait islanders and other diverse groups within a broad Diversity Action Plan. Specific actions for CALD groups were retained. It is too early to see whether this approach leads to further improvements for CALD populations.[43]

# Chapter 18

# Concluding Observations and Future Prospects

The historical development of nineteenth century lunatic and benevolent asylums in the Australian colonies were reactive to the needs of a growing population. Neither type of asylum was specifically designed for older people but each in its own way had a higher proportion of older people than resided in the general community. This has been the pattern of service development for older people with dementia and mental disorders until recent years; an acceptance that 'something needs to be done' due to the ageing population with mental incapacity, but with service developments that have usually involved inappropriately designed institutions that are inadequately resourced with insufficient and poorly trained care staff. That there have been repeated reports of abuses leading to inquiries and Royal Commissions into both the aged care and mental health system across the country since the 1850s is hardly surprising given the failure thus far of any Government response to adequately address the issues at hand.

Each ageing cohort brings with it the life experiences of its generation. Characteristics of the ageing population have repeatedly contributed to the challenges of meeting the needs of those with mental incapacities, particularly in the absence of extended family. In the nineteenth century, it was the ageing of former convict paupers in Tasmania, while in Victoria, NSW and Western Australia it was the ageing of single male migrant gold miners, and in South Australia the ageing of free emigrants ill-chosen to be pioneer colonists. After the Second World War, the marked increase in the number of older people with dementia was one of the major driving forces in the growth of mental hospitals across the country as until the 1960s there was no affordable alternative long-term residential care available. Then from the 1980s onwards the ageing of the post-war migrants from Europe and later from Asia, as well as more recently Aboriginal and Torres Strait Islanders, has brought to the fore the need to better meet the needs of a diverse ageing population.

To add to this the 'baby boomer' generation from the increased birth rates after the Second World War between 1946 and 1964 and which first reached the age of 65 in 2011 is already bringing about changes. The baby boomers are healthier than their predecessors and can be expected to have a longer life expectancy. Life expectancy at birth has increased from around 47 years in the 1880s to nearly 81 years in 2017–19 for males and from nearly 51 years in the 1880s to 85 years in 2017–19 for females, with a narrowing gap between males and females.[1,2] Importantly, older people are living longer. In the period 2016–2018, at age 65 males could expect to live another 19.9 years and females another 22.6 years, ranking sixth overall in the world for life expectancy.[3] The combination of the increased life expectancy and large numbers of baby boomers has fuelled the ageing population and in June 2020 nearly 4.2 million Australians (16.4 per cent of the Australian population) were aged 65 years and over.[4]

The baby boomer generation is healthier than previous generations and is the first generation to have an expectation of a decade or more healthy living after retirement, and according to the Ageing Baby Boomers in Australia project good health is one of the defining characteristics of their retirement expectations.[5] Those in good health do not see themselves as being old. On health measures, although 73 per cent of older people reported their health as good to excellent in 2014–15, only 35 per cent reported sufficient physical activity according to national guidelines, while 72 per cent were overweight or obese. There has been a significant reduction in the proportion of older people with disabilities between 1998 and 2015, particularly in those aged 85 years and over.[6] While baby boomers are consuming less tobacco than their predecessors, this has been counter-balanced by an increase in risky alcohol consumption and cannabis use with increased numbers of presentations to drug and alcohol services.[7,8]

The baby boomers have brought social changes with them to the ageing population. This was a non-conformist generation that during the 1960s and 1970s experimented with drugs, were sexually liberated, expressed concerns about the environment, recognised women's rights, and had political views that were more liberal when they were young but have become more conservative as they have aged. They were more likely to travel overseas for holidays as 'jumbo jets' dominated the skies and continue to do so in late life often exploring more adventurous destinations than previous generations. Baby boomers have embraced technology and change; the Internet being a prime example evolving from a 1990s mid-life novelty to an old age fixture used daily for entertainment, shopping, banking, and searching for information.[9] The number of older people participating in the workforce has increased with baby boomers delaying their retirement, often by having part-time careers in a different field, and have more disposable income. A lower proportion of older people receive an aged pension while superannuation funded retirement is increasing.[10]

Yet this obscures the common experience that older job seekers report of age discrimination in the workplace, where from midlife onwards it becomes harder to secure employment. This led to the Howard Government appointing Pru Goward in 2005 as the first Age Discrimination Commissioner in the Australian Human Rights Commission. The extent of the problem was quantified in a 2015 Australian Human Rights Commission report on age discrimination in the workplace that found 27 per cent of workers aged 50 years and over reported age discrimination in the previous two years and in 80 per cent of cases it had a negative impact.[11] Concerns about ageism remain but research in 2016 by Josh Healy and Ruth Williams at the University of Melbourne found that less than 10 per cent of one thousand people surveyed were resolutely ageist. Ageist views were more common in younger males. However succession-based and stereotypical ageist views were present in over 30 per cent suggesting intergenerational tensions, with the perception that older Australians were not relinquishing their societal roles or resources quickly enough.[12] There are also mounting concerns about the abuse of older people (elder abuse) which resulted in a National Plan in 2019. Abuses include physical, sexual, financial, psychological or emotional, and neglect, some of which have been linked with ageism. While the mandatory reporting of elder abuse in a similar fashion to child abuse was not addressed, the importance of strengthening safeguards was part of the five year, five part plan.[13]

The Ageing Baby Boomers in Australia project found that personal autonomy and economic resources were two of their defining characteristics of the generation.[14] Yet, while many baby boomers have acquired wealth, often through property ownership, others have struggled. Home ownership has decreased to around 75 per cent of older people and a higher proportion of older people are still paying off a mortgage. Women are more likely to be pensioners and have less superannuation accumulated. Low income earners may have to work beyond retirement age out of necessity and are unhappy about it. Or they are unable to secure employment at all. The number of older people who are carers is increasing and although the majority of older carers are female, with age the proportion of male carers increases. For many, caring for grandchildren is an expectation although there are mixed views about the responsibility with most looking forward to it but a sizable minority wishing to avoid it.[15,16]

In 2021, it was estimated that there were 472,000 Australians living with dementia, with 28,300 having young onset dementia (YOD). In the absence of a medical breakthrough, the number of Australians living with dementia is projected to increase to 590,000 by 2028. In 2018, dementia was estimated to cost $15 billion, increasing to $18.7 billion by 2025. Dementia is the major cause of disability in older people, with 52 per cent of those in residential aged care facilities having dementia.[17] Baby boomers have expectations of receiving quality health and aged care and for the next few decades will be the major consumers of health and aged care services.[18] Arguably, they were the generation that drove the complaints and utilised technology to film the abuses of their relatives in residential aged care facilities that resulted in the Aged Care Royal Commission. Irrespective of whatever changes ensue from the Royal Commission recommendations, their expectations will likely be greater than what is delivered, at least in the short to medium term.

The Royal Commission into Aged Care Quality and Safety handed down its final report in February 2021 with 148 recommendations, being tabled in parliament in March 2021. Commissioners Lynelle Briggs and Tony Pagone (who replaced Richard Tracey when he died) recommended a new Aged Care Act that provided a broad definition of aged care with an aged care system based on a universal human rights approach. The rights of older people receiving aged care were defined along with 21 principles under which the new Act should be administered. An integrated system of long-term support and care of older people was recommended that included welfare support, community services to enhance social participation, affordable and appropriate housing, high quality health care and aged care. This would be achieved through a new National

Cabinet Reform Committee on Ageing and Older Australians to be established between the Australian and State and Territory Governments. It recommended that an independent office of the Inspector-General of Aged Care should be established to investigate, monitor, and report on the administration and governance of the aged care system.[19] These recommendations were accepted in the Australian Government's response.[20]

Notably there was disagreement between the two Commissioners on a number of the recommendations particularly those related to governance of the proposed new aged care system. Commissioner Pagone favoured the establishment of a new independent Australian Aged Care Commission, while Commissioner Briggs favoured that the combined Department of Health and Aged Care should be responsible and that it report to a Cabinet Minister.[21] The Government accepted Commissioner Briggs' recommendations which included the establishment of a Council of Elders to advise the Minister and the Department, the abolition of the Aged Care Quality and Safety Commission to be replaced by an independent Aged Care Safety and Quality Authority, and that the role of the Independent Hospital Pricing Authority be expanded to include Aged Care.[22]

While the recommendations were essentially focused on the aged care program, there were specific recommendations about dementia care and regarding access to older people's mental health services for those receiving residential aged care or personal care at home. Recommendation 15 was to establish a comprehensive, clear and accessible post-diagnosis dementia support pathway for people living with dementia, their carers and families. This was largely about ensuring that GPs and geriatricians (no mention of other specialties such as psychiatrists or neurologists) have information and material about the pathways and refer them at the point of diagnosis. The pathways would include information about dementia, services, and the aged care system along with various support services, education and care planning. In other words, in large part it was about better navigation of the system.[23] The recommendation was accepted and the Government response envisaged a nationally consistent local support pathways that would be incorporated within a new National Framework for Action on Dementia.[24] Hopefully one outcome of this will be to broaden the scope of the pathway to include pre-diagnosis and diagnosis, particularly as a large proportion of dementia diagnoses occur during an aged care system assessment. Dementia Australia in its Roadmap to Quality Dementia Care also recommended the establishment of dementia support pathways but with two key differences; it recognised that the pathway needed to commence pre-diagnosis, and to minimise the challenges of service navigation, a single centralised national dementia access point managed by Dementia Australia that would complement My Aged Care.[25] It is debatable whether such a centralised separate national dementia pathway is the best way forward as in seeking simplicity it appear to add complexity by having to integrate the full range of local services, most run by other organisations, at a national level.

Another recommendation that was also accepted by the Government related to Specialist Dementia Care Services and the need to determine whether the number and capacity of the new Specialist Dementia Care Units is adequate to address the needs of those 'people exhibiting extreme changed behaviour' and whether the units are suitable for short stay respite admissions. It also recommended that Australian Government funded specialist dementia services provide treatment to those with comorbid mental health conditions.[26] This recommendation is consistent with the ongoing development and evaluation of this program. Both of the dementia recommendations are to be achieved by January 2023.

Two recommendations were about increased regulation of restrictive practices and antipsychotic drug prescription in residential aged care facilities. In both instances, the former involving an accredited independent expert with behaviour support plans lodged with the Quality Regulator reviewed quarterly, and the latter either a psychiatrist or geriatrician, the involvement of a specialist to authorise the intervention will be required. Both recommendations were accepted by the Government, although the prescription of antipsychotics was referred to the Pharmaceutical Benefits Advisory Committee (PBAC).[27] While efforts to reduce antipsychotic drugs in residential aged care are required, a number of potential concerns arose out of this proposed regulation. These include the failure to distinguish between antipsychotic drugs used to treat serious mental illness such as schizophrenia, bipolar disorder or severe recurrent depression from those used for control of dementia behavioural disturbances. As the authority for GPs to continue to prescribe antipsychotics would only be for a 12 month period irrespective of the mental condition of the resident, a review would be required and there was no guarantee that in a person with chronic serious mental illness that the most appropriate specialist, a psychiatrist, undertook that review. The potential for the inappropriate cessation of essential maintenance medication was of concern. Fortunately, in November 2021, the PBAC determined that this recommendation was 'not implementable at present due to substantial risk of unintended consequences'.[28] A related concern is the failure to consider the potential that other sedative drugs could be substituted for antipsychotic drugs. Increased access to medication management reviews by a pharmacist was another recommendation but not directly tied to antipsychotic drugs.[29] The Aged Care Quality and Safety Commission released the regulatory changes to the *Aged Care Act 1997* about restrictive practices that were announced in July 2021 to commence on September 1 2021. These covered chemical restraints (drugs used primarily to control behaviour), environmental restraints (such as locked doors), mechanical restraints (such as lap belts and bed rails), physical restraint (using force to primarily influence behaviour), and seclusion. For each of these a detailed behaviour support plan will need to be developed, although the independent expert assessment recommended by the Royal Commission appears to have been diluted. Chemical restraint, which is broader than antipsychotic drugs, appropriately excluded treatment of mental illness, physical disorders and end of life care in its definition. As chemical restraint would require consent by a guardian with powers to authorise restrictive practice, it can be expected that some 'gaming' of the system might occur.[30]

The other recommendation specific to mental health, which was accepted in principle by the Australian Government pending a new National Mental Health and Suicide Prevention agreement, was regarding increased access to State and Territory older people's mental health services for those in residential and community aged care with the introduction of performance measures and benchmarks and standardised eligibility criteria that do not exclude dementia. One issue not mentioned here, and which has been a source of confusion to aged care and mental health service providers, relates to the interface between Dementia Support Australia than manages DBMAS and the Severe Behaviour Response Teams and the State and Territory older people's mental health services. The recommendations appear to add to the confusion by suggesting that both services should include persons with dementia and comorbid mental disorders within their eligibility criteria but without giving guidance as to how that interface should occur. Given the wide disparity in capacity across State and Territory older people's mental health to provide these services, this might provide an opportunity for States and Territories (and regions within those jurisdictions) to develop their services. There is also the danger that without service enhancements the State and Territory older people's mental health services might be pressured into prioritising recipients of services from the Commonwealth aged care program over other clients rather than on mental health risk parameters.[31,32]

The other two focus areas included in Dementia Australia's roadmap, building workforce capability and dementia-friendly design for residential aged care facilities, were also featured in the Royal Commission final report with a degree of similarity that suggests that the Royal Commission recommendations drew heavily on Dementia Australia's submissions. The need to increase training in dementia for health and care workers was recognised including a review of curricula ensuring that there is adequate coverage of dementia topics. Similarly, developing standards of dementia-friendly design that could be applied to both large and 'small household' facilities was seen as the first step. These recommendations were accepted in the government response. The challenge with each of these areas will be how quickly they can be enacted and rolled out.[33,34,35]

The evolving development of services to better meet the needs of a diverse older population in an inclusive and culturally safe manner has been a feature of the past decade. The Australian Government's Diversity Action Plan of 2019 includes Lesbian, Gay, Bisexual, Transgender and Intersex (LGBTI) populations as well as CALD and Aboriginal and Torres Strait Islander populations.[36] While there was a broad Royal Commission recommendation about system design for diversity, difference, complexity, and individuality, a whole chapter with seven recommendations was devoted to addressing the specific needs of the Aboriginal and Torres Strait Islander populations. Key elements of the Aboriginal and Torres Strait Islander recommendations, all of which were accepted in the Australian Government response, were consistent with the suggestions made by the National Advisory Group for Aboriginal and Torres Strait Islander Aged Care in their submission. These include an Aboriginal and Torres Strait Islander aged care pathway with culturally safe and trauma-informed assessment care provided in a flexible manner, with Aboriginal and Torres Strait Islander organisations given priority to becoming service providers. Another recommendation was for regular training on cultural safety and trauma-informed care for all those who provide assessment and care in the aged care system. An Aboriginal and Torres Strait Islander Aged Care Commissioner was proposed and the employment and training of an Aboriginal and Torres Strait Islander aged care workforce. Funding cycle and program stream recommendations to facilitate these changes were also accepted by the Australian Government.[37,38]

One recommendation accepted by the Government was for there to be no persons under the age of 65 living in residential aged care by January 2025 with no new admissions from January 2022, although there was a caveat that an exception would be if it was demonstrably in their best interests with the examples given that they are close to their 65th birthday or have relatives living nearby. It was also recommended that alternative accommodation be developed for younger people with some contribution by the Commonwealth.[39] This segues neatly with changes associated with the National Disability Insurance Scheme (NDIS). The NDIS has been responsible for funding disability support services for YOD in recent years and while this has in general been well-received by consumers, service gaps still exist with lack of integration of health and NDIS funded services.[40] But importantly, having dementia more formally accepted as a disability has opened the door to services that focus on enablement rather than just support to cope with deficits. This approach to dementia services should herald a direction that services for older people with dementia should take including therapies such as cognitive rehabilitation and occupational therapy interventions as standard components of care.

The implementation phase of the Australian Government response to the Royal Commission will be crucial. In the 2020–21 Federal budget, $17.7 billion was allocated over five years to address the Royal Commission findings with a large focus on extra home care packages, with $229.4 million to meet many of the specific dementia-related recommendations ranging from enhancements to the National Dementia Support Program to dementia training initiatives.[41] But will this be enough to achieve the desired system change? Estimates made by the Australia Institute suggest that it would require at least an extra $10 billion per year for the 148 Royal Commission recommendations to be fulfilled, leaving the Government budgetary response only meeting approximately a third of what is needed. The two proposed funding mechanisms made by the Royal Commissioners were not accepted by the Government (Medicare-style Aged Care levy or adjustments to personal tax rates), while three other possible funding mechanisms were suggested by the Australia Institute. Without the additional funding, the danger is that the improvements will not adequately address the wide-ranging problems that exist.[42] Historically, this has been the pattern of previous inquiries and Royal Commissions into institutional abuses in mental health and aged care; acceptance of a need for change but inadequate resourcing to achieve all of the changes recommended. The Government response avoided increasing individual contributions to fund the aged care system and this would appear to be a political response as added taxes or levies would likely be unpopular.

The NHMRC National Institute of Dementia Research that was established in 2015 under the Boosting Dementia Research Initiative and delivered by Dementia Australia, closed in June 2020 having, according to the NHMRC, achieved its remit in targeting and coordinating the strategic expansion of dementia research. Three research roadmaps are its legacy – a Strategic Roadmap for Dementia Research and Translation, a CALD Dementia Research Action Plan, and an Aboriginal and Torres Strait Islander Roadmap for Dementia Research translation.[43] The overall strategic roadmap had several areas immediately relevant to provision of dementia services. The first involved improving dementia diagnosis and prevention and here the establishment of the Australian Dementia Network (ADNeT) was a key achievement as it brings together researchers, clinicians and consumers. Through ADNeT the first Australian dementia clinical quality registry has been established which allow the tracking, benchmarking and reporting on the clinical care of people with dementia. Another element has been to establish consistent best practice guidelines for the diagnosis and treatment of dementia in memory clinics. There is also a link to facilitate participants in clinical trials for new anti-dementia drugs.[44,45] These initiatives in benchmarking certainly allow for monitoring of variation in dementia care and outcomes for those attending one of the fifteen institutions involved in ADNeT, although at this stage this will not include the many people with dementia who are diagnosed and managed outside of these settings. It will be some years before the impact of ADNeT can be properly evaluated. Other strategic research areas immediately relevant to service delivery were in improving the quality of life and quality of care for people with dementia and a strengths-based and healing-centred approach to research into dementia in the Aboriginal and Torres Strait Islander population.[46]

In 2020 Alzheimer's Disease International released a Dementia Innovation Readiness Index that analysed the readiness of 30 cities globally in promoting innovation readiness for the treatment, prevention, risk reduction, and care of dementia. Sydney was the only Australian city in the Index and it was rated eighth overall, with the top three cities located in the UK. There were five domains in the Index with Sydney performing better on the 'access to care' and 'business environment' domains but less well on the other domains 'strategy and commitment', 'early detection and diagnosis' and 'community support'. The extent to which these ratings are specific to Sydney or can be regarded as an indicator for Australia is unclear. However, the broad findings from around the world was that even the top performing cities had significant gaps in their readiness.[47]

The COVID-19 pandemic that struck Australia in 2020, which is still active in mid-2022, brought significant challenges to the aged care system, older people in general, and in particular, those with dementia and other mental disorders. The Aged Care Royal Commission released a special report about COVID-19 and its impact on the aged care system, making six recommendations about it. Those residing in residential aged care have a high risk of adverse outcomes with COVID-19 as noted by the 685 deaths out of 2049 infections by the end of 2020, a one third mortality as compared with the overall COVID-19 mortality of less than 3 per cent. The impact in residential aged care facilities went well beyond those who became infected with all facilities having to stop family visits for months at a time putting the residents in isolation with its deleterious impacts on their health and well-being. The Royal Commission noted that levels of depression, loneliness, anxiety, suicidality and confusion had increased amongst residents along with fear of contracting the virus. Aged care workers were severely challenged, being at increased risk of contracting COVID-19 and exposing their lack of skills and training in infection control. The Royal Commission recommendations, all accepted by the Australian Government, addressed issues of family visits, access to allied health through new Medicare numbers, having a national aged care plan for COVID-19, and measures to improve infection control.[48] Similar concerns have also been expressed by older people's mental health services in the UK regarding the challenges of infection control in inpatient units and the provision of physical and social care in the community.[49]

For older people with dementia, particularly those with more severe dementia in residential aged care facilities, there have been particular challenges. Beyond the isolation from the outside world has been the dilemma of how to maintain social distancing within facilities for individuals who are unable to understand what is required and the reasons for it, as well as the curbs being placed on their physical activity that is difficult to achieve for those who are 'wanderers' in whom standard contemporary management practice is to allow them as much freedom as possible within the facility. In facilities where COVID-19 occurred, it became necessary to further isolate such residents within the facility as they were key vectors enabling spread. Concerns have been expressed by Alzheimer's Disease International (ADI) to the World Health Organisation that mortality from COVID-19 might be higher in people with dementia,[50] a concern later confirmed in England and Wales where mortality of dementia during the pandemic was three times higher than what would have been expected.[51] ADI was also concerned that the impact of social distancing on people with dementia would accelerate cognitive decline by reducing their access to social stimulation. COVID-19 has also had an impact upon dementia diagnosis globally as fewer people attend clinics for assessment.[52] In Australia, ADNeT released a perspectives paper early in the pandemic on the operation of memory clinics in Australia during the pandemic and noted that most had ceased to operate beyond the most urgent face-to-face consultations. Telehealth was being utilised for screening assessments and liaison with primary care increased in this process. It noted that neuropsychologists were adapting their practice to conduct web-based assessments and that Dementia Australia were offering carer support groups online.[53] A rapid literature review of the impact of COVID-19 on the well-being of people with dementia that was undertaken after nearly a year of the pandemic confirmed that people with dementia, dementia services, and research had been disproportionately affected across all domains including prevention, diagnosis, ongoing management and care with increased use of antipsychotic drugs, and negative impacts on carers. Mixed reactions in the use of telehealth for assessment and care were noted.[54]

The pandemic has facilitated the use of technology in old age mental health assessments beyond that described for dementia care. With face-to-face assessments being minimised during periods of lockdown, most mental health assessments have been undertaken using telehealth, a process facilitated in private practice by the creation of Medicare Benefits items. Although videoconferencing is preferred over teleconferencing for mental health and cognitive assessments, some older people have found that challenging due to lack of familiarity with the technology or limitations imposed by their mental or cognitive state. The assistance of a family member or carer can facilitate the process. In addition technological limitations affecting the quality of the video and concerns regarding privacy and confidentiality still need to be addressed but experience to date during the pandemic has been generally positive offering opportunities to improve accessibility in rural and remote Australia. Future mental health service developments for older people are almost certainly going to include a significant telehealth component post-pandemic.[55] Currently there is Australian research being led by Viviana Wuthrich at Macquarie University on which the author is an investigator, exploring the use of phone- or web-based cognitive behaviour therapies for the treatment of older people referred to older people's mental health services for treatment of anxiety and depression. If such stepped-care approaches are effective, this is another direction that service development could take with or without the use of technology.[56]

With the Aged Care Royal Commission there has been a lot of recent activity at a Commonwealth level that impacts upon services for older people with dementia and mental disorders, but generally only if they are recipients of Commonwealth funded aged care services. In contrast developments in State and Territory older people's mental health services have stalled in most jurisdictions. South Australia is an exception and has emerged from the Oakden scandal with a Statewide plan with $48 million funding to support the new developments in the 2021–22 State budget in the north eastern Adelaide suburbs.[57] While NSW has a well-developed State plan, there has been limited funding enhancements to accompany it and the state remains below the national average for acute inpatient units for older people. The Royal Commission in Victoria gave scant attention to Aged Persons Mental Health services beyond stating they needed parity with adult services and although Victoria probably continues to have the most well-developed comprehensive services there is little evidence of new development. Queensland lacks a State plan for older people's mental health and although there have been some enhancements of acute bed numbers, the state remains well below the national average on this parameter. Western Australia potentially has a good model of care developed by the Northern Metropolitan Older Adult Mental Health Service but efforts to turn it into a Statewide model have been thwarted. Tasmania, the ACT and the Northern Territory lack plans for older people's mental health service, with the ACT moving towards a 'whole of life' approach to governance that potentially has a negative impact on integrated mental health care for older people.

Why has the development of older people's mental health services across the country appeared to have stagnated when the population continues to age? Perhaps part of the answer relates to the focus of successive National Mental Health Plans on child and adolescent mental health and the lack of reasonable consideration of the needs of older people, including in the area of suicide prevention despite older men having the highest suicide rates. This clearly influences Commonwealth and State mental health funding directions in mental health. One of the recurrent dilemmas that older people's mental health services have faced is that it tends to fall in the gap between mental health and aged care at senior Commonwealth and State levels of health planning. Until this is resolved the issue will be ongoing.

Does it matter whether an older person is managed in an older people's mental health service as opposed to an adult mental health service? The consensus of evidence is that it does matter on a whole range of parameters including accessibility, acceptability, safety, quality of care, and outcomes. Staff working in adult mental health services have skills that are more focused towards younger to middle-aged adults and often find working with older adults a challenge. Older people often find the pace and activities available in adult mental health settings geared towards the young.[58]

One aspect of older people's mental health services that has been a recurring feature has been the tendency for inpatient facilities to be 'hand-me downs' from other uses. This is gradually changing with most new wards in the past decade being new builds. While there is a dearth of literature on the design of acute older people's inpatient mental health units, there is sufficient evidence to indicate that more attention needs to be given to design elements that might reduce the risk of falls, self-harm and violence while providing a pleasant environment that is visually appealing, allows for privacy, and has adequate indoor and outdoor leisure areas.[59]

The historical use of the age of 65 to delineate between adult and older people's mental health services was largely based on this being the statutory pension age rather than any specific health parameter. The Commonwealth uses the age of 70 to plan for aged care services and many hospital geriatric medical services use the age of 75 or 80 as their cut-off. Arguably, particularly in the absence of adequate funding enhancements, the lifting of the pension age, and the better health of those aged 65–75 years, the age of entry to older people's mental health services should be lifted to either 70 or 75 years. There are also two models of application of the age cut-off with adult services that has funding implications. The model adopted in Victoria and some other states follows that in the UK with all persons aged 65 years and over managed in their Aged Persons Mental Health services. The other model used in NSW and most other states, while still using the age of 65 for new presentations, leaves those older people with chronic serious mental illness or relapses and no significant accompanying aged-related conditions in adult services. However it should be noted that many individuals with chronic serious mental illness or long standing addictions have significant physical health issues and limited social supports at a relatively young age and are often best managed in an older people's mental health service.[60,61] Whatever model is followed, an older age of separation from adult services should still capture the essence of what older people's mental health services provide that is not well covered by adult services, which is largely related to complexity fuelled by physical and/or cognitive health issues, social circumstances, cultural diversity, and the need for age-appropriate interventions and environments provided by clinicians skilled in working with older people.

Broader movements in the style of mental health service delivery to adults have also been taken up by older people's mental health services in recent years. The 'recovery model' of care is one example that has become the dominant paradigm in adult mental health services with its focus on an individual's strengths rather than deficits. The recovery model aims to restore hope and achieve well-being through psychosocial interventions. For older people there are barriers to the recovery model including those related to deteriorating physical health and the effects of dementia. Yet, with adaptation and a person-centred approach to care, older people's mental health services have been increasingly adopting the model by including interventions such as falls prevention, interventions involving carers, and well-being groups.[62] In NSW a recovery-oriented practice improvement project commenced in 2015 and developed resources for NSW older people's mental health services.[63]

Mental health peer support workers are now a standard feature of adult mental health services but have been slower in uptake in older people's mental health. Peer workers have lived experience of mental illness and recovery and use that experience in providing direct care in hospital and community settings. They are employed by the mental health service. In my experience, older people are less inclined to be interested in becoming paid peer workers and are more inclined to provide voluntary service. Despite the slow uptake, it is likely that peer support workers will eventually become a standard feature of older people's mental health services. There is also a move to have consumer-led mental health services but this is embryonic in adult mental health and has had limited evaluation. In the main such services are those populated by individuals with chronic serious mental illness and whether such an approach would ever be applicable in older people's mental health services is unclear.[64]

The separation of basic dementia care from mental health care that commenced in the 1960s and was accelerated in the 1980s was long overdue and had been suggested by the Inspector Generals of the Insane a century earlier. There remains a need for continued mental health service provision for the minority of people with dementia with significant mental and or behavioural comorbidity along the lines suggested in the seven-tiered model.[65] The same model applied to the broad range of mental disorders in late life particularly mood disorders and psychoses is also relevant to older people's mental health service development particularly with regards to prevention and stepped care interventions instituted in primary care where it is expected there will be greater investment.[66]

Whether the concerted national effort to develop services for dementia will be complemented by similar efforts to provide appropriate services for older people with mental disorders is yet to be seen, but perhaps the Aged Care Royal

Commission has taken the first steps in that regard with its recommendation for increased access to older people's mental health services for those in the aged care system. This is where the National Mental Health Service Planning Framework for older people needs to result in a coordinated national strategy to improve older people's mental health services.

# Appendix

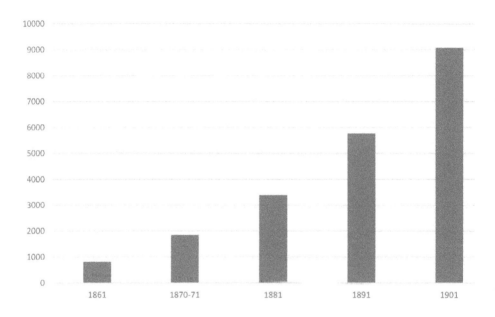

**Fig. 1:** Estimated Number of Persons with Dementia in Australia 1861–1901. Population data extracted from 'Australian Bureau of Statistics. Australian Historical Population Statistics, Cat. No. 3105.0.65.001 Canberra, Commonwealth of Australia, 2006'; Dementia prevalence data based on Table D2.4, 'Dementia in Australia' (2012), p. 210. Figure originally published in Draper B, *Dementia in Nineteenth-Century Australia*, Health and History, 23 (1), 38–60, 2021. Used with permission.

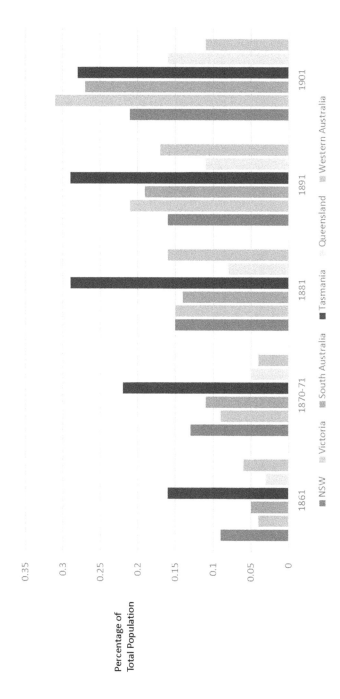

**Fig. 2:** Estimated Proportion of the Total Population with Dementia, Australian Colonies/States 1861–1901. Population data extracted from 'Australian Bureau of Statistics. Australian Historical Population Statistics, Cat. No. 3105.0.65.001 Canberra, Commonwealth of Australia, 2006'; Dementia prevalence data based on Table D2.4, 'Dementia in Australia' (2012), p. 210. Number of people with dementia presented as the proportion of the total population. Figure originally published in Draper B, *Dementia in Nineteenth-Century Australia*, Health and History, 23 (1), 38-60, 2021. Used with permission.

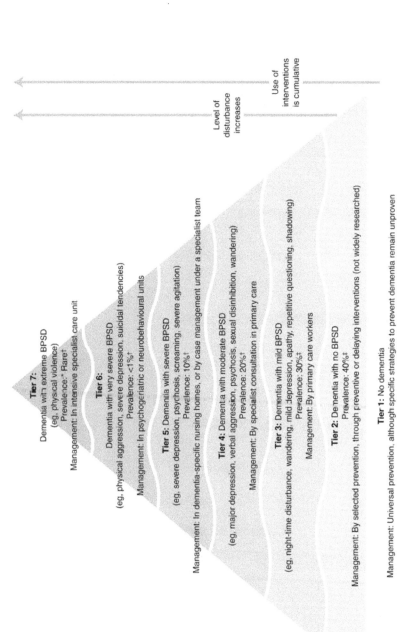

**Fig. 3:** 7-Tiered Model of Service Delivery for Behavioural and Psychological Symptoms of Dementia. Brodaty H, Draper B, Low L-F, *Behavioural and Psychological Symptoms of Dementia – a 7 tiered Model of Service Delivery*, Medical Journal of Australia, 178, 231–234, 2003. Used with permission.

# Endnotes

## 1 Mental Health and Dementia in Old Age: a brief overview of international influences on colonial Australia

1  Thane P, *Social Histories of Old Age and Aging*, Journal of Social History, 37 (1), Special Issue, 93–111, 2003.

2  Nusteling HPH, 'The population of England, 1539–1873: an issue of demographic homeostasis', *Histoire & Mesure*, VIII-1/2, 59–92, 1993.

3  Ottaway SR, *The Decline of Life: Old Age in Eighteenth-Century England,* Cambridge University Press, Cambridge, 2004.

4  Ibid.

5  Williams S, *Support for the elderly during the 'crisis of the Old Poor Law', c.1790–1834,* Population, economy, and welfare, 1200–2000, Cambridge, September 2011. https://www.campop.geog.cam.ac.uk/events/richardsmithconference/papers.html (accessed 27 May 2020).

6  Ibid.

7  Thane P, *Old Age in English History: Past Experiences, Present Issues,* Oxford University Press, Oxford, 2000, p. 193. Thane comments that neither the demography of the late eighteenth century nor labour market changes were sufficient to explain the focus on the aged poor. Rather it was the efforts to look for explanations of poverty and other social issues such as unemployment and housing that brought older people into focus.

8  Ibid. 3 Ottaway examined the social history of ageing in the eighteenth century and intentionally avoided taking a 'pathological' view of the ageing process. But of course it is difficult to avoid mentioning the age-related deterioration in health that increased older people's functional decline and need for increased family support or institutional care. Within that context it is remarkable that cognitive change was barely mentioned, even though at the time such change would have been regarded as a normal accompaniment of ageing.

9  Berrios GE, *Dementia during the seventeenth and eighteenth centuries: a conceptual history*, Psychological Medicine, 17, 829–837, 1987.

10  Prichard JC, *A Treatise on Insanity and other disorders affecting the mind,* London, Sherwood, Gilbert and Piper, 1835.

11  Ibid.

12  Ibid. 9.

13  Förstl H, Howard R, Burns A, Levy R, *'The strange mental state of an old man who thought he would be slaughtered' – an early report of dementia with delusion (1785)*, Journal of the Royal Society of Medicine, 84, 432–434, 1991.

14  Ibid. 10, pp. 88–89. Berrios notes that it was Willis in the seventeenth century who first proposed that dementia was acquired and not congenital.

15  Ibid. 10, p. 92.

16  Ridley N, Draper B, Withall A, *Alcohol-related Dementia: an update of the evidence*, Alzheimer's Research & Therapy, 5: 3. doi:10.1186/alzrt157, 2013.

17  Ibid. 10, pp. 83–100.

18  Ibid. 9, Amentia was a diagnosis commonly used in Tasmania until the mid-1860s.

19  Anonymous, *Mental exercise conducive of health and happiness*, South Australian Register, Wednesday 11 June 1845, p. 3.

20  Sweetser W, *Mental hygiene, or, an examination of the intellect and passions*, New York, J & HG Langley, 1843, p. 27.

21  American Psychiatric Association, *Diagnostic and Statistical Manual of Mental Disorders. Fifth Edition*, Arlington VA, American Psychiatric Association, 2013.

22  Australian Institute of Health and Welfare, *Dementia in Australia*. Cat No. Age 70, Canberra, AIHW, 2012.

23  Nitrini R, *A cure of one of the most frequent types of dementia: a historical parallel*, Alzheimer's Disease and Associated Disorders, 19, 156–158, 2005.

24  Davis G, *The most deadly disease of asylumdom: general paralysis of the insane and Scottish psychiatry c.1840–1940*, Journal of the Royal College of Physicians of Edinburgh, 42, 266–273, 2012.

25  Stewart M, Debattista J, Fitzgerald L, Williams O, *Syphilis, General Paralysis of the Insane, and Queensland asylums*, Health and History, 19 (1), 60–79, 2017.

26  Ibid. 24.

27  Ibid. 23.

28  Berrios GE, *'Depressive pseudodementia' or 'melancholic dementia': a nineteenth century view*, Journal of Neurology, Neurosurgery, and Psychiatry, 48, 393–400, 1985.

29  Berrios GE, *J.C. Prichard and the concept of 'moral insanity'*, History of Psychiatry, 10, (37), 111–126, 1999.

30  Whitlock FA, *Prichard and the concept of 'moral insanity'*, Australian & New Zealand Journal of Psychiatry, 1, 72–79, 1967.

31  Berrios GE, *Historical aspects of psychoses: 19th century issues*, British Medical Bulletin, 43, (3), 484–498, 1987.

32  Ibid. 10, p. 12.

33   Ibid. 10, p. 6.

34   Ibid. 21.

35   Ibid. 10, pp. 72–73.

36   Berrios GE, *Melancholia and depression during the nineteenth century: a conceptual history*, British Journal of Psychiatry, 153, 298–304, 1988.

37   Willmuth LR, *Medical views of depression in the elderly: historical notes,* Journal of the American Geriatrics Society, 27 (2), 495–499, 1979.

38   Kiloh LG, *Pseudo-dementia,* Acta Psychiatrica Scandinavica, 37: 336–351, 1961.

39   Ibid. 28.

40   Ibid. 10, pp. 26–30.

41   Ibid. 21.

42   Clinical Epidemiology and Health Service Evaluation Unit, Melbourne Health., *Clinical Practice Guidelines for the Management of Delirium in Older People,* Melbourne, Victorian Government Department of Human Services, October 2006.

43   Berrios GE, *Delirium and confusion in the nineteenth century: a conceptual history,* British Journal of Psychiatry, 139, 439–449, 1981.

44   Ibid. p. 439.

45   Ibid. 10, p. 168.

46   Andrews ES, *Senility before Alzheimer: Old age in British psychiatry, c.1835–1912,* Doctoral thesis, University of Warwick, April 2014, pp. 46–50.

47   Kosky R, *From morality to madness: a reappraisal of the asylum movement in psychiatry, 1800–1940,* Australian and New Zealand Journal of Psychiatry, 20, 180–187, 1986. As previously noted in the foreword, I have used the terminology that reflected usage in the era under discussion and recognise words such as 'lunatics' are not acceptable in contemporary discussions of mental disorders.

48   Cummins CJ, *A History of Medical Administration in NSW 1788–1973,* 2nd edition, Sydney, NSW Department of Health, 2003.

49   Ibid. 47.

50   Ibid. 48.

51   Ibid. 47.

52   Ibid. 1.

53   Andrews ES, *Institutionalising senile dementia in 19th century Britain,* Sociology of Health & Illness, 39 (2), 244–257, 2017.

54   Yorston G, Haw C, *Old and mad in Victorian Oxford: a study of patients aged 60 and over admitted to the Warneford and Littlemore Asylums in the nineteenth century,* History of Psychiatry, 16(4), 395–421, 2005.

55   Ibid. 53, The experience in Great Britain was understandably the most important influence on the organisation of lunatic asylums in colonial Australia and of the views of key asylum administrators during the nineteenth century.

56  Fox P, *From senility to Alzheimer's disease: The rise of the Alzheimer's disease movement,* The Milbank Quarterly, 67 (1), 58–102, 1989, p. 61.

57  Ibid. 53, p. 244.

58  Anonymous, *Report of the Thirty-Seventh Annual Meeting of the Medico-Psychological Association,* Journal of Mental Science, 28, 460, 1882.

59  Blashfield RK, *Pre-Kraepelin names for mental disorders,* Journal of Nervous and Mental Disease, 207, 726–730, 2019.

60  Rybakowski JK, *120th anniversary of the Kraepelinian dichotomy of psychiatric disorders,* Current Psychiatry Reports, 21, 65, 2019.

61  Berrios GE, 'The insanities of the third age: a conceptual history of paraphrenia', *Journal of Nutrition, Health & Ageing,* 7 (6), 394–399, 2003.

## 2 The Early Colonial Days and First Asylums in NSW

1  Harris J, *Hiding the bodies: the myth of the humane colonisation of Aboriginal Australia,* Aboriginal History, 27, 79–104, 2003.

2  Irish P, *Hidden in Plain View: The Aboriginal people of coastal Sydney,* NewSouth, Sydney, 2017, 19.

3  Gillen M, *The Founders of Australia: a biographical dictionary of the First Fleet,* Sydney, Library of Australian History, 1989.

4  Cummins CJ, *A History of Medical Administration in NSW 1788–1973,* 2nd edition, Sydney, NSW Department of Health, 2003.

5  Collins D, *An Account of the English Colony in New South Wales – Volume 1,* London, Cadell & Davies, 1798, Project Gutenberg 2004.

6  Ibid. p. 120.

7  Flynn M, *The Second Fleet – Britain's Grim Convict Armada of 1790,* Sydney, Library of Australian History, 2001.

8  Robson L, *The Convict Settlers of Australia,* Melbourne, Melbourne University Press, 1973.

9  Thane P, 'Social Histories of Old Age and Aging, *Journal of Social History,* 37 (1), Special Issue, 93–111, 2003.

10  Australian Bureau of Statistics, *Australian Historical Population Statistics, Cat. No. 3105.0.65.001,* Canberra, Commonwealth of Australia, 2006.

11  Ibid. 7.

12  Grimshaw P, Willett G, *Family Structure in colonial Australia,* Australia 1888, No. 4 May, 5–27, 1980.

13  Davison G, 'Our youth is spent and our backs are bent': The origins of Australian ageism, In: Walker D, Garton S (eds) Ageing, Australian Cultural History 14, Geelong, Deakin University, 1995, 40–62.

14  Ibid. 10.

15   Ibid. 5.

16   Tench W, *Chapter 13, April 1791*, In: *A Complete Account of the Settlement at Port Jackson,* London, 1793, Project Gutenberg, January 2013.

17   Dowd BT, *Alt, Augustus Theodore (1731–1815),* Australian Dictionary of Biography, National Centre of Biography, Australian National University, http://adb.anu.edu.au/biography/alt-augustus-theodore-1702/text1845, published first in hardcopy 1966 (accessed online 18 January 2020).

18   Fletcher BH, *Phillip, Arthur (1738–1814),* Australian Dictionary of Biography, National Centre of Biography, Australian National University, http://adb.anu.edu.au/biography/phillip-arthur-2549/text3471, published first in hardcopy 1967 (accessed online 1 June 2020).

19   Gray AJ, *Brewer, Henry (1739–1796),* Australian Dictionary of Biography, National Centre of Biography, Australian National University, http://adb.anu.edu.au/biography/brewer-henry-1825/text2095, published first in hardcopy 1966 (accessed online 9 January 2020).

20   Rumsey HJ, *The Pioneers of Sydney Cove*, Sydney, Sunnybrook Press, 1937.

21   Ibid. 5.

22   Hughes R, *The Fatal Shore: A History of the Transportation of Convicts to Australia 1787–1868,* London, Vintage, 2003, p. 73. Hughes gives no reference for his claim that Dorothy Handland, who was also known as Dorothy Gray, had died by suicide. Hughes also claimed that she was aged 82, most likely based on the inaccurate journal of Arthur Bowes, as her age was in her 60s. There were no coroner's inquests into deaths in the early days of the colony thus accurate records of suicides are lacking. David Collins mentions a number of suicides in his journal for these years and it is likely that this is the most accurate record.

23   Ibid. 5, p. 297.

24   Ibid. 5, p. 23.

25   Ibid. 4.

26   Bostock J, *The Dawn of Australian Psychiatry 1788–1850*, Sydney, Australasian Medical Publishing Company, 1968.

27   *Sydney Gazette and New South Wales Advertiser*, p. 2, 9 October 1808.

28   *Sydney Gazette and New South Wales Advertiser*, p. 2, 15 October 1809.

29   Ibid. 4.

30   First Fleet OnLine, http://firstfleet.uow.edu.au/objectv.html (accessed 23 January 2020).

31   Garton S, *Out of Luck: Poor Australians and Social Welfare 1788–1988,* Sydney, Allen & Unwin, 1990.

32   Ibid. 30.

33  Ibid. 4, p. 25.

34  Ibid. 4, p. 34.

35  Shea P, *Defining Madness*. Sydney, Hawkins Press, 1999, p. 22.

36  Parkinson JP, *The Castle Hill Lunatic Asylum (1811–1826) and the Origins of Eclectic Pragmatism in Australian Psychiatry*, Australian and New Zealand Journal of Psychiatry, 15, 319–322, 1981.

37  Neil WD, *The lunatic asylum at Castle Hill: Australia's first psychiatric hospital 1811–1826*, Sydney, Dryas, 1992.

38  Raeburn T, Liston C, Hickmott J, Cleary M, *Liverpool 'lunatic asylum': a forgotten chapter in the history of Australian health care*, Collegian, 25, 347–353, 2018.

39  Dickey B, *No Charity There: a short history of social welfare in Australia*, Sydney, Allen & Unwin, 1980, p. 7.

40  *Sydney Gazette*, 1 June 1811, p. 1.

41  Ibid. 36.

42  Ibid. 37.

43  Ibid. 36.

44  Ibid. 37.

45  Ibid. 36.

46  Ibid. 4, p. 35.

47  Rathbone R, *A very present help – caring for Australians since 1813: The History of the Benevolent Society of NSW*, Sydney, State Library of NSW Press, 1994.

48  Cummins CJ, *The Development of the Benevolent (Sydney) Asylum 1788–1855*, Sydney, Department of Health, 1971.

49  Ibid. 39.

50  Earnshaw B, *The lame, the blind, the mad, the malingerers: sick and disabled convicts within the colonial community*, Journal of the Royal Australian Historical Society, 81, part 1, 1995.

51  Ibid. 48, p. 6.

52  Ibid. 7, p. 487–488.

53  Karskens G, *Declining life: on the Rocks in early Sydney*, In: Walker D & Garton S (eds) Ageing, Australian Cultural History 14, Geelong, Deakin University, 1995, pp. 63–75.

54  Ibid.

55  Ibid.

56  'A Gentleman in Sydney', *On the comfort and happiness of the labouring classes in the colony of New South Wales, compared with the same classes in Great Britain*, Sydney Gazette and New South Wales Advertiser, Thursday 29 July 1830, p. 4.

57  Ibid. 20.

58   Ibid. 7, p. 216–217.

59   Dunk J, *Bedlam at Botany Bay*, Sydney, NewSouth Publishing, 2019, 158–179.

60   The History of Parliament Trust, *Mills, George Galway (1765–1828)*, History of Parliament online, https://www.historyofparliamentonline.org/volume/1790–1820/member/mills-george-galway-1765-1828 (accessed 9 November 2020).

61   Ibid. 59.

62   Anonymous, 'Coroner's Inquest on the body of G.G. Mills esq', *Sydney Gazette and New South Wales Advertiser*, 15 February 1828, p. 2.

63   R Darling to Hay, 15 February 1828, Historical Records of Australia, Series 1, vol. xiii, p. 784.

64   Ibid. 62.

65   Ibid. 38.

66   Sainty MR, Johnson KA (eds), *Census of New South Wales – November 1828*, Sydney, Public Library of Australian History, 1980.

67   Raeburn T, Liston C, Hickmott J, Cleary M, *Colonial surgeon Patrick Hill (1794–1852): unacknowledged pioneer of Australian mental health care*, History of Psychiatry, 30 (1), 90–103, 2019 .

68   Ibid. 3.

69   Ibid. 66.

70   Ibid. 26, p. 37.

71   Barnard M, *A History of Australia*, 2nd edition, Sydney, Angus & Robertson, 1963, p. 145.

72   Ibid. 26.

73   Ibid. 26.

74   Ibid. 38.

75   Ibid. 38.

76   Steven M, *Birnie, James (1762–1844)*, Australian Dictionary of Biography, National Centre of Biography, Australian National University, http://adb.anu.edu.au/biography/birnie-james-1783/text2007 published first in hardcopy 1966 (accessed online 14 September 2019).

77   Ibid. 59, pp. 145–146.

78   Ibid 66.

79   Considering the Benevolent Society's well established views against providing assistance to alcoholics, possibly his community status and connections overrode those concerns.

80   Ibid. 7, p. 521–522.

81   Tampke J, *The Germans in Australia*, Melbourne, Cambridge University Press, 2006, p. 22.

82  Ibid. 7, p. 522.

83  Ibid. 81.

84  Ibid. 7, p. 522.

85  Walsh GP, *Divine, Nicholas (1769–1830)*, Australian Dictionary of Biography, National Centre of Biography, Australian National University, http://adb.anu.edu.au/biography/divine-nicholas-1979/text2399, published first in hardcopy 1966, (accessed online 15 September 2019).

86  Murphy M, *Newtown Ejectment Case*, https://www.newtownproject.com.au/portfolio-items/newtown-ejectment-case/ (accessed 9 November 2020).

87  *Sydney Gazette and New South Wales Advertiser*, 25 November 1824, p. 2.

88  Ibid. 86.

89  Ibid. 85.

90  Cologon 'JH, Nicholas Devine, Catholic pioneer and Free-Man'. *Catholic Weekly*, 6 November 1952, p. 1.

91  Norman LG, *Historical notes on Newtown*, Sydney, Council of the City of Sydney, 1963.

92  Ibid. 86.

93  Ibid. 90.

94  Ibid. 85.

95  Ellis MH, *John Macarthur*, Penrith, Discovery Press, 1972, pp. 21–25.

96  Steven M, *Macarthur, John (1767–1834)*, Australian Dictionary of Biography, National Centre of Biography, Australian National University, http://adb.anu.edu.au/biography/macarthur-john-2390/text3153 published first in hardcopy 1967, (accessed online 17 September 2019).

97  Ibid. 95, p. 451.

98  Ibid. 95, pp. 498–499.

99  Ibid. 95, pp. 526–527.

100 Reynolds, Emma. *Madman on the money: How Australian pioneer John Macarthur died in obscurity after being declared a lunatic*. Finance, News.com.au, 27 January 2015.

101 Ibid. 96.

102 Ibid. 71, p. 144.

103 Dunk J, *Work, paperwork and the imaginary Tarban Creek Lunatic Asylum, 1846*, Rethinking History, 22:3, 326–355, 2018.

104 Ibid. 4, p. 35.

105 Ibid. 26, p. 38.

106 Ibid. 103.

107 Ibid. 4, p. 36.

108 Ibid. 4, p. 35.

109 Blaxland J, *Mr Blaxland's protests,* Sydney Monitor and Commercial Advertiser, Wednesday 10 October 1838, p. 1.

110 Gunson N, *Oakes, Francis (1770–1844),* Australian Dictionary of Biography, National Centre of Biography, Australian National University, http://adb.anu.edu.au/biography/oakes-francis-2513/text3397 published first in hardcopy 1967, (accessed online 14 September 2019).

111 Ibid. 59, p. 147.

112 Ibid. 48, p. 19.

113 Ibid. 26, p. 80.

114 McDonald DI, *Campbell, Francis Rawdon (1798–1877),* Australian Dictionary of Biography, National Centre of Biography, Australian National University, http://adb.anu.edu.au/biography/campbell-francis-rawdon-3156/text4715 published first in hardcopy 1969 (accessed online 3 June 2020).

115 Ibid. 103, p. 342.

116 Ibid. 26, p. 118.

117 Ibid. 26, pp. 115–116.

118 Ibid. 26, pp. 169–209.

119 McDonald DI, *Gladesville Hospital: the formative years 1838–1850,* Journal Royal Australian Historical Society, 51, 273–295, 1965.

120 Jervis J, *The Mental Hospital, Parramatta,* Royal Australian Historical Society Journal and Proceedings, 19, 191–196, 1933.

121 Ibid. 114.

122 Ibid. 120.

123 Ibid. 47.

124 Ibid. 48.

125 Ibid. 47.

126 Ibid. 2, p. 19–23.

127 Butlin NG, *Our original aggression: Aboriginal populations of southeastern Australia, 1788–1850,* Sydney, Allen and Unwin, 1983, p. 176.

128 Ibid. 2, p. 88.

129 Ibid. 2, p. 112.

130 Saggers S, Gray D, *Explanations of Indigenous alcohol use,* In: Gray, D. & Saggers, S. (eds) Indigenous Australian alcohol and other drug issues: Research from the National Drug Research Institute. Curtin University of Technology, Perth, 2002, p. 175.

131 Ibid. 2, p. 42.

## 3 Population Ageing and Growth of the Asylums: 1851–1900

1   Australian Bureau of Statistics, *Australian Historical Population Statistics, Cat. No. 3105.0.65.001*, Canberra, Commonwealth of Australia, 2006.

2   Histpop – the online historical population reports website, *Census of England and Wales, 1861* http://www.histpop.org/ohpr/servlet/Show?page=Home (accessed 17 June 2020).

3   Gilleard C, *The other Victorians: age, sickness and poverty in 19th-century Ireland*, Ageing & Society, 36, 1157–1184, 2016.

4   Barnard M, *A History of Australia*, 2nd edition, Sydney, Angus & Robertson, 1963, p. 411–412.

5   Jalland P, *Old Age in Australia: A History*, Melbourne, Melbourne University Press, 2015, p. 14.

6   Ibid.

7   Report of the Inspector of Lunatic Asylums or the Hospitals for the Insane, for the year ending 31 December 1881, Melbourne, Government Printer, 1883, p. 15.

8   Vreugdenhil AJ, *Out of Sight, Out of Mind. Senile dementia in nineteenth century Launceston*, In: Effecting a Cure: Aspects of Health and Medicine in Launceston, P.A.C. Richards, B. Valentine, T. Dunning (eds), Launceston, Myola House of Publishing, 74–87, 2006.

9   Draper B, *Dementia in nineteenth-century Australia*, Health and History, 23(1), 38–60, 2021.

10  Australian Institute of Health and Welfare, *Dementia in Australia. Cat No. Age 70*, Canberra, AIHW, 2012, Table D2.4, p. 210.

11  Prince M, Ali GC, Guerchet M, Prina AM, Albanese E, Wu YT, *Recent global trends in the prevalence and incidence of dementia, and survival with dementia*, Alzheimer's Research & Therapy, 8, 23, 2016, DOI 10.1186/s13195-016-0188-8.

12  Hendricks S, Peetoom K, Bakker C, *et al.*, *Global prevalence of young-onset dementia. A systematic review and meta-analysis*, JAMA Neurology, 78(9), 1080–1090, doi:10.1001/jamaneurol.2021.2161.

13  Ridley N, Draper B, Withall A, *Alcohol-related Dementia: an update of the evidence*, Alzheimer's Research & Therapy, 5, 3, 2013, DOI 10.1186/alzrt157.

14  Nitrini R, *A cure of one of the most frequent types of dementia: a historical parallel*. Alzheimer's Disease and Associated Disorders, 19, 156–158, 2005.

15  Butlin NG, *Our original aggression: Aboriginal populations of southeastern Australia, 1788–1850*, Sydney, Allen and Unwin, 1983, p. 175.

16  Manning FN, *Insanity in Australian Aborigines with a brief analysis of 32 cases*, Intercolonial Medical Congress of Australasia, 4, 857–860, 1889.

17  Brewer GJ, *Copper-2 ingestion, plus increased meat eating leading to increased copper*

*absorption, are major factors behind the current epidemic of Alzheimer's disease,* Nutrients, 7, 10053–10064, 2015.

18 Ibid. 10.

19 By applying the estimated dementia prevalence to the total population rather than just the aged population the relative impact of dementia across the colonies is better emphasised.

20 Davison G, '*Our youth is spent and our backs are bent': The origins of Australian ageism.* In: Walker D & Garton S (eds) Ageing, Australian Cultural History 14, Geelong, Deakin University, 1995, pp. 40–62.

21 Ibid. 5, pp. 15–34.

22 Garton S, *Out of Luck: Poor Australians and Social Welfare 1788–1988,* Sydney, Allen & Unwin, 1990, p. 99.

23 Ibid. 5, p. 31.

24 The information about the growth of the number of patients in lunatic asylums and the number of lunatic asylums between 1850 and 1900 was compiled from multiple sources. Victorian data for 1850 was obtained from Darebin Heritage. 'Yarra Bend Lunatic Asylum,' Darebin Libraries, http://heritage.darebinlibraries.vic.gov.au/article/631 (accessed 6 July 2020) and for 1900 from the 'Report of the Inspector of Lunatic Asylums, for the year ending 31st December, 1900.' Melbourne, Government Printer, 1901. For NSW, data for 1850 was obtained from John Bostock, *The Dawn of Australian Psychiatry 1788–1850,* Sydney, Australasian Medical Publishing Company, 1968 and for 1900 from the 'Annual Report, Inspector General of the Insane for the Year 1900,' Legislative Assembly, NSW, July 1901. For Queensland the information was obtained from Queensland Health. *The Road to Recovery – a history of mental health services in Queensland 1859–2009,* Queensland Government, 2013. Tasmanian data for 1850 was extracted from Susan Piddock, 'A Space of their Own: Nineteenth century lunatic asylums in England, South Australia and Tasmania'. (PhD thesis Flinders University of South Australia, 2003) Table 8.4 and for 1900 from Ralph W Gowlland, *Troubled asylum: the history of…the Royal Derwent Hospital.* New Norfolk, Tasmania, 1981, 161. South Australian data for 1850 was extracted from Piddock, Table 4 and for 1900 from the 'Report for the Hospitals of the Insane, for the Year 1900', Adelaide, Government Printer 1901. Western Australian data was extracted from Roger Virtue, 'Lunacy and Social Reform in Western Australia 1886–1903', *Studies in Western Australia History,* 1, (1977): 29–65.

25 Brunton W, 'At variance with the most elementary principles': the state of British colonial lunatic asylums in 1863, History of Psychiatry, 26 (2), 147–165, 2015.

26 Richards J, *Going up the Line to Goodna – a History of Woogaroo Lunatic Asylum, Goodna Mental Hospital, and Wolston Park Hospital 1865–2015,* Queensland Government, 2017, p. 20.

27  Lewis M, *Managing Madness: Psychiatry and Society in Australia, 1788–1980,* Australian Government Publishing Service, Canberra, 1988, pp. 12–13.

28  Garton S, *Medicine and Madness: A Social history of insanity in New South Wales, 1880–1940,* New South Wales University Press, Kensington, 1988, p. 172.

29  Edwards GA, *Restraint in the treatment of the mentally ill in the late 19th century,* Australian and New Zealand Journal of Psychiatry, 4, 201–205, 1970.

30  Roth DT, *Life, Death and Deliverance at Callan Park Hospital for the Insane 1877–1923,* Doctoral thesis, Australian National University, May 2020.

31  Seitz D, Lawlor B, *Module 6 – Pharmacological management.* In: Draper B, Brodaty H, Finkel S. (eds) The IPA Complete Guides to Behavioral and Psychological Symptoms of Dementia (BPSD), International psychogeriatric Association, Chicago, 2015.

32  Ibid. 29.

33  Burnham JC, *The Royal Derwent Hospital in Tasmania: historical perspectives on the meaning of community psychiatry,* Australian & New Zealand Journal of Psychiatry, 9, 163–167, 1975.

34  Ibid. 28.

35  Anonymous, *A Senile Judge,* Queanbeyan Observer Friday 31 July 1896, p. 2.

36  Anonymous, *An old identity,* Clarence and Richmond Examiner, Saturday 1 January 1898, p. 4.

37  Ibid. 20.

38  Ibid. 16.

39  Ibid. 16, p. 858.

40  Ibid. 16, p. 859.

41  Ibid. 16, p. 858.

42  Ibid. 16, p. 859.

43  Irish P, *Hidden in Plain View: The Aboriginal people of coastal Sydney,* NewSouth, Sydney, 2017, pp. 88–89.

44  Karskens G, *The Colony: a history of early Sydney,* Allen & Unwin, Sydney, 2009, pp. 529–531.

45  Ibid. 43, p. 82.

46  Pybus C, *Truganini – Journey through the apocalypse,* Allen & Unwin, Sydney, 2020.

## 4 New South Wales 1851–1900

1  Cummins CJ, *A History of Medical Administration in NSW 1788–1973,* 2nd edition, Sydney, NSW Department of Health, 2003, pp. 36–37.

2  Smith TG, *'With tact, intelligence and a special acquaintance with the insane'. A history of the development of mental health care (nursing) in NSW Australia, from colonisation to federation, 1788–1901,* Doctoral thesis, University of Western Sydney, 2005, pp. 231–232.

3    Ibid. pp. 216–219.

4    Ibid. 1, p. 38.

5    Ibid. 2, pp. 206–214.

6    Ibid. 2, pp. 225–228.

7    Conway J, *Blaxland, Gregory (1778–1852)*, Australian Dictionary of Biography, National Centre of Biography, Australian National University, http://adb.anu.edu.au/biography/blaxland-gregory-1795/text2031, published first in hardcopy 1966 (accessed online 14 September 2019).

8    Blaxland Wine Group, *Gregory Blaxland.* https://blaxwine.com.au/gregory-blaxland/ (accessed 21 September 2020).

9    Anonymous, *Parramatta,* Sydney Morning Herald, Tuesday 4 January 1853, p. 2.

10   McDonald DI, *Frederic Norton Manning, 1839–1903,* Journal Royal Australian Historical Society, 58, 190–201, 1972.

11   Manning FN, *Report on Lunatic Asylums,* Thomas Richards, Governor Printer, Sydney, 1868.

12   Ibid. 10.

13   Ibid. 1, p. 39.

14   Garton S, *Medicine and Madness: a Social history of insanity in New South Wales, 1880–1940,* New South Wales University Press, Kensington, 1988, p. 30.

15   Ibid. 10, pp. 192–193.

16   Manning FN, *The Hospital for the Insane, Gladesville,* Sydney Morning Herald, Thursday 14 March 1878, p. 6.

17   Ibid. 1, p. 40.

18   Manning FN, *Lunacy Reports,* Sydney Morning Herald, Wednesday 18 April 1877, p. 7 (2).

19   Ibid.

20   Ibid. 1, p. 40.

21   Luke S, *Callan Park: Hospital for the Insane,* Australian Scholarly Publishing Pty Ltd, Sydney, 2018, p. 213.

22   A Pilgrim, *Parramatta Lunatic Asylum,* Freeman's Journal, Saturday 25 August 1877, p. 17.

23   Ibid. 10, pp. 195–196.

24   Inspector General of the Insane, *Report for the year ending December 31, 1885.* New South Wales Parliament, 1886.

25   Ibid. 1, pp. 46–47.

26   Ibid. 14, p. 27.

27   Manning FN, *Report of the Inspector General of the Insane,* Sydney Morning Herald, Saturday 8 May 1880, p. 3.

28 Inspector General of the Insane, *Report for the year ending December 31, 1882*, New South Wales Parliament, 1883, Table 3.

29 Ibid. p. 9.

30 Inspector General of the Insane, *Report for the year ending December 31, 1892*, New South Wales Parliament, 1893, p. 8.

31 Inspector General of the Insane, *Report for the year ending December 31, 1887*, New South Wales Parliament, 1888.

32 Inspector General of the Insane, *Report for the year ending December 31, 1893*, New South Wales Parliament, 1894.

33 Inspector General of the Insane, *Report for the year ending December 31, 1884*, New South Wales Parliament, 1885, p. 5.

34 Hume SH, *Hume, Hamilton (1797–1873)*, Australian Dictionary of Biography, National Centre of Biography, Australian National University, http://adb.anu.edu.au/biography/hume-hamilton-2211/text2869, published first in hardcopy 1966 (accessed online 15 September 2019).

35 Draper B, *Older people in hospitals for the insane in New South Wales, Australia, 1849–1905*, History of Psychiatry, 32 (4), 436–448, 2021, doi.org/10.1177/0957154X211029479.

36 Ibid.

37 NSW State Archives, Gladesville Mental Hospital Medical Casebook 12, 4/8141, Case 232.

38 NSW State Archives, Callan Park Mental Hospital Medical Casebook 2, 3/4652, Case 210.

39 NSW State Archives, Gladesville Mental Hospital Medical Casebook 23, 4/8151, Case 283.

40 NSW State Archives, Gladesville Mental Hospital Medical Casebook 17, 4/8146, Case 349.

41 NSW State Archives, Callan Park Mental Hospital Medical Casebook 8, 3/4657, Case 248.

42 NSW State Archives, Gladesville Mental Hospital Medical Casebook 11, 4/8140, Case 228.

43 NSW State Archives, Gladesville Mental Hospital Medical Casebook 5, 4/8138, Case 180.

44 NSW State Archives, Gladesville Mental Hospital Medical Casebook 5, 4/8138, Case 179.

45 NSW State Archives, Gladesville Mental Hospital Medical Casebook 11, 4/8140, Case 229.

46 NSW State Archives, Callan Park Mental Hospital Medical Casebook 2, 3/4652, Case 196.

47 NSW State Archives, Callan Park Mental Hospital Medical Casebook 2, 3/4652, Case 199.

48 NSW State Archives, Callan Park Mental Hospital Medical Casebook 9, 3/4658, Case 270.

49 Anonymous, *The Tichborne Case – death of William Creswell,* Daily Telegraph, Tuesday 13 December 1904, p. 5.

50 Anonymous, *The Tichborne Case,* Daily Telegraph, Saturday 19 January 1895, p. 10.

51 Anonymous, *Monday October 23 1871,* Argus, Monday 23 October 1871, p. 4 (7).

52 Jackson JDD, *Orton-Tichborne evidence,* Australian Town and Country Journal, Saturday 12 April 1884, p. 23.

53 Anonymous, *The Tichborne mystery*, Evening News, Wednesday 14 February 1900, p. 3.

54 Ibid. 49.

55 NSW Office of Environment and Heritage, *Rydalmere Hospital Precinct (former).* https://www.environment.nsw.gov.au/heritageapp/ViewHeritageItemDetails. aspx?id=5000658 (accessed 1 September 2020).

56 Anonymous, *Report of the Thirty-Seventh Annual Meeting of the Medico-Psychological Associatio*n, Journal of Mental Science, 28, 460, 1882.

57 Andrews ES, *Senility before Alzheimer: Old age in British psychiatry, c1835–1912,* Doctoral thesis, University of Warwick, April 2014, p. 200.

58 Inspector General of the Insane, *Report for the year ending December 31, 1891*, New South Wales Parliament, 1892.

59 Ibid. 1, p. 52.

60 Rathbone R, *A very present help – caring for Australians since 1813. The History of the Benevolent Society of NSW*, Sydney, State Library of NSW Press, 1994.

61 Ibid. 1, p. 53.

62 Ibid. 60, p. 65.

63 Dickey B, *No Charity There: a short history of social welfare in Australia*, Sydney, Allen & Unwin, 1980, p. 47.

64 Ibid. 1, pp. 53–54.

65 Garton S, *Out of Luck: Poor Australians and Social Welfare 1788–1988,* Sydney, Allen & Unwin, 1990, p. 54.

66 Elyard W, Walker G, *Lunatic Asylums,* Sydney Mail, Saturday 30 January 1864, p. 10.

67 NSW State Archives, Gladesville Mental Hospital Medical Casebook 19, 4/8148, Case 407.

68 NSW State Archives, Gladesville Mental Hospital Medical Casebook 9, 4/10566, Case 378.

69 NSW State Archives, Gladesville Mental Hospital Medical Casebook 9, 4/10566, Case 379.

70 NSW State Archives, Gladesville Mental Hospital Medical Casebook 17, 4/8146, Case 353.

71 Ibid. 1, pp. 199–200.

72 Ibid. 63, p. 78.

73 Ibid. 1, p. 55.

74 O'Brien A, *Poverty's Prison: The poor in NSW 1880–1918,* Carlton, Victoria, Melbourne University Press, 1988.

75 Report of the Government Asylums Inquiry Board to NSW Legislative Assembly, Charles Potter, Government Printer, Sydney May 1887.

76 Ibid. p. 14.

77 Ibid. p. 36.

78 Jalland P, *Old Age in Australia: A History,* Melbourne, Melbourne University Press, 2015, p. 21.

79 Ibid. 75, p. 36.

80 Ibid. 78, p. 20.

81 Ibid. 75, p. 39.

82 Ibid. 78, p. 32.

83 Ibid. 60.

84 Many people are unaware that suicide and attempted suicide remained on the criminal statutes in NSW until 1983 although prosecutions had long since ceased.

85 Anonymous, *Parramatta Police Court,* Cumberland Argus and Fruitgrowers Advocate, Saturday 31 March 1894, p. 4.

86 Anonymous, *Parramatta,* Sydney Evening News, Monday 10 August 1891, p. 6.

87 Anonymous, *The Bathurst Assizes,* Sydney Daily Telegraph, Thursday 24 April 1884, p. 5.

88 Anonymous, *Attempted Suicide,* Sydney Daily Telegraph, Tuesday 24 November 1896, p. 2.

## 5 Tasmania: an Ageing Nineteenth Century Convict Colony

1 Barnard M, *A History of Australia,* 2nd edition, Sydney, Angus & Robertson, 1963, p. 176.

2 Garton S, *Out of Luck: Poor Australians and Social Welfare 1788–1988,* Sydney, Allen & Unwin, 1990, p. 17.

3 Brown JC, *'Poverty is not a Crime'. The development of social services in Tasmania, 1803–1900,* Hobart, Tasmanian Historical Research Association, 1972, p. 6.

4 Ibid. pp. 12–14.

5 Anonymous, *Beggars,* Launceston Advertiser, Wednesday 4 April 1832, p. 109.

6 Piddock S, *Convicts and the free: nineteenth century lunatic asylums in South Australia and Tasmania (1830–1883),* Australasian Historical Archaeology, 19, 84–96, 2001.

7   Vreugdenhil A, *'Incoherent and violent if crossed': The admission of older people to the New Norfolk Lunatic Asylum in the nineteenth century*, Health and History, 14, (2), 91–111, 2012.

8   Ibid. 3, p. 48.

9   Ibid. 6.

10  Ibid. 3, p. 51.

11  Ibid. 7.

12  Ibid. 3, p. 19.

13  Ibid. 3, pp. 38–39.

14  Ibid. 7.

15  Ibid. 3, p. 53.

16  Trollope A, *Trollope's Australia*, edited by Hugh Dow. Thomas Nelson, Melbourne, 1966, p. 54.

17  Ibid. 2, p. 55.

18  Ibid. 3, p. 89.

19  Ratcliffe E, Kirkby K, *Psychiatry in Tasmania: from old cobwebs to new brooms*, Australasian Psychiatry, 9 (2), 128–132, 2001.

20  Burnham JC, *The Royal Derwent Hospital in Tasmania: historical perspectives on the meaning of community psychiatry*, Australian & New Zealand Journal of Psychiatry, 9, 163–167, 1975.

21  Ibid. 2, p. 49.

22  Ibid. 6.

23  Piper A, *Admission to charitable institutions in colonial Tasmania: from individual failing to social problem*, Tasmanian Historical Studies, 9, 43–62, 2004, p. 49.

24  Ibid. pp. 51–52.

25  Ibid. 6, p. 93.

26  Ibid. 7.

27  Ibid. 6, p. 93.

28  Ibid. 20, p. 163.

29  Ibid. 6, p. 94.

30  Piddock S, *A space of their own: Nineteenth century lunatic asylums in England, South Australia and Tasmania*, doctoral thesis, Flinders University of South Australia, October 2002, p. 327.

31  Ibid. 3, pp. 97–98.

32  Gowlland RW, *Troubled asylum: the history of…the Royal Derwent Hospital*, New Norfolk, Tasmania, 1981, p. 72.

33  Ibid. p. 74.

34  Ibid. 3, p. 103.

35  Ibid. 32, p. 85.

36  Ibid. 6, p. 94.

37  Ibid. 32, p. 112.

38  Ibid. 7.

39  Ethics committee approval was obtained from the University of New South Wales Human Research Ethics Committee (#190705) and approval was obtained from Libraries Tasmania to use the medical casebooks in de-identified form.

40  Libraries Tasmania, Archives Series, *Royal Derwent Hospital, TA465*, volume 17, folio 119.

41  Libraries Tasmania, Archives Series, *Royal Derwent Hospital, TA465*, volume 19, folio 287.

42  Libraries Tasmania, Archives Series, *Royal Derwent Hospital, TA465*, volume 16, folio 23.

43  Libraries Tasmania, Archives Series, *Royal Derwent Hospital, TA465*, volume 19, folio 297.

44  Libraries Tasmania, Archives Series, *Royal Derwent Hospital, TA465*, volume 19, folio 151.

45  Libraries Tasmania, Archives Series, *Royal Derwent Hospital, TA465*, volume 19, folio 304.

46  Vreugdenhil AJ, *Out of Sight, Out of Mind. Senile dementia in nineteenth century Launceston*, In: Effecting a Cure: Aspects of Health and Medicine in Launceston, Myola, P.A.C. Richards, B. Valentine, T. Dunning (ed), South Launceston, pp. 74–87, 2006.

47  Piper A, *Beyond the convict system: the aged poor and institutionalisation in colonial Tasmania*, Doctoral thesis, University of Tasmania, 2003, pp. 54–55.

48  Ibid. 30, p. 192.

49  Ibid. 16, p. 156.

50  Ibid. 3, p. 89.

51  Libraries Tasmania, Archives Series, *Hospital for the Insane, Cascades. Case Book HSD54.* This case book has the notes of all of the patients transferred to the Cascades Hospital.

52  Libraries Tasmania, Archives Series, *Royal Derwent Hospital, TA465*.

53  Jalland P, *Old Age in Australia: a History*, Melbourne, Melbourne University Press, 2015, p. 19.

54  Ibid. 20, pp. 56–57.

55  Hargrave J, *A pauper establishment is not a jail: old crawlers in Tasmania 1856–1895.* Master's thesis, University of Tasmania, 1993, pp. 23–24.

56  Ibid. 46.

57  Ibid. 3, pp. 102–105.

58 Special Correspondent, *The Invalid Depot, New Town,* Hobart Mercury, Saturday 27 December 1884, p. 3.

59 Ibid. 3, p. 103.

60 Ibid. 3, p. 157.

61 Ibid. 52.

62 Libraries Tasmania, Archives Series, *Royal Derwent Hospital, TA465*, Volume 30, Folio 70.

63 Libraries Tasmania, Archives Series, *Royal Derwent Hospital, TA465*, Volume 30, Folio 96.

64 Ibid. 3 p. 51.

65 Ibid. 23.

66 Australian Bureau of Statistics, *Australian Historical Population Statistics, Cat. No. 3105.0.65.001,* Canberra, Commonwealth of Australia, 2006.

67 Kippen R, *Death in Tasmania: using civil death registers to measure nineteenth century cause-specific mortality,* Doctoral thesis, Australian National University, January 2002, p. 199.

68 Ibid. p. 211.

69 Anonymous, *Attempted Suicide,* Launceston Daily Telegraph, Thursday 15 May 1890, p. 2.

70 Our own Correspondent, *Launceston,* Tasmanian News, Thursday 15 May 1890, p. 2.

71 Moyle H, *Tasmania in the 19th and early 20th centuries,* In 'Australia's Fertility Transition', pp. 41–62, ANU Press, 2020.

72 Ibid. 3, p. 161.

**6 The Ageing Effects of a Gold Rush: Victoria in the Nineteenth Century**

1 Australian Bureau of Statistics, *Australian Historical Population Statistics, Cat. No. 3105.0.65.001,* Canberra, Commonwealth of Australia, 2006.

2 Davison G, 'Our youth is spent and our backs are bent': The origins of Australian ageism', in: Walker D & Garton S (eds) Ageing, Australian Cultural History 14, Geelong, Deakin University, 1995, pp. 40–62.

3 Darebin Heritage, *Yarra Bend Lunatic Asylum.* Darebin Libraries, http://heritage. darebinlibraries.vic.gov.au/article/631 (accessed 6 July 2020).

4 Dax EC, 'The first 200 years of Australian psychiatry', *Australian and New Zealand Journal of Psychiatry*, 23, 103–110, 1989.

5 Willis E, … *of 'unsound mind'*, Historic Environment, 14, No. 2, 1999.

6 Ibid. 4.

7 Bonwick R, *The history of Yarra Bend Lunatic Asylum, Melbourne,* Masters thesis, University of Melbourne, Melbourne, November 1995, pp. 33–35.

8   Report of the Inspector of Asylums on the Hospitals for the Insane for the Year 1868, Government Printer, Melbourne, 1869.

9   Brothers CRD, *Early Victorian Psychiatry*, Government Printer, Melbourne, 1962.

10  Craig DA, *The Lion of Beechworth*, Beechworth, Victoria, 2000.

11  Day C, *Magnificence, misery, and madness. A history of the Kew Asylum 1872–1915*, Doctoral thesis, University of Melbourne, 1998, p. 35.

12  Kirkby KC, *History of Psychiatry in Australia, pre-1960*, History of Psychiatry, 10, 191–204, 1999.

13  The Lunacy Statute, 1867, *Victorian Government Gazette*, Supplement 10 September 1867.

14  Ibid. 8.

15  Anonymous, The Argus, Saturday 10 June 1865, p. 4.

16  Ibid. 8, p. 5.

17  Report of the Inspector of Asylums on the Hospitals for the Insane for the Year 1870, Government Printer, Melbourne, 1871.

18  Report of the Inspector of Asylums on the Hospitals for the Insane for the Year 1872, Government Printer, Melbourne, 1873, p. 8.

19  Ibid.

20  Ibid. 11, pp. 36–39.

21  Report of the Inspector of Asylums on the Hospitals for the Insane for the Year 1877, Government Printer, Melbourne, 1878.

22  Public Record Office of Victoria. VPRS 7680 P1 Register of Patients (VA2840), Kew 1871–1919, Units 1–4.

23  Report of the Inspector of Asylums on the Hospitals for the Insane for the Year 1888, Government Printer, Melbourne, 1889.

24  Ibid. 7, p. 51.

25  Ibid. 21.

26  Thomas J, *The Vagabond papers: Sketches of Melbourne Life in Light and …* George Robertson, Melbourne, 1877, p. 95.

27  Report of the Inspector of Asylums on the Hospitals for the Insane for the Year 1879, Government Printer, Melbourne, 1880, p. 22.

28  Anonymous, *The Chronicle,* Camperdown Chronicle, Tuesday 29 April 1879, p. 2 (4).

29  Report of the Inspector of Asylums on the Hospitals for the Insane for the Year 1880, Government Printer, Melbourne, 1881.

30  Report of the Inspector of Asylums on the Hospitals for the Insane for the Year 1881, Government Printer, Melbourne, 1882, p. 14.

31  Report of the Inspector of Asylums on the Hospitals for the Insane for the Year 1882, Government Printer, Melbourne, 1883, p. 24.

32   Ibid. 7, pp. 54–55.

33   Coleborne C, *The 'scientific management' of the insane and the problem of 'difference' in the asylum in Victoria 1870s–1880s*, Australasian Victorian Studies Journal, 2 (1), 126–137, 1996.

34   Ibid. 12.

35   Crowther A, *Administration and the Asylum*, In: Coleborne, C. & MacKinnon, D. (eds), 'Madness' in Australia: histories, heritage, and the asylum. St Lucia, Queensland, Queensland University Press, 2003, pp. 93–95.

36   Report of the Inspector of Asylums on the Hospitals for the Insane for the Year 1885, Government Printer, Melbourne, 1886, p. 14.

37   Ibid. p. 15.

38   Ibid. 22, unit 4, male register 2773, register entry 29 September 1885.

39   Ibid. 22, unit 4, male register 2937, register entry 25 September 1886.

40   Ibid. 22, unit 4, male register 2935, register entry 17 November 1886.

41   Ibid. 22.

42   Report of the Inspector of Asylums on the Hospitals for the Insane for the Year 1886, Government Printer, Melbourne, 1887.

43   Ibid. 23.

44   Report of the Inspector of Asylums on the Hospitals for the Insane for the Year 1890, Government Printer, Melbourne, 1891.

45   Anonymous, *Castlemaine Police Court, Lunacy*, Mount Alexander Mail, Saturday 8 October 1887, p. 2.

46   Report of the Inspector of Asylums on the Hospitals for the Insane for the Year 1893, Government Printer, Melbourne, 1894.

47   Report of the Inspector of Asylums on the Hospitals for the Insane for the Year 1891, Government Printer, Melbourne, 1892.

48   Report of the Inspector of Asylums on the Hospitals for the Insane for the Year 1900, Government Printer, Melbourne, 1901.

49   Anonymous, *Death of a Lunatic*, Ovens and Murray Advertiser, Saturday 26 November 1892, p. 8.

50   Ibid. 11, pp. 151–154.

51   Ibid. 22.

52   Report of the Inspector of Asylums on the Hospitals for the Insane for the Year 1887, Government Printer, Melbourne, 1888.

53   Draper B, *Richard Mahony: the Misfortunes of Younger Onset Dementia*, Medical Journal of Australia, 190, 94–95, 2009.

54   Kehoe M, *The Melbourne Benevolent Asylum, Hotham's Premier Building*, Hotham History Project, 1998, p. 14.

55 Dickey B, *No Charity There: a short history of social welfare in Australia*, Sydney, Allen & Unwin, 1980.

56 Anonymous, *The Benevolent Asylum,* Argus, Friday 13 June 1856, p. 4.

57 Ibid. 54, p. 84.

58 Jalland P, *Old Age in Australia: a History,* Melbourne, Melbourne University Press, 2015, p. 16.

59 Garton S, *Out of Luck: Poor Australians and Social Welfare 1788–1988,* Sydney, Allen & Unwin, 1990, p. 56.

60 Ibid. 58.

61 Ibid. 54, p. 43.

62 Anonymous, *Police Court Friday March 12,* Geelong Advertiser, Saturday 13 March 1875, p. 3.

63 Ibid. 58, p. 17.

64 Anonymous, *Castlemaine Police Court, Tuesday Sept 11th*, Mount Alexander Mail, Wednesday 12 September 1888, p. 2.

65 Ibid. 59, p. 58.

66 Anonymous, *Melbourne Hospital Committee,* The Age, Wednesday 2 August 1882, p. 6.

67 Anonymous, *The Melbourne Hospital,* The Argus, Wednesday 2 August 1882, p. 11 – I have removed the man's name from the quote.

68 Anonymous, The Argus, Monday 12 July 1875, page 1 (5) – I have removed the man's name from the quote.

69 Anonymous, *Inquests,* The Age, Saturday 4 December 1886, p. 9.

70 Anonymous, *News and Notes in a Nutshell,* Melbourne Herald, Tuesday 2 April 1895, p. 1.

71 Cooke S, *'Terminal old age': Ageing and suicide in Victoria 1841–1921, In*: Walker D & Garton S (eds) Ageing, Australian Cultural History 14, Geelong, Deakin University, 1995, pp. 76–91.

72 Draper B, *Suicidal behaviour and suicide prevention in later life,* Maturitas, 79(2), 179–183, 2014.

73 Ibid. 71.

74 Hone JA, *Chirnside, Thomas (1815–1887),* Australian Dictionary of Biography, National Centre of Biography, Australian National University, http://adb.anu.edu.au/biography/chirnside-thomas-3203/text4815, published first in hardcopy 1969, (accessed online 15 September 2019).

75 Anonymous, *The suicide of Mr Thomas Chirnside,* Ballarat Star, Tuesday 28 June 1887, p. 3.

76 Anonymous, *Suicide of Mr Chirnside,* Warragul Guardian and Buln Buln and Narracan Shire Advocate, Tuesday 28 June 1887, p. 3.

## 7 Nineteenth Century South Australia, Western Australia and Queensland

1    Piddock S, *Convicts and the free: nineteenth century lunatic asylums in South Australia and Tasmania (1830–1883),* Australasian Historical Archaeology, 19, 84–96, 2001.

2    Goldney R, *Lessons from history: the first 25 years of psychiatric hospitals in South Australia,* Australasian Psychiatry, 15 (5), 368–371, 2007.

3    Bostock J, *The Dawn of Australian Psychiatry 1788–1850*, Sydney, Australasian Medical Publishing Company, 1968, p. 153.

4    Piddock S, *Possibilities and realities: South Australia's asylums in the 19th Century,* Australasian Psychiatry, 12 (2), 172–175, 2004.

5    Shlomowitz E, Garton S, 'How much more generally applicable are remedial words than medicines': Care of the Mentally Ill in South Australia, 1858–1884*, Journal of Australian Colonial History, 4(1), 81–103, 2002.

6    Whitridge W, *Statistics of insanity in South Australia,* South Australian Register, Monday 17 October 1859, p. 3.

7    Australian Bureau of Statistics. *Australian Historical Population Statistics, Cat. No. 3105.0.65.001,* Canberra, Commonwealth of Australia, 2006.

8    Ibid. 6.

9    Lunacy Act 1847. South Australia Parliament. https://dspace.flinders.edu.au/xmlui/handle/2328/2048 (accessed 20 July 2020).

10   Ibid. 5.

11   Ibid. 5, pp. 84–87.

12   The Lunatics Act 1864. South Australia Parliament. https://dspace.flinders.edu.au/xmlui/handle/2328/2485 (accessed 20 July 2020).

13   Ibid. 5.

14   Paterson A, *The Lunatic Asylum*, South Australian Chronicle and Weekly Mail, Saturday 11 March 1871, p. 11.

15   Ibid. 4.

16   Ibid. 14.

17   Anonymous, *Our insane asylums Dr Cleland's report*, Adelaide Observer, Saturday 6 July 1901, p. 43.

18   Ibid. 4.

19   An Eye-witness, *the Adelaide Hospital for the Insane No. 1,* South Australian Register, Wednesday 27 November 1878, p. 5.

20   Ibid. 5, p. 91.

21   Report on the Hospitals for the Insane for the Year 1886, Government Printer, Adelaide, 1887.

22   Cleland WL, *Lunatic Asylums Annual Report*, Adelaide Observer, Saturday 2 June 1900, p. 15 (2).

23 Bell M, *From the 1870s to the 1970s: the changing face of public psychiatry in South Australia*, Australasian Psychiatry, 11 (1), 79–86, 2003.

24 Jalland P, *Old Age in Australia: a History*, Melbourne, Melbourne University Press, 2015, p. 18.

25 Garton S, *Out of Luck: Poor Australians and Social Welfare 1788–1988*, Sydney, Allen & Unwin, 1990, p. 47.

26 Ibid. 24.

27 Anonymous, *Report of the Destitute Commission*, Express and Telegraph, Wednesday 21 October 1885, p. 6 (2).

28 Ibid. 24.

29 Lindsay A, *The Destitute Board Annual Departmental Report*, Adelaide Observer, Saturday 15 September 1900, p. 16.

30 Ibid. 21.

31 Anonymous, *Enquiry by the Board, Statements of Officials*, Adelaide Observer, Saturday 14 July 1894, p. 41 (2).

32 Ibid. 24.

33 Anonymous, *Social Evils, the Destitute Asylum*, South Australian Advertiser, Wednesday 25 April 1860, p. 5.

34 Special Reporter, *Our Aged Poor, the Destitute Asylum*, Adelaide Advertiser, Friday 13 May 1898, p. 6 (2).

35 Special Correspondent, *The Destitute Asylum*, Weekly Herald, Saturday 5 November 1898, p. 9 (3).

36 Anonymous, *Coroner's Inquest, Determined Suicide*, Evening Journal, Monday 6 December 1880, p. 2.

37 Anonymous, *Coroner's Inquests, Suicide at the Destitute Asylum*, Adelaide Observer, Saturday 9 November 1889, p. 33.

38 Anonymous, *Inquest on Suicide*, South Australian Register, Wednesday 10 March 1875, p. 6.

39 Anonymous, *Law and Criminal Courts, De Lunatico Inquirendo*, Adelaide Observer, Saturday 22 November 1873, p. 5.

40 Skerritt P, Ellis A, Prendergast F, Harrold C, Blackmore H, Derham B, *Psychiatry in Western Australia since Federation: an eloquent testimony*, Australasian Psychiatry, 9 (3), 226–228, 2001.

41 Hetherington P, *Paupers, Poor Relief & Poor Houses in Western Australia 1829–1910*, UWA Publishing, Crawley, 2009, pp. 21–25.

42 States Records Office of WA. https://archive.sro.wa.gov.au/index.php/various-records-mental-health-hospitals-au-wa-s4867 (accessed 3 November 2019).

43 Hall J, *'May they rest in peace': The History and Ghosts of the Fremantle Lunatic Asylum*, Hesperian Press, Carlisle WA, 2013, p. 5.

44  Ibid. 40.

45  Ibid. 43, p. 5.

46  Ibid. 43, p. 6.

47  Virtue R, *Lunacy and Social Reform in Western Australia 1886–1903,* Studies in Western Australia History, 1, 29–65, 1977.

48  Ibid.

49  Ibid. 7.

50  Ibid. 40.

51  Ibid. 47, p. 33.

52  Ibid. 43, p. 11–12.

53  Ibid. 47, pp. 33–34.

54  Ibid. 43, p. 41.

55  Ibid. 47, p. 37.

56  Ibid. 43, p. 41.

57  Ibid. 47, p. 40.

58  Ibid. 47, p. 43.

59  Ibid. 47, p. 48.

60  Ibid. 43, p. 15.

61  State Records Office of Western Australia, *Register of male/female patients and admissions Fremantle Asylum, S4507-Cons 1120 25.*

62  Tamblyn M, *Johns, Joseph Bolitho (1827–1900),* Australian Dictionary of Biography, National Centre of Biography, Australian National University, http://adb.edu.au/biography/johns-joseph-bolitho-3859/text6139, published first in hardcopy 1972 (accessed online 15 September 2019).

63  Ibid. 43, p. 17.

64  Anonymous, *Suicide in Wellington Street, an old man shoots himself,* Western Mail, Saturday 28 April 1894, p. 23.

65  Anonymous, *The suicide in Wellington Street, the wife's story,* Daily News, Friday 27 April 1894, p. 3.

66  Dickey B, *No Charity There: a short history of social welfare in Australia,* Sydney, Allen & Unwin, 1980, p. 55.

67  Ibid. 41, p. 70.

68  Ibid. 7.

69  Ibid. 41, pp. 70–86.

70  Anonymous, *Vigilans et Audax,* West Australian, Friday 13 August 1886, p. 3.

71  Evans RL, *Charitable Institutions of the Queensland Government to 1919,* Masters Thesis, University of Queensland, 1969, p. 19.

72  Lawrence J, *A Century of Psychiatry in Queensland,* Australasian Psychiatry, 10 (2), 155–161, 2002.

73 NSW State Archives, Gladesville Mental Hospital Medical Casebook 10, 4/8139, Case 188.

74 Ibid. 71, pp. 26–31.

75 Queensland Health, *The road to recovery – a history of mental health services in Queensland 1859-2009,* Queensland Government, 2013, p. 4.

76 Ibid. 71, p. 39.

77 Richards J, *Going up the Line to Goodna – a History of Woogaroo Lunatic Asylum, Goodna Mental Hospital, and Wolston Park Hospital 1865–2015,* Queensland Government, 2017, p. 21.

78 Ibid. 75, p. 4.

79 Ibid. 71, pp. 85–90.

80 Ibid. 75, p. 4.

81 Ibid. 71, p. 277.

82 Ibid. 71, pp. 118–120.

83 Ibid. 77, pp. 70–71.

84 Ibid. 71, p. 16.

85 Woogaroo Commission, *Present condition and management of reception houses and the Woogaroo Asylum,* Brisbane Week, Saturday 19 May 1877, p. 20.

86 Ibid. 75, p. 5.

87 Finnane M, *Wolston Park Hospital, 1865–2001: a Retrospect,* Queensland Review, 15 (2), 39–58, 2008, p. 52.

88 Ibid. 7.

89 Anonymous, *Notes and News,* Gympie Times and Mary River Mining Gazette, Thursday 24 September 1896, page 3 (3).

90 Anonymous, *Shocking suicide at Maryborough,* Queensland Times, Ipswich Herald and General Advertiser, Saturday 27 October 1888.

91 Ibid. 71, pp. 147–168.

92 Ibid. 71, p. 46.

93 Patrick R, *The Case of Dr Jonathan Labatt,* John Oxley Journal: a bulletin for historical research in Queensland, 1 (6), 7–15, 1980.

94 Ibid. 71, p. 47.

95 Ibid. 71, p. 48.

96 Ibid. 71, pp. 153–154.

97 Ibid. 71, pp. 153–154.

98 Ibid. 24, p. 19.

## 8 From Federation to the Second World War

1 Australian Bureau of Statistics, *Australian Historical Population Statistics, Cat. No. 3105.0.65.001,* Canberra, Commonwealth of Australia, 2006.

2    Jalland P, *Old Age in Australia: A History*, Melbourne, Melbourne University Press, 2015, pp. 30–31.

3    Davison G, *'Our youth is spent and our backs are bent': The origins of Australian ageism*, In: Walker D, Garton S (eds) Ageing, Australian Cultural History 14, Geelong, Deakin University, 1995, pp. 40–62.

4    In NSW, the hospitals for the insane were rebadged as mental hospitals in 1910 by the Inspector General Eric Sinclair. He changed his title from Inspector General of the Insane to Inspector General of Mental Hospitals in 1918 (see Cummins, CJ. *A History of Medical Administration in NSW 1788–1973*. 2nd edition, Sydney, NSW Department of Health, 2003 p. 102).

5    Report of the Inspector General of Mental Hospitals for the Year Ended 30 June 1935, Government Printer, Sydney, New South Wales.

6    Report of the Inspector General of Mental Hospitals for the Year Ended 30 June 1941, Government Printer, Sydney, New South Wales.

7    Dax EC, *The evolution of community psychiatry*, Australian and New Zealand Journal of Psychiatry, 26, 295–301, 1992.

8    Garton S, *Out of Luck: Poor Australians and Social Welfare 1788–1988,* Sydney, Allen & Unwin, 1990, p. 104.

9    Ibid. 1.

10   State Records Office of Western Australia, Register of male/female patients and admissions Fremantle Asylum AU WA S4507 – cons 1120 25.

11   Anonymous, *Treatment of the Insane*, West Australian, 5 February 1915, p. .3.

12   Report of the Inspector General of the Insane for the year ended 31 December 1919, Fred Wm. Simpson, Government Printer, Perth, 1920.

13   Hetherington P, *Paupers, Poor Relief & Poor Houses in Western Australia 1829–1910*, UWA Publishing, Crawley, 2009, pp. 147–156.

14   Anonymous, *Old Men's Home Inquiry,* Kalgoorlie Western Argus, 6 June 1916, p. 13.

15   Anonymous, *Old Men's Home Inquiry. Commissioner's Findings,* Western Mail, 7 July 1916, p. 40.

16   Anonymous, *Old Men's Home Inquiry. Minister criticised,* Daily News, 14 July 1916, p. 1.

17   Anonymous, *Old Men's Home Inmate's Point of View,* West Australian, 11 August 1916, p. 9.

18   Report of the Inspector of Lunatic Asylums for the Year ending 31 December 1901, J Kemp, Government Printer, Melbourne, 1902.

19   Report of the Inspector General of the Insane for the Year ending 31 December 1907, J Kemp, Government Printer, Melbourne, 1908.

20   Report of the Inspector General of the Insane for the Year ending 31 December 1905, J Kemp, Government Printer, Melbourne, 1906.

21 Report of the Inspector-General of the Insane for the Year 1901, Legislative Assembly NSW, 9 October 1902.

22 Report of the Inspector-General of Mental Hospitals for the Year 1918, Legislative Assembly NSW, 16 October 1919.

23 Garton S, *Medicine and Madness: A Social history of insanity in New South Wales, 1880–1940,* New South Wales University Press, Kensington, 1988, p. 168.

24 Inspector General of the Insane Report for the Year 1913, Legislative Assembly, NSW, 1914.

25 Aftercare. *Aftercare: Our Journey 1907–2017,* Sydney, Australia. www.aftercare.com.au (accessed 8 April 2019).

26 Ibid. 2, p. 32.

27 Cummins CJ, *A History of Medical Administration in NSW 1788–1973,* 2nd edition, Sydney, NSW Department of Health, 2003, p. 200.

28 Gowlland RW, *Troubled asylum: the history of...the Royal Derwent Hospital,* New Norfolk, Tasmania, 1981, pp. 121–137.

29 Parkside Lunatic Asylum, Royal Commission's Report, Adelaide Advertiser, 27 August 1909, p. 6.

30 Bell M, *From the 1870s to the 1970s: the changing face of public psychiatry in South Australia,* Australasian Psychiatry, 11 (1), 79–86, 2003.

31 Cleland WL, *Insane at Parkside. Interesting Annual Report,* Daily Herald, 28 June 1912, p. 8.

32 Inspector-General of Hospitals, *Mental Defectives. Report by Inspector General.* Adelaide Register, 15 September 1916, p. 9 (2).

33 Inspector-General of Hospitals, *Mental Hospital Inspector's Annual Report,* Daily Herald, 18 September 1918, p. 8.

34 Anonymous, *Old People's Home,* Adelaide Register, 27 January 1917, p. 8.

35 Queensland Health, *The Road to Recovery – a history of mental health services in Queensland 1859–2009,* Queensland Government, 2013.

36 Inspector of Hospitals for the Insane, *Hospitals for the Insane, Facts for 1910,* Brisbane Telegraph, 27 October 1911, p. 3.

37 Lawrence J, *A Century of Psychiatry in Queensland,* Australasian Psychiatry, 10 (2), 155–161, 2002.

38 Lewis M, *Managing Madness: Psychiatry and Society in Australia, 1788–1980,* Australian Government Publishing Service, Canberra, 1988, p. 47.

39 Ibid. 35.

40 Evans RL, *Charitable Institutions of the Queensland Government to 1919,* Master's Thesis, University of Queensland, 1969, p. 104.

41 Ibid. 37.

42 Ibid. 38.

43 Ibid. 35.

44 Inspector of Hospitals for the Insane, *Hospitals for the Insane. Medical Superintendent's Report,* Daily Standard, 10 October 1917, p. 3.

45 Ibid. 40, pp. 190–202.

46 Norris R, *Deakin, Alfred (1856–1919),* Australian Dictionary of Biography, National Centre of Biography, Australian National University, http://adb.anu.edu.au/biography/deakin-alfred-5927/text10099, published first in hard copy 1981, (accessed online 10 October 2019).

47 Draper B, Withall A, *Young onset dementia,* Internal Medicine Journal, 46(7), 779–786, 2016.

48 Ibid. 46.

49 Alfred Deakin Prime Ministerial Library, *Alfred Deakin.* https://www.deakin.edu.au/library/special-collections/alfred (accessed 17 November 2020).

50 Ibid. 46.

51 National Archives of Australia, *Alfred Deakin: after office.* https://www.naa.gov.au/explore-collection/australias-prime-ministers/alfred-deakin/after-office (accessed 17 November 2020).

52 Ibid. 45.

53 Coleman W, *Six problems in the biography of Alfred Deakin,* Agenda, 25, (1), ANU Press, Canberra, 2018.

54 Toole JF, *Dementia in world leaders and its effects upon international events: the examples of Franklin D Roosevelt and T Woodrow Wilson,* European Journal of Neurology, 6, 115–119, 1999.

55 Ibid. 2, p. 81.

56 Anonymous, *The Aged Insane, Remarkable Cases at Parkside,* Adelaide Mail, 11 December 1920, p. 2.

57 Piggin S, *Abbott, William Edward (Wingen) (1844–1924),* Australian Dictionary of Biography, National Centre of Biography, Australian National University, http://adb.anu.edu.au/biography/abbott-william-edward-wingen-6/text8233, published first in hardcopy 1979 (accessed online 25 September 2019).

58 Van der Poorten, HM, *Darrell, George Frederick Price (1851–1921),* Australian Dictionary of Biography, National Centre of Biography, Australian National University, http://adb.anu.edu.au/biography/darrell-george-frederick-price-3369/text5089, published first in hardcopy 1972 (accessed online 10 October 2019).

59 Ibid.

60 Ibid. 57.

61 Ibid. 26, p. 114.

62 These data were extracted from the NSW Inspector General of Mental Hospitals Annual Reports from 1920 through to 1939/40.

63 NSW Inspector General of Mental Hospitals, Annual Report for the Year ended 30 June 1928, p. 10.

64 Ibid. 2, pp. 82–86.

65 Anonymous, *Newington's Cold Charity*, Truth, 2 September 1928, p. 21.

66 Anonymous, *Pitiful Scenes Lidcombe Hospital*, Sydney Morning Herald, 1 February 1928, p. 16.

67 Ibid.

68 Ibid. 2, pp. 82–86.

69 Ibid. 62.

70 Anonymous, *The Mental Hospital Services*, Medical Journal of Australia, June 20, 678–680, 1925.

71 Anonymous, *The Mental Hospital Services*, Medical Journal of Australia, November 20, 705–706, 1926.

72 Anonymous, *The Mental Hospital Services*, Medical Journal of Australia, November 26, 755–758, 1927.

73 Higgs WG, *'Help the Insane'*, Melbourne Herald, 20 December 1928, p. 21.

74 Holt AG, *Hillcrest Hospital: the first 50 years*, Victoria, the Hillcrest Hospital Heritage Committee, 1999.

75 Ibid. 37, p. 43.

76 Ibid. 62.

77 Report of the Inspector General of Mental Hospitals for the Year ended 30 June 1940, Government Printer, Sydney 1941, p. 5.

78 Ibid. 22, p. 168.

79 Ibid. 37, p. 43.

80 Report of the Inspector General of Mental Hospitals for the Year ended 30 June 1938, Government Printer, Sydney 1939.

81 Report of the Inspector General of Mental Hospitals for the Year ended 30 June 1937, Government Printer, Sydney 1938.

82 Ford R, *Sexuality and 'Madness': regulating women's gender deviance through the asylum, the Orange Asylum in the 1930s,* In: Coleborne, C. & MacKinnon, D. (eds), 'Madness' in Australia: histories, heritage, and the asylum. St Lucia, Queensland, Queensland University Press, 2003, pp. 109–119.

83 Hughes M, *Providing responsive services to LGBT individuals with dementia,* In: Westwood S, Price E, (Eds.), Lesbian, gay, bisexual and trans individuals living with dementia: Concepts, practice and rights. London, England, Routledge New York, 2016.

84    Peisah C, Burns K, Edmonds S, Brodaty H, *Rendering visible the previously invisible in health care: the ageing LGBTI communities*, Medical Journal of Australia, 209(3), 106–108, 2018.

85    Anonymous, *Mental Cases, Overcrowded Homes,* Weekly Times, 14 November 1936, p. 32.

86    Jones WE, *Mental Hygiene, Former Director's Report,* The Age, 1 December 1937, p. 6.

87    Anonymous, *Insanity Ratio, Grave Official Review,* The Age, 23 November 1938, p. 6.

88    Annual Reports of the Inspector General of Hospitals for the Insane 1937/38 to 1941/42, Government Printer, Brisbane 1939–1943, Queensland State Archives, Item ID436477.

89    Anonymous, *Plan for New State Home for Aged at Lota,* Brisbane Telegraph, 26 January 1938, p. 1.

90    Anonymous, *The Hospital Board,* Brisbane Week, 21 March 1930, p. 11.

91    Anonymous, *Inmates at Dunwich,* Brisbane Telegraph, 15 October 1940, p. 13.

92    Anonymous, *Minister to Inquire on Dunwich conditions,* Courier-Mail, 10 July 1944, p. 3.

93    Anonymous, *Suicide indicts Dunwich in Farewell Letter,* Brisbane Telegraph, 7 July 1944, p. 2.

94    Ibid. 74, p. 38.

95    Director-General Medical Services, *Says Mental Homes Should Be Improved,* Adelaide News, 21 October 1941, p. 3.

96    Anonymous, *Mental Hospital to be Improved,* Adelaide News, 4 August 1937, p. 7.

97    Anonymous, *Old Folks are not at Home,* Adelaide Mail, 22 May 1943, p. 11.

98    Whyntie A, *The History of Sunset Hospital,* Perth, B&S Printing, 1999.

99    State Records Office of Western Australia, S675 Cons752 1933/0564 Annual Report of the Inspector General of the Insane for the Year ended 31 December 1932.

100   State Records Office of Western Australia, S4410 Cons1067 1941/114 Report of the Inspector General of the Insane for the Year ended 31 December 1940.

101   Harris J, *Hiding the bodies: the myth of the humane colonisation of Aboriginal Australia.* Aboriginal History, 27, 79–104, 2003.

102   Rowley CD, *Outcasts in White Australia, Melbourne,* Pelican Books, 1973, p. 9.

103   O'Shane P, *The Psychological Impact of White Colonialism on Aboriginal People,* Australasian Psychiatry, 3 (3), 149–153, June 1995.

104   Ibid. 101.

105   Maynard J, *Australian history – Lifting Haze or Descending Fog?* Aboriginal History, 27, 139–145, 2003.

106   Ibid. 10.

107   Anonymous, *Patient's Death,* Hobart Mercury, 12 October 1932, p. 5.

## 9 International influences in the Twentieth Century

1    Robinson RA, *The Evolution of Geriatric Psychiatry,* Medical History, 16(2), 184–193, 1972.

2    Roth M, *The natural history of mental disorders in old age,* Journal of Mental Science, 101, 281–301, 1955.

3    Beveridge W, *Social insurance and allied services – a report,* London, HM Stationery Office, November 1942.

4    Goedert M, *Oskar Fischer and the study of dementia,* Brain, 132, 1102–1111, 2009.

5    Maurer K, Volk S, Gerbaldo H, *Auguste D and Alzheimer's disease,* The Lancet, 349, May 24, 1546–1549, 1997.

6    Ibid. 4.

7    Fox P, *From senility to Alzheimer's disease: The rise of the Alzheimer's disease movement,* The Milbank Quarterly, 67, (1), 58–102, 1989, p. 61.

8    Ibid. 1.

9    Ibid. 7.

10   Davis G, *The most deadly disease of asylumdom: general paralysis of the insane and Scottish psychiatry c1840–1940,* Journal of the Royal College of Physicians of Edinburgh, 42, 266–273, 2012.

11   Nitrini R, *A cure of one of the most frequent types of dementia: a historical parallel,* Alzheimer's Disease and Associated Disorders, 19, 156–158, 2005.

12   Ibid. 1.

13   Rybakowski JK, *120th anniversary of the Kraepelinian dichotomy of psychiatric disorders,* Current Psychiatry Reports, 21, 65, 2019.

14   Schwartz MF, Stark JA, *The distinction between Alzheimer's disease and senile dementia: Historical Considerations,* Journal of the History of the Neurosciences, 1 (3), 169–187, 2009.

15   Inspector-General of Mental Hospitals, *Report for the year ended 30 June 1931,* Legislative Assembly, NSW, 1932.

16   Ibid. 1.

17   Ibid. 2.

18   Mayer-Gross W, *Electric convulsion treatment in patients over 60,* Journal of Mental Science, 91, 101–103, 1945.

19   Kay DWK, Beamish P, Roth M. *Old age mental disorders in Newcastle upon Tyne Part 1: A study of prevalence,* British Journal of Psychiatry, 110, 146–158, 1964.

20   Kay DWK, Beamish P, Roth M. *Old age mental disorders in Newcastle upon Tyne Part 2: A study of possible social and medical causes,* British Journal of Psychiatry, 110, 668–682, 1964.

21   Kiloh LG, *Pseudo-dementia,* Acta Psychiatrica Scandinavica, 37, 336–351, 1961.

22 Wilson K, Mottram P, Sivanranthan A, Nightingale A, *Antidepressants versus placebo for the depressed elderly*, Cochrane Database of Systematic Reviews 2001, Issue 1. Art. No.: CD000561. DOI: 10.1002/14651858.CD000561.

23 Cuijpers P, Karyotaki E, Pot AM, Park M, Reynolds III, CF, *Managing depression in older age: Psychological interventions,* Maturitas, 79, 160–169, 2014.

24 Miller MD, Mark D, *Using Psychoanalytically Oriented Psychotherapy with the Elderly,* Jefferson Journal of Psychiatry, 4 (1), 13–21, 1986.

25 American Psychiatric Association, *Diagnostic and Statistical Manual of Mental Disorders. Third Edition,* Washington DC, American Psychiatric Association, 1980.

26 American Psychiatric Association. *Diagnostic and Statistical Manual of Mental Disorders, Fifth Edition.* Arlington VA, American Psychiatric Association, 2013.

27 McKhann G, Drachman D, Folstein M, Katzman R, Price D, Stadlan EM, *Clinical diagnosis of Alzheimer's disease: report of the NINCDS-ADRDA Work Group under the auspices of the Department of Health and Human Services Task Force on Alzheimer's disease*, Neurology, 34(7), 939–944, 1984.

28 McKhann GM, Knopman DS, Chertkow H, *et al.*, *The diagnosis of dementia due to Alzheimer's disease: recommendations from the National Institute on Aging-Alzheimer's Association workgroups on diagnostic guidelines for Alzheimer's disease,* Alzheimer's and Dementia 7(3), 263–269, 2011.

29 Knopman DS, Petersen RC, Jack Jr CR, *A brief history of 'Alzheimer's disease': Multiple meanings separated by a common name,* Neurology, 92(22), 1053–1059, 2019.

30 Massoud F, Gauthier S, *Update on the pharmacological treatment of Alzheimer's disease,* Current Neuropharmacology, 8, 69–80, 2010.

31 National Institute for Health and Care Excellence, *Donepezil, galantamine, rivastigmine and memantine for the treatment of Alzheimer's disease* www.nice.org.uk/guidance/ta217 (accessed 12 January 2021).

32 Brodaty H, Ames D, Snowdon J, *et al.*, *A randomized placebo-controlled trial of risperidone for the treatment of aggression, agitation and psychosis of dementia,* Journal of Clinical Psychiatry, 64, 134–143, 2003.

33 Gurwitz JH, Bonner A, Berwick DM, *Reducing excessive use of antipsychotic agents in nursing homes.* JAMA, 318(2), 118–119, 2017.

34 Draper B, Low LF, *What is the effectiveness of old age mental health services?* World Health Organization Regional Office for Europe Health Evidence Network. Copenhagen, Denmark, 2004.

35 Rollett C, Parker J, *Population and Family*, In: Halsey AH, (ed) Trends in British Society since 1900. UK, Palgrave MacMillan, 1972, pp. 20–63.

36 US Bureau of the Census, *65+ in the United States*, Current Population Reports, Special Studies, P23–190, Washington DC, US Government Printing Office, 1996.

37  Australian Bureau of Statistics, *Australian Historical Population Statistics, Cat. No. 3105.0.65.001,* Canberra, Commonwealth of Australia, 2006.

38  Hicks J, Allen G, *A Century of Change: Trends in UK statistics since 1900,* Research Paper 99/111, Social and General Statistics Section, House of Commons Library, 21 December 1999 http://www.parliament.uk (accessed 19 May 2020).

39  Ibid. 36.

40  Age UK, *Our history.* https://www.ageuk.org.uk/about-us/people/our-history/ (accessed 28 May 2020).

41  Ibid. 3.

42  Ibid. 37.

43  Office for National Statistics, *Living longer: is age 70 the new age 65?* November 2019 https://www.ons.gov.uk/peoplepopulationandcommunity/birthsdeathsandmarriages/ ageing/articles/livinglongerisage70thenewage65/2019-11-19 (accessed 21 May 2020).

44  Nascher I, *Geriatrics,* New York Medical Journal, 90, 358–359, 1909.

45  Denham M, *A Brief History of the Care of the Elderly.* British Geriatrics Society, June 2016  https://www.bgs.org.uk/resources/a-brief-history-of-the-care-of-the-elderly (accessed 6 May 2020).

46  Thane P, *Old Age in English History. Past Experiences, Present Issues,* Oxford University Press, Oxford, 2000, pp. 436–438.

47  Ibid. 45.

48  Webster C, *The elderly and the early National Health Service,* In: Life and Death and the Elderly ed. Pelling M, Smith R, London, Routledge, 1991, 165–193.

49  Ibid. 45.

50  Ibid. 46, pp. 445–446.

51  Hilton C, *Psychogeriatrics in England in the 1950s: greater knowledge with little impact on the provision of services,* History of Psychiatry, 27(10), 3–20, 2016.

52  Hilton C, *Psychogeriatrics in England: Its route to recognition by the government as a distinct medical specialty c1970–89,* Medical History, 60(2), 206–228, 2016.

53  Shepherd M, *Lewis, Sir Aubrey Julian (1900–1975),* Australian Dictionary of Biography, National Centre of Biography, Australian National University, http:/adb. anu.edu.au/biography/lewis-sir-aubrey-julian-10823/text19201, published first in hardcopy 2000 (accessed 13 January 2021).

54  Ibid. 51.

55  Sanders A, *Dax, Eric Cunningham (1908–2008),* Obituaries Australia, National Centre of Biography, Australian National University, http://oa.anu.edu.au/obituary/ dax-eric-cunningham-13941/text24835 (accessed 13 January 2021).

56  Cook L, Dax E, Maclay W, *The geriatric problem in mental hospitals,* Lancet, 259, 377–382, 1952.

57  Ibid. 52, p. 213.

58  Arie T, *The first year of the Goodmayes psychiatric service for old people,* Lancet ii, 1179–1182, 1970.

59  Hilton C, *The development of psychogeriatric services in England from circa 1940 until 1989,* Doctoral thesis, King's College, London, 2014, p. 189.

60  Ibid. 52.

61  Ibid. 59, p. 254.

62  Ibid. 52.

63  Chester TE, *The Guillebaud Report,* Public Administration. 34 (2), 199–210, June 1956.

64  Thane P, *History of Social Care in England,* Memorandum submitted to the House of Commons' Health Committee Inquiry: Social Care, October 2009 https://publications.parliament.uk/pa/cm200809/cmselect/cmhealth/1021/1021we49.htm (accessed 28 May 2020).

65  Ibid. 59, pp. 266–267.

66  Peace SM, *The development of residential and nursing home care in the United Kingdom,* In: Katz, JS, Peace SM, eds. End of Life in Care Homes: a Palliative Approach. Oxford, Oxford University Press, pp. 15–42, 2003.

67  Arie T, Dunn T, *A 'Do-it-yourself' psychiatric-geriatric joint patient unit,* Lancet, ii, 1313–1316, 1973.

68  Hilton C, *Joint geriatric and old-age psychiatric wards in the UK, 1940s to early 1990s: a historical study,* International Journal of Geriatric Psychiatry, 29, 1071–1078, 2014.

69  Ibid. 67, p. 1315.

70  Ibid. 68.

71  Ibid. 59, p. 307.

72  Wattis J, Wattis L, Arie T, *Psychogeriatrics: A National Survey of a New Branch of Psychiatry,* British Medical Journal, 282, 1529–33, 1981.

73  Ibid. 59, p. 275–283.

74  Ibid. 52.

75  Ibid. 64.

76  Mary Marshall eFestchrift, Personal Social Services Unit, University of Manchester, 2005. Microsoft Word – marymarshall eFestschrift booklet web.doc (pssru.ac.uk) (accessed 18 January 2021).

77  Fleming R, Zeisel J, Bennett K, *World Alzheimer Report 2020 Design Dignity Dementia: dementia-related design and the built environment Volume 1,* London, England, Alzheimer's Disease International, 2020.

78  McSherry W, *Dignity in care: meanings, myths and the reality of making it work in practice,* Nursing Times, 106(40), 20–23, 2010.

79  Report of the Mid Staffordshire NHS Foundation Trust Public Inquiry, London: The Stationery Office, 2013. www.midstaffspublicinquiry.com (accessed 20 March 2017).

80  Ibid. 77.

81  Laver K, Cumming R, Dyer S, *et al.*, *Clinical Practice Guidelines for Dementia in Australia*, Medical Journal of Australia, 204(5), 191–193, 2016.

82  Ibid. 46, p. 455.

83  Hilton C, Arie T, *The Development of Old Age Psychiatry in the UK,* In: Abou-Saleh MT, Katona C, Kumar A, (Eds) Principles and Practice of Geriatric Psychiatry, 3rd ed, John Wiley, 2011, pp. 7–11.

84  Australian Government Department of Health, *Psychological Treatment Services for people with mental illness in Residential Aged Care Facilities,* Canberra, Australian Government Department of Health, 2018.

85  Joint Commissioning Panel for Mental Health, *Guidance for commissioners of older people's mental health services* May 2013 http://www.jcpmh.info/wp-content/uploads/jcpmh-olderpeople-guide.pdf (accessed 19 January 2021).

86  World Health Organisation, *Mental Health Problems of Aging and the Aged,* Geneva: WHO, 1959.

87  World Health Organisation, *Psychogeriatrics*, Geneva, WHO, 1972, pp. 10–11.

88  World Health Organisation and GPWorldPA, *Organisation of care in psychiatry of the elderly – a technical consensus statement,* Aging and Mental Health, 2, 246–252, 1998.

89  Alzheimer's Disease International, *About Us.* https://www.alzint.org/about-us/ (accessed 18 January 2021).

90  Alzheimer's Disease International, *Our History.* https://www.alzint.org/our-history/ (accessed 18 January 2021).

91  Fejer I, *From Robin Hood to the Pharaohs – History of the Forming Phase of IPA,* The International Psychogeriatric Association Newsletter, 8(1), 24–28, 1991.

92  Folstein ME, Folstein SE, McHugh PR, *Mini-Mental State: a practical method for grading the state of patients for the clinician,* Journal of Psychiatric Research, 12, 189–198, 1975.

93  Basic D, Rowland JT, Conforti DA, *et al.*, *The validity of the Rowland Universal Dementia Assessment Scale (RUDAS) in a multicultural cohort of community-dwelling older persons with early dementia,* Alzheimer's Disease and Associated Disorders, 23,124–129, 2009.

94  LoGiudice D, Smith K, Thomas J, *et al.*, *Kimberley Indigenous Cognitive Assessment tool (KICA): Development of a cognitive assessment tool for older Indigenous Australians,* International Psychogeriatrics, 18, 269–280, 2006.

95  Wilson D, *Quantifying the quiet epidemic: Diagnosing dementia in late 20th Century Britain,* History of the Human Sciences, 27(5), 126–146, 2014.

96  Mace N, Rabins P, *The 36-Hour Day: A family guide to caring for persons with Alzheimer's disease, related dementing illnesses, and memory loss in later life*, 1st ed, Johns Hopkins University Press, Baltimore, 1981.

## 10 National Developments after the Second World War to 1980

1   Australian Bureau of Statistics, *Australian Historical Population Statistics, Cat. No. 3105.0.65.001*, Canberra, Commonwealth of Australia, 2006.

2   Jalland P, *Old Age in Australia: a History*, Melbourne, Melbourne University Press, 2015, pp. 126–128.

3   Hetherington J, *Is old age a crime?* Melbourne Herald, 7 October 1950, p. 15.

4   Ibid. 2, p. 129.

5   Ibid. 2, pp. 171–186.

6   Australian Association of Gerontology, *Our History*, Our History – Australian Association of Gerontology (aag.asn.au) (accessed 4 February 2021).

7   Ibid. 2 pp. 150–151.

8   Hutchinson B, *Old People in a Modern Australian Community: A social Survey*, MUP Carlton 1954.

9   Stoller A, *Growing Old – Problems of Old Age in the Australian Community*, Melbourne, Cheshires, 1960.

10  Ibid. 8.

11  Sax S, *How it all began – geriatric medicine in Australia*, Australian Journal on Ageing, 13 (1), 5–7, 1994.

12  Ibid. 2, pp. 196–199.

13  Ibid. 11.

14  Ibid. 11, p. 6.

15  Ibid. 2, pp. 204–207.

16  Ibid. 11.

17  Hunter C, *Nursing and care for the aged in Victoria: 1950s to 1970s*, Nursing Inquiry, 12, 278–286, 2005.

18  Ibid. 11.

19  Ibid. 17.

20  Ibid. 11.

21  Ibid. 2, pp. 208–209.

22  Ibid. 11.

23  Ibid. 11.

24  Hunter CE, *Doctoring old age. A social history of geriatric medicine in Victoria*, Doctoral thesis, University of Melbourne, February 2003, p. 291.

25  Warner D, *Kew Conditions 'Horrifying'*, Melbourne Herald, 14 December 1946, p. 4.

26  Ibid.

27  Ibid.

28  Rubinstein WD, Rubinstein HL, *Menders of the Mind. A History of the Royal Australian and New Zealand College of Psychiatrists, 1946–1996,* Oxford, Oxford University Press, 1996, p. 12.

29  Stafford BFR, *Division of Mental Hygiene Annual Report 1950–51,* QS 201/1, 1937–1963. Brisbane, AH Tucker Government Printer, 1951, p. 2.

30  Tipping EW, *There's a lot to be done yet out at Kew,* Melbourne Herald, 2 October 1954, p. 5.

31  Stoller A, Arscott KW, *Report on Mental Health Facilities and Needs of Australia,* Canberra, Commonwealth of Australia, 1955.

32  InflationTool, *Value of 1955 Australian dollars today,* Value of 1955 Australian Dollars today – Inflation Calculator (inflationtool.com) (accessed 6 May 2022).

33  Ibid. 31, p. 169.

34  Roth M, *The natural history of mental disorders in old age,* Journal of Mental Science, 101, 281–301, 1955.

35  Cummins CJ, *A History of Medical Administration in NSW 1788–1973,* 2nd edition, Sydney, NSW Department of Health, 2003, p. 115.

36  McClemens, the Honourable Mr. Justice, *Report of the Callan Park Mental Hospital Royal Commission,* Sydney, Government Printer, 1961, p. 244.

37  Daniels D, *Social security payments for the aged, people with disabilities and carers 1901 to 2010,* Canberra, Parliament of Australia, 2011.

38  Dax EC, *The evolution of community psychiatry,* Australian and New Zealand Journal of Psychiatry, 26, 295–301, 1992.

39  Lewis M, Garton S, *Mental Health in Australia, 1788–2015: A History of Responses to Cultural and Social Challenges,* In: Minas H, Lewis M, (eds) Mental Health in Asia and the Pacific. Historical and Cultural Perspectives, New York, Springer Nature, 2017, pp. 289–313.

40  Ibid. 38.

41  Ibid. 39.

42  Ibid. 39.

43  Peterson BH, *The Age of Ageing,* Australian and New Zealand Journal of Psychiatry, 7, 9–15, 1973.

44  Ibid. 37.

45  Ibid. 2, p. 215.

46  Ibid. 11.

47  Parliament of Australia, *Residential care for the aged: an overview of Government policy from 1962 to 1993,* Social Policy Group, Department of the Parliamentary Library, Canberra, Commonwealth of Australia, 1993.

48  Ibid. 2, pp. 218–222.

49 Ibid. 24, pp. 192–195.

50 Burvill P, *Psychiatric population of nursing homes,* Australian and New Zealand Journal of Psychiatry, 3, 75–79, 1969.

51 Sax S, *Report for the Consultative Committee for the Care of the Aged,* NSW Department of Public Health, August 1965.

52 Ibid. 2, p. 219.

53 Lefroy RB, *Permanent Care of Elderly People in Institutions,* Medical Journal of Australia, 4 October, 707–12, 1969.

54 Healy J, *Community services: long term care at home?* In: Kendig HL, McCallum J (eds) Grey Policy: Australian policies for an ageing society. Sydney, Allen & Unwin, 1990, pp. 127–149.

55 Ibid. 47.

56 Ibid. 54.

57 Ibid. 47.

58 Howe AL, *From states of confusion to a national action plan for dementia care: the development of policies for dementia care in Australia,* International Journal of Geriatric Psychiatry, 12, 165–171, 1997.

59 Carter J, *States of confusion: Australian policies and the elderly confused,* Social Welfare Research Centre Report Proceedings, No. 4, University of New South Wales, Sydney, 1981.

60 Ibid. 58.

## 11 State Developments after the Second World War to 1980

1 Dax EC, *Asylum to Community. The Development of the Mental Hygiene Service in Victoria, Australia,* Melbourne, FW Cheshire, 1961, p. 15.

2 Section of Mental Hygiene, *Report under Section 4 of 'The Mental Hygiene Act of 1938' for 1944/45,* Queensland Government, 1946.

3 Division of Mental Hygiene, *Annual Report for year ending 30th June 1955,* Brisbane, AH Tucker Government Printer, 1956.

4 Inspector-General of Mental Hospitals. *Report of the Inspector-General of Mental Hospitals for the year ending 30th June 1945,* Sydney, Thomas Henry Tennant Government Printer, 1947.

5 Inspector-General of Mental Hospitals, *Report of the Inspector-General of Mental Hospitals for the year ending 30th June 1956,* Sydney, AH Pettifer Government Printer, 1957.

6 Ibid. 4.

7 Inspector-General of Mental Hospitals, *Report of the Inspector-General of Mental Hospitals for the year ending 30th June 1946,* Sydney, Thomas Henry Tennant Government Printer, 1947.

8    Inspector-General of Mental Hospitals, *Report of the Inspector-General of Mental Hospitals for the year ending 30th June 1947*, Sydney, AH Pettifer Acting Government Printer, 1948.

9    Inspector-General of Mental Hospitals, *Report of the Inspector-General of Mental Hospitals for the year ending 30th June 1948*, Sydney, AH Pettifer Acting Government Printer, 1949.

10   Inspector-General of Mental Hospitals. *Report of the Inspector-General of Mental Hospitals for the year ending 30th June 1949*, Sydney, AH Pettifer Acting Government Printer, 1950.

11   Stoller A, Arscott KW, *Report on Mental Health Facilities and Needs of Australia*. Canberra, Commonwealth of Australia, 1955, p. 82.

12   Cook L, Dax E, Maclay W, *The geriatric problem in mental hospitals*, Lancet, 259, 377–382, 1952.

13   Ibid. 1 pp. 19–20.

14   Bower H, *Dr Herbert Bower – Psychiatrist 19/12/1914 – 29/8/2004*, Australasian Psychiatry, 12(4), 430–432, 2004.

15   Mental Hygiene Authority, *Report of the Mental Hygiene Authority for the year ended 30th June 1955*, Melbourne, WM Houston Government Printer, 1956.

16   Mental Hygiene Authority, *Report of the Mental Hygiene Authority for the year ended 31st December, 1956*, Melbourne, WM Houston Government Printer, 1957.

17   Bower HM, *The Beattie-Smith Lectures – Part 1. Old Age in Western Society*, Medical Journal of Australia, II(8), 285–292, 1964, p. 285.

18   Ibid.

19   Bower HM, *The Beattie-Smith Lectures – Part 2. Old Age in Western Society*, Medical Journal of Australia, II(9), 325–332, 1964.

20   Ibid. 1, pp. 134–137.

21   Hunter CE, *Doctoring old age. A social history of geriatric medicine in Victoria*, Doctoral thesis, University of Melbourne, February 2003, pp. 195–196.

22   Teltscher B, *Misreferral of patients to a geriatric hospital*, The Medical Journal of Australia, i: 218–219, 1968.

23   Mental Hygiene Authority, *Report of the Mental Hygiene Authority for the year ended 31st December, 1957*, Melbourne, WM Houston Government Printer, 1958, p. 53.

24   Mental Hygiene Authority, *Report of the Mental Hygiene Authority for the year ended 31st December, 1958*, Melbourne, WM Houston Government Printer, 1959, p. 53.

25   Mental Hygiene Authority, *Report of the Mental Hygiene Authority for the year ended 31st December, 1959*, Melbourne, WM Houston Government Printer, 1960.

26   Bower HM, *Sensory stimulation and the treatment of senile dementia*, Medical Journal of Australia, i(22), 1113–1119, 1967.

27    Robson B, *From mental hygiene to community mental health: psychiatrists and Victorian public administration from the 1940s to 1990s,* Provenance: The Journal of Public Record Office Victoria, issue 7, 2008, ISSN 1832–2522.

28    Bower HM, *The first psychogeriatric day-centre in Victoria,* Medical Journal of Australia, i(May 17), 1047–1050, 1969.

29    Ibid. 14.

30    Anonymous, *Bower praised as Australian doyen,* IPA Bulletin, Winter 1995 – Spring 1996, p. 12.

31    Mental Hygiene Authority, *Report of the Mental Hygiene Authority for the year ended 31st December, 1962,* Melbourne, AC Brooks Government Printer, 1963.

32    Davies GV, *The geriatric population of a mental hospital,* The Medical Journal of Australia, I, 181–184, 1965.

33    Davies GV, *Female geriatric admissions to a mental hospital,* The Medical Journal of Australia, ii, 309–312, 1965.

34    Mental Hygiene Authority, *Report of the Mental Hygiene Authority for the year ended 31st December, 1968,* Melbourne, Government Printer, 1969.

35    Mental Hygiene Authority, *Report of the Mental Hygiene Authority for the year ended 31st December, 1972,* Melbourne, Government Printer, 1973.

36    Harrison AW, *Assessment and accommodation of demented patients in the community,* Australian and New Zealand Journal of Psychiatry, 15, 53–55, 1981.

37    Draper B, *G Vernon Davies: Unsung pioneer of old age psychiatry in Victoria,* Australasian Psychiatry, 30(2), 203–205, 2022.

38    Walter J, *Davies, Alan Fraser (1924–1987),* Australian Dictionary of Biography, National Centre of Biography, Australian National University, https://adb.anu.edu.au/biography/davies-alan-fraser-12406/text22303 published first in hardcopy 2007 (accessed online 2 February 2021).

39    Ibid. 16.

40    Ibid. 23 p. 57.

41    Davies V, *Clinical advances in geriatric psychiatry,* The Medical Journal of Australia, ii, 43–46, 1959.

42    Ibid. 25.

43    Mental Hygiene Authority, *Report of the Mental Hygiene Authority for the year ended 31st December, 1961,* Melbourne, AC Brooks Government Printer, 1962.

44    Davies GV, *The relation of physical and mental disease in later life,* Medical Journal of Australia, July 22, 48(2), 152–154, 1961.

45    Ibid. 30.

46    Ibid. 37.

47    Davies GV, *Family relationships of elderly mental hospital patients,* Australian and New

Zealand Journal of Psychiatry, 2, 264–271, 1968.

48   Davies GV, Teltscher B, Davies B, *Senile and arteriosclerotic dementia – a study of personal, social and family data*, Australian and New Zealand Journal of Psychiatry, 3, 398–400, 1969.

49   Davies GV, *Correspondence to Honorary Secretary RANZCP,* RANZCP Archives, 17 December 1973.

50   Mental Health Authority, *Mental Health Services in Victoria, 1975,* Melbourne, Mental Health Authority, 1975, p. 18–19.

51   Ibid. 1 p. 135.

52   Craig DA, *The Lion of Beechworth*, Beechworth, Victoria, 2000, p. 164.

53   Ibid. 21, p. 281.

54   Inspector-General of Mental Hospitals, *Report of the Inspector-General of Mental Hospitals for the year ending 30th June 1953,* Sydney, AH Pettifer Government Printer, 1954.

55   Ibid. 11 p. 53.

56   Inspector-General of Mental Hospitals, *Report of the Inspector-General of Mental Hospitals for the year ending 30th June 1955,* Sydney, AH Pettifer Government Printer, 1956.

57   Inspector-General of Mental Hospitals, *Report of the Inspector-General of Mental Hospitals for the year ending 30th June 1957,* Sydney, Victor CN Blight, Government Printer, 1958.

58   Cummins CJ, *A History of Medical Administration in NSW 1788–1973,* 2nd edition, Sydney, NSW Department of Health, 2003, p. 111.

59   Director of State Psychiatric Services, *Report of the Director of State Psychiatric Services for the Year ended June 30 1961,* Sydney, Victor CN Blight, Government Printer, 1962.

60   Health Commission of NSW, *Inpatient statistics of psychiatric hospitals 1973–74,* Sydney, Health Commission of NSW, 1975.

61   Ibid. 58.

62   Health Advisory Council, *Report on Care of the Aged – plans based on the proposals. NRS-5170,* NSW State Archives, 1963.

63   McClemens, the Honourable Mr. Justice, *Report of the Callan Park Mental Hospital Royal Commission,* Sydney, Government Printer, 1961, pp. 313–314.

64   NSW Association for Mental Health, '*Mental Health of the Aged Standing Committee*', Australasian Psychiatric Bulletin, 1(1), 18–19, 1960.

65   NSW Association for Mental Health, '*Mental Health of the Aged Standing Committee*', Australasian Psychiatric Bulletin, 3(1), 18–19, 1962.

66   NSW Association for Mental Health, '*Mental Health of the Aged Standing Committee*',

Australasian Psychiatric Bulletin, 4(1), 1963.

67  NSW Association for Mental Health, *'Mental Health of the Aged Standing Committee'*, Australasian Psychiatric Bulletin, 5(3), 1964.

68  Director of State Psychiatric Services, *Report of the Director of State Psychiatric Services for the Year ended June 30 1963,* Sydney, Victor CN Blight, Government Printer, 1964.

69  Director of State Psychiatric Services, *Report of the Director of State Psychiatric Services for the Year ended June 30 1964,* Sydney, Victor CN Blight, Government Printer, 1966.

70  Sax S, *Report for the Consultative Committee for the Care of the Aged,* NSW Department of Public Health, August 1965.

71  Director of State Psychiatric Services, *Reports of the Director of State Psychiatric Services for the Years ended 30 June 1965 and 30 June 1966,* Sydney, Victor CN Blight, Government Printer, 1967.

72  Dobbie JA, *A survey of older admissions to psychiatric hospitals in Sydney,* Australian and New Zealand Journal of Psychiatry, 1, 80–85, 1967.

73  Director of State Psychiatric Services, *Report of the Director of State Psychiatric Services for the Year ended 30 June 1969,* Sydney, Victor CN Blight, Government Printer, 1970.

74  Merlin M, *The development of a psychogeriatric service at Parramatta,* Unpublished lecture notes, Clinicians Conference, Sydney, 19 June 1981.

75  Ibid.

76  Ibid. 73.

77  Williams S, *What is psychogeriatrics in NSW?* Unpublished lecture notes, Clinicians Conference, Sydney, 19 June 1981.

78  Director of State Psychiatric Services, *Report of the Director of State Psychiatric Services for the Year ended 30 June 1971,* Sydney, Victor CN Blight, Government Printer, 1972.

79  Ibid. 77.

80  Goodall JB, *Whom nobody owns: The Dunwich Benevolent Asylum, an Institutional biography 1866–1946,* Doctoral thesis, Department of History, University of Queensland, 1992.

81  Stafford BFR, *Division of Mental Hygiene Annual Report 1950–51,* QS 201/1, 1937–1963. Brisbane, AH Tucker Government Printer, 1951.

82  Stafford BFR, *Division of Mental Hygiene Annual Report 1952–53,* QS 201/1, 1937–1963. Brisbane, AH Tucker Government Printer, 1953.

83  Stafford BFR, *Division of Mental Hygiene Annual Report 1953–54,* QS 201/1, 1937–1963. Brisbane, AH Tucker Government Printer, 1954.

84 Stafford BFR, *Division of Mental Hygiene Annual Report for the year ended 30thJune 1961,* QS 201/1, 1937–1963. Brisbane, SG Reid Government Printer, 1961.

85 Stafford BFR, *Division of Mental Hygiene Annual Report for the year ended 30thJune 1960,* QS 201/1, 1937–1963. Brisbane, SG Reid Government Printer, 1960.

86 Stafford BFR, *Division of Mental Hygiene Annual Report for the year ended 30thJune 1962,* QS 201/1, 1937–1963. Brisbane, SG Reid Government Printer, 1962.

87 Noble HN, *The Management of the Elderly Mentally Frail (abstract),* Australasian Psychiatric Bulletin, 2(2), 23–24, 1961.

88 Queensland Health, *The Road to Recovery – a history of mental health services in Queensland 1859–2009,* Queensland Government, 2013.

89 Daniel R, *A two-year study of geriatric admissions in a Queensland mental hospital,* The Medical Journal of Australia, I, 1034–1039, 1968.

90 The Prince Charles Hospital, *TPCH History: Home.* Home – TPCH History – LibGuides at The Prince Charles Hospital (accessed 18 February 2021).

91 Bell M, *From the 1870s to the 1970s: the changing face of public psychiatry in South Australia,* Australasian Psychiatry, 11 (1), 79–86, 2003.

92 Holt AG, *Hillcrest Hospital: the first 50 years,* Victoria, the Hillcrest Hospital Heritage Committee, 1999.

93 Kay HT, *1870–1970. Commemorating the Centenary of Glenside Hospital,* Netley, SA, Griffin Press, 1970.

94 Dibden WA, *A biography of psychiatry: The story of events and the people involved in the development of services for the psychiatrically ill in South Australia 1939–1989,* Adelaide, University of Adelaide Library, 2001, p. 242.

95 Ibid. p. 239.

96 Martyr P, *Claremont Hospital for the Insane has a Shadowy Past,* MeDeFacts, University of Western Australia, September 2010, pp. 12–13.

97 Hills N, *Asylum to Mainstream. The Closure and Replacement of Swanbourne Hospital 1979–1985,* Unpublished 2nd edition, 2019.

98 State Records Office of WA, *Sunset Hospital, Nedlands.* AU WA A810 – SUNSET HOSPITAL, NEDLANDS – State Records Office of WA (sro.wa.gov.au) (accessed 1 March 2021).

99 State Records Office of WA, *Claremont Mental Hospital.* AU WA A543 – CLAREMONT MENTAL HOSPITAL – State Records Office of WA (sro.wa.gov. au) (accessed 19 February 2021).

100 Ellis AS, *Eloquent Testimony.* Perth, UWA Press, 1983, p. 154.

101 Ibid. 97, p. 39.

102 Hills NF, *Promise and practice: WA psychiatry for the elderly,* Australasian Psychiatry, 3(4), 260–262, 1995.

103 Ratcliffe E, Kirkby K, *Psychiatry in Tasmania: from old cobwebs to new brooms*, Australasian Psychiatry, 9 (2), 128–132, 2001.

## 12 National developments in dementia services: 1980–2020

1    Australian Bureau of Statistics, *Australian Historical Population Statistics, Cat. No. 3105.0.65.001,* Canberra, Commonwealth of Australia, 2006.

2    Australian Bureau of Statistics, *Australian Demographic Statistics, June 2020*, National, state and territory population, June 2020 | Australian Bureau of Statistics (abs.gov. au) (accessed 4 February 2021).

3    Australian Institute of Health and Welfare, *Older Australia at a glance* Cat No AGE 87, Canberra, AIHW, 2018.

4    Parliament of Australia, *Residential care for the aged: an overview of Government policy from 1962 to 1993,* Social Policy Group, Department of the Parliamentary Library, Canberra, Commonwealth of Australia, 1993.

5    Healy J, *Community services: long term care at home?* In: Kendig HL, McCallum J (eds) Grey Policy: Australian policies for an ageing society, Sydney, Allen & Unwin, 1990, pp. 127–149.

6    Parliament of Australia, *In a home or at home? Home care and accommodation for the aged*, Report of the House of Representatives Standing Committee on Expenditure. Chair: LB McLeay, Canberra, Australian Government Publishing Service, 1981.

7    Ibid. 4.

8    Howe AL, *From states of confusion to a national action plan for dementia care: the development of policies for dementia care in Australia*, International Journal of Geriatric Psychiatry, 12, 165–171, 1997.

9    Henderson AS, *The Coming Epidemic of Dementia*, Australian and New Zealand Journal of Psychiatry, 17, 117–127, 1983.

10   Henderson AS, Jorm AF, *Dementia in Australia. Aged and Community Care Service Development and Evaluation Reports, Number 35,* Canberra, Australian Government Publishing Service, 1998.

11   Parliament of Australia, *Private Nursing Homes in Australia: Their Conduct, Administration and Ownership. Report by the Senate Select Committee on Private Hospitals and Nursing Homes,* Australian Government Publishing Service, Canberra, 1985, p. 61.

12   Department of Community Services and Health, *Nursing Home and Hostels Review*, Canberra, Australian Government Publishing Service, 1986.

13   Ibid. 8.

14   Department of Community Services and Health, *Living in a Nursing Home. Outcome Standards for Australian Nursing Homes,* Canberra, Australian Government Publishing Service, 1987.

15  Ibid. 4.

16  Ibid. 4.

17  Carter J, *States of confusion: Australian policies and the elderly confused*, Social Welfare Research Centre Report Proceedings, No. 4, University of New South Wales, Sydney, 1981.

18  McKay R, Draper B, *Is it too late to prevent a decline in mental health care for older Australians?* Medical Journal of Australia, 197(2), 87–88, 2012.

19  Ibid. 5.

20  Warne R, *Issues in the development of geriatric medicine in Britain and Australia*, Medical Journal of Australia, 146, 139–141, 1987.

21  Lefroy RB, *The development of geriatric medicine in Australia*, Medical Journal of Australia, 161, 18–20, 1994.

22  I worked in the Lidcombe Hospital memory clinic in 1985 and it had been operational for some years before that.

23  Brodaty H, *Low diagnostic yield in a memory disorders clinic*, International Psychogeriatrics, 2(2), 149–159, 1990.

24  Ames D, Flicker L, Helme R, *A memory clinic at a geriatric hospital: rationale, routine and results from the first 100 patients*, Medical Journal of Australia, 156, 618–622, 1992.

25  Hall K, *Memory Clinics in Victoria*, IPA Bulletin, 16(4), 12–14, 1999.

26  Ibid. 8.

27  Hunter C, Doyle C, *Dementia policy in Australia and the 'social construction' of infirm old age*, Health and History, 16(2), 44–62, 2014.

28  NSW Association for Mental Health, *Minutes of the Governing Council, 8 December 1981*, NSW Association for Mental Health Archives.

29  NSW Association for Mental Health, *Minutes of the Governing Council, 8 June, 1982*, NSW Association for Mental Health Archives.

30  Australian National Association for Mental Health, *Annual Report 1982–83*, ANAMH, Melbourne, 1983.

31  Brodaty H, *Correspondence to John Snowdon, President NSW Association for Mental Health*. NSW Association for Mental Health Archives, 1989.

32  Ibid. 8.

33  Ibid. 8.

34  Department of Health, Housing and Community Services, *Mid-term Review of the Aged Care Reform Strategy Report*, Canberra, Australian Government Publishing Service, 1991, p. 128.

35  Ibid. 8.

36  Draper B, Hudson C, Peut A, Karmel R, Chan C, Gibson D, *Hospital Dementia*

*Services Project: Aged care and dementia services in NSW hospitals,* Australasian Journal on Ageing, 33(4), 237–243, 2014.

37   Cations M, Withall A, White F, et al., *Why aren't people with young onset dementia and their caregivers using formal services? Results from the INSPIRED study,* PLOS ONE, 12(7), e0180935, 2017.

38   Thane P, *The Cultural History of Old Age,* In: Walker D & Garton S (eds) Ageing, Australian Cultural History 14, Geelong, Deakin University, 1995, p. 27.

39   Ibid. 8.

40   Department of Health, Housing, and Community Services, *Putting the Pieces Together: a National Action Plan for Dementia Care,* Canberra, Australian Government Publishing Service, 1992.

41   Ibid. 8.

42   Jorm AF, Mackinnon AJ, Henderson AS, et al., *The Psychogeriatric Assessment Scales: a multidimensional alternative to categorical diagnoses of dementia and depression in the elderly,* Psychological Medicine, 25, 447–460, 1995.

43   Department of Health and Family Services, *Mid-plan report of the National Action Plan for Dementia Care.* Canberra, Australian Government Publishing Service, 1996.

44   Ibid. 8.

45   Ibid. 40.

46   Human Rights and Equal Opportunities Commission, *Human Rights and Mental Illness: Report of the National Inquiry into the Human Rights of People with Mental Illness – Part III.* Canberra, Australian Government Publishing Service, 1993.

47   Ibid. 8.

48   Department of Health and Ageing, *Report to the Minister for Ageing on Residential Care and People with Psychogeriatric Disorders,* Canberra, Australian Government Publishing Service, 2008.

49   Rosewarne R, Opie J, Bruce A, et al., *Care Needs of People with Dementia and Challenging Behaviour Living in Residential Facilities,* Canberra, Australian Government Publishing Service, 1997.

50   Brodaty H, Draper B, Miller J, et al., *Randomised controlled trial of different models of care for nursing home residents with dementia complicated by psychosis or depression,* Journal of Clinical Psychiatry, 64, 63–72, 2003.

51   Ibid. 43.

52   Ibid. 27.

53   Australian Institute of Health and Welfare, *Older Australia at a Glance,* Canberra, Australian Government Publishing Service, 1997.

54   Department of Health and Ageing, *Community Packaged Care Guidelines.* Canberra, Australian Government Publishing Service, 2007.

55  Gray L, *Two year review of aged care reforms*, Canberra, Commonwealth of Australia, 2001.

56  Draper B, *Understanding Alzheimer's and Other Dementias*. Sydney, Longueville Media, p. 127, 2011.

57  Brodaty H, Ames D, Boundy KL, et al., *Pharmacological treatment of cognitive deficits in Alzheimer's disease*, Medical Journal of Australia, 175, 324–329, 2001.

58  Wood P, *Restrictions on dementia drugs dropped*, Australian Doctor, 24 April 2013 www.australiandoctor.com.au/news/latest-news/restrictions-on-dementia-drugs-dropped (accessed 25 April 2013).

59  Australian Institute of Health and Welfare, *Dementia in Australia Cat no. age 70*, Canberra, AIHW, 80–86, 2012.

60  Although the PBS indication for the prescription of the cholinesterase inhibitor drugs was limited to Alzheimer's disease, there is evidence that dementia due to Lewy body disease which includes Parkinson's disease can also benefit and in the US rivastigmine is able to be used for those indications. In Australia, clinicians are able to get around that issue by quite correctly stating that the patient has 'possible Alzheimer's disease' as post-mortem neuropathological studies show that there is often comorbidity of Alzheimer's disease and Lewy body disease and of course in the main these are clinical diagnoses. A similar approach is often taken with vascular dementia although benefits are much less frequently obtained.

61  Myer Foundation, *2020: a vision for aged care in Australia*, Melbourne, Myer Foundation, 2002.

62  Department of Health and Ageing, *A New Strategy for Community Care: The Way Forward*, Canberra, DOHA, August 2004.

63  Ibid. 27.

64  Access Economics, *The Dementia Epidemic: Economic impact and positive solutions for Australia*, Canberra, Alzheimer's Australia, March 2003.

65  Ibid. 27.

66  Ibid. 48.

67  Brodaty H, Gresham M, *Effect of a training programme to reduce stress in carers of patients with dementia*, British Medical Journal, 2;299(6712), 1375–9, 1989.

68  Brodaty H, Gresham M, Luscombe G, *The Prince Henry Hospital dementia caregivers' training programme*, International Journal of Geriatric Psychiatry, 12(2), 183–92, 1997.

69  Ibid. 48.

70  Brodaty H, Cumming A, *Dementia services in Australia*, International Journal of Geriatric Psychiatry, 25, 887–895, 2010.

71  Ibid. 48.

72  According to a 2007 report on 'Australia's Welfare', the breakdown of ownership of residential aged care providers was 61% 'not-for-profit', 27% private for profit, 12% State and local governments (Australian Institute of Health and Welfare, *Australia's Welfare,* Canberra, AIHW, 2007).

73  Pritchard RJ, *Psychogeriatric nursing in Victoria, Australia,* IPA Bulletin, 8(1), 19–20, 1991.

74  Snowdon J, Vaughan R, Miller R, Burgess E, Tremlett P, *Psychotropic drug use in Sydney nursing homes,* Medical Journal of Australia, 163, 70–72, 1995.

75  Snowdon J, *A follow-up survey of psychotropic drug use in Sydney nursing homes,* Medical Journal of Australia, 170, 293–294, 1999.

76  Draper B, Brodaty H, Low L-F, et al., *Use of psychotropic drugs in Sydney nursing homes: Associations with depression, psychosis and behavioural disturbances,* International Psychogeriatrics, 13(1), 107–120, 2001.

77  The Mental Health Foundation of Australia and the Australian National Association for Mental Health, *Media Release 12-87/88– Elderly use most medications for mental illness,* RANZCP Archives, 1987.

78  Snowdon J, *Medication use by elderly persons in Sydney,* Australian Journal on Ageing, 12(2), 14–21, 1993.

79  Brodaty H, Ames D, Snowdon J, et al., *A randomized placebo-controlled trial of risperidone for the treatment of aggression, agitation, and psychosis of dementia,* Journal of Clinical Psychiatry, 64, 134–143, 2003.

80  Schneider LS, Tariot PN, Dagerman KS, et al., *Effectiveness of atypical antipsychotic drugs in patients with Alzheimer's disease,* New England Journal of Medicine, 355(15), 1525–38, 2006.

81  NSW Ministry of Health and the Royal Australian and New Zealand College of Psychiatrists, *Assessment and Management of People with Behavioural and Psychological Symptoms of Dementia (BPSD),* North Sydney, NSW Ministry of Health, May 2013.

82  Ford AH, *Neuropsychiatric aspects of dementia,* Maturitas, 79, 209–215, 2014.

83  Brodaty H, Draper B, Low L-F, *Behavioural and Psychological Symptoms of Dementia – a 7 tiered Model of Service Delivery,* Medical Journal of Australia, 178, 231–234, 2003. The term BPSD has come under criticism in recent years because some regard it as a demeaning term that objectifies and disempowers people. It is a term meant to be used to guide the planning and provision of clinical care and there are likely more acceptable terms, such as 'responsive behaviours' or 'changed behaviours' that might better reflect the lived experience of dementia.

84  Ibid. 69.

85  Ibid. 48.

86  Ministerial Conference on Ageing, *Communique,* 15 December 2010.

87 I gave a presentation on behalf of the Psychogeriatric Expert Reference Group to the Commonwealth Mental Health Standing Committee on 18 September 2009.

88 Department of Health and Ageing, *Review of the Aged Care Funding Instrument,* Canberra, DOHA, 2011.

89 Mark Gaukroger was the Director of Dementia Policy with DOHA and he issued the email invitations to attend the Round Table on 22 August 2012 and the follow-up meeting on 24 September 2012. I attended the latter meeting.

90 Australian Medical Association, *The Rudd Government's plans for a national health system.* Australian Medicine, 2 May 2010, https://ama.com.au/ausmed/its-final-last (accessed 28 May 2020).

91 Access Economics, *Caring Places: planning for aged care and dementia 2010-2050,* Canberra, Access Economics, July 2010.

92 Ibid. 70.

93 KPMG, *Dementia services pathways – an essential guide to effective service planning,* KPMG, February 2011.

94 Productivity Commission, *Caring for Older Australians, Inquiry Report No 53,* Canberra, Australian Government, 2011.

95 Ibid. 48.

96 Australian Institute of Health and Welfare, *Dementia in Aged Care Residents 2011, AIHW Aged Care Series Statistics No 32,* Canberra, AIHW, 2011.

97 Department of Health and Ageing, *The Dementia and Veterans' Supplements in Aged Care, Consultation Paper,* Canberra, DOHA, April 2013.

98 Department of Social Services, *Phase one – Severe Behaviour Response Teams Operational Guidelines,* Canberra, DSS, May 2015.

99 Masso M, Duncan C, Grootematt P, et al., *Specialist dementia care units: an Evidence Check rapid review,* brokered by the Sax Institute (www.saxinstitute.org.au) for the Commonwealth Department of Health, 2017.

100 Department of Health, *Specialist Dementia Care Program Framework,* Canberra, Department of Health, December 2018.

101 Groves A, Thomson D, McKellar D and Procter N, *The Oakden Report,* Adelaide, South Australia, SA Health, Department for Health and Ageing, 2017.

102 ABC Four Corners, *Who Cares?* Posted 17 September 2018, Who Cares? – Four Corners (abc.net.au) (accessed 15 April 2021).

103 Royal Commission into Aged Care Quality and Safety, *Interim Report: Neglect,* Canberra, Commonwealth of Australia, 2019.

104 Department of Health, *Specialist Dementia Care Program,* Specialist Dementia Care Program (SDCP) | Australian Government Department of Health (accessed 15 April 2021).

105 Royal Commission into Aged Care Quality and Safety, *Background Paper 1. Navigating the maze: an overview of Australia's current aged care system,* Canberra, Commonwealth of Australia, February 2019.

106 Department of Health, *Geriatric Medicine 2016 Fact Sheet,* Canberra, Commonwealth of Australia, 2017 https://hwd.health.gov.au/webapi/customer/documents/factsheets/2016/Geriatric%20medicine.pdf (accessed 28 May 2020).

107 Woodward MC, Woodward E, *A national survey of memory clinics in Australia,* International Psychogeriatrics, 21(4), 696–702, 2009.

108 Ibid. 103.

## 13 National Developments in Old Age Psychiatry 1980–2020

1 The terminology used to describe mental health services for older people has varied over time and between jurisdictions to this day. Historically the most frequently used term was 'psychogeriatric services' but for many people the word 'psychogeriatric' has pejorative connotations. It is the term used until this point in the book to retain historical accuracy. These days the most frequently used term is 'older people's mental health services' and this is the term I have chosen to use, except when describing specific developments or in reporting publications that have used other terms.

2 Snowdon J, *The early days of old age psychiatry in New South Wales,* PGNA Newsletter, November 2020, pp. 4–5.

3 Snowdon J, *Psychiatric services for the elderly,* Australian and New Zealand Journal of Psychiatry, 21, 131–136, 1987.

4 Snowdon J, Draper B, *The Faculty of Psychiatry of Old Age,* Australasian Psychiatry, 7(1), 30–32, 1999.

5 Chiu E, *Correspondence to Dr Joan Lawrence, RANZCP President,* RANZCP Archives, 7 December 1987.

6 Carter PH (Registrar, RANZCP), *Correspondence to Dr Ed Chiu,* RANZCP Archives, 17 May 1988.

7 Ibid. 4.

8 Chiu E, *SPOA Report to General Council RANZCP October 1988,* RANZCP Archives, August 1988.

9 Ames D, *Edmond Chiu installed as President of IPA,* IPA Bulletin, 16(3), 1, 1999.

10 Chiu E, *Cane toads, jacarandas, headstones and the MCG – a very fortunate journey,* FPOA News, March 2005, 11–13.

11 Chiu E, Ames D, Hassett A, *Old Age Psychiatry in the Department,* In: Chiu E & Preston J (eds) The Department of Psychiatry at the University of Melbourne 1964–2009: personal reminiscences. University of Melbourne, 2010, pp. 180–184.

12 Ibid.

13 I did a podcast interview with David Ames in December 2019 that contributed to

this biography, available at History of psychiatry of old age podcast | RANZCP.

14  Draper B, Snowdon J, *Psychiatry of old age: from Section to Faculty,* Australian and New Zealand Journal of Psychiatry, 33, 785–788, 1999.

15  Ames D, *SPOA Report to General Council RANZCP,* RANZCP Archives, March 1991.

16  Ibid. 11.

17  Ibid. 8.

18  RANZCP Position Statement 22, *Psychiatric Services for the Elderly,* RANZCP Archives, May 1987.

19  Psychogeriatrics Working Party, Ministerial Implementation Committee on Mental Health and Developmental Disability (Chair WA Barclay), *Report to the Minister for Health, Volume Three,* Sydney, NSW Minister for Health, November 1988.

20  Broadbent R, *Correspondence from RANZCP Registrar to Honorary Secretary RANZCP Branches on 'Proposed Statement on Geriatric Psychiatry Services',* RANZCP Archives, 9 November 1992.

21  RANZCP Position Statement 29, *Relationships between Geriatric and Psychogeriatric Services,* RANZCP Archives, May 1990.

22  Ibid. 20 It is noteworthy that Noel Wilton was the NSW Director of Mental Health in the mid-90s, a period in which efforts to develop old age mental health services in NSW had stalled in large part due to attitudes within the Mental Health Branch of the NSW Department of Health about funding old age mental health services, which were believed to be better located in the aged care program (see Snowdon J, *Psychiatry of Old Age,* Australasian Psychiatry, 3(6): 431–435, 1995).

23  Snowdon J, Ames D, Chiu E, Wattis J, *A survey of psychiatric services for elderly people in Australia,* Australian and New Zealand Journal of Psychiatry, 29, 207–214, 1995.

24  Draper B, *Psychogeriatric services in Australia,* IPA Bulletin, 11(2), 19–20, Winter 1994.

25  Draper B, *Psychogeriatric training in Australia and New Zealand: a survey of psychiatry trainees and training program coordinators,* Australian and New Zealand Journal of Psychiatry, 28, 121–128, 1994.

26  Ibid. 11.

27  I have worked with Henry Brodaty since 1992 in clinical, research and advocacy roles and have observed his impact in these areas. Details of his achievements and areas of work were extracted from his CV as well as from a podcast interview that can be accessed from the RANZCP website History of psychiatry of old age podcast | RANZCP.

28  Levy R, *President's Report. A Precedent-setting success: Congress brings 1300 to Sydney,* IPA Bulletin, 12 (2), 1–2, Winter 1995 – Spring 1996.

29 Chiu E, *Spirit in Ageing, 7th Congress Chairman's Report,* IPA Bulletin, 12 (2), 10, Winter 1995 –Spring 1996.

30 Turner J, *Letter to the Editor,* PGNA Newsletter, 8–9, November 2020.

31 Ibid. 4.

32 Ibid. 14.

33 The information covered here is distilled from a podcast interview I did with John Snowdon in 2019. The interview can be accessed from the RANZCP website History of psychiatry of old age podcast | RANZCP.

34 I was the Chair of the advanced training committee from 1999 to 2005 and have kept the statistics for that period. The 2021 data was provided to me by the RANZCP Manager of Training and Development on May 7 2021.

35 Draper B, Reutens S, Subau D, *Workforce and advanced training survey of the RANZCP Faculty of Psychiatry of Old Age: issues and challenges for the field,* Australasian Psychiatry, 18, 142–145, 2010.

36 This information was obtained by email from the RANZCP administrative officer for Faculties, Sections and Networks on 22 April 2021.

37 The information about the early years of FPOA was gleaned from various FPOA archival records retained by the author as he was a member of the FPOA executive from 1999 to 2011.

38 McKay R, *From the Chair,* Faculty of Psychiatry of Old Age Newsletter, April, 2–3, 2013.

39 RANZCP Position Statement 81, *Use of antidepressants to treat depression in dementia,* RANZCP Archives, January 2015.

40 The information about the involvement of Australians in IPA was gleaned from various IPA publications retained by the author.

41 Ibid. 35.

42 Draper B, Low L-F, *Psychiatric services for the 'old' old,* International Psychogeriatrics, 22, 582–588, 2010.

43 O'Connor D, Melding P, *A survey of publicly funded aged psychiatry services in Australia and New Zealand,* Australian and New Zealand Journal of Psychiatry, 40, 368–373, 2006.

44 Department of Health and Ageing, *National Mental Health Report 2005, Table A-9,* Canberra, 2005.

45 Department of Health and Ageing, *National Mental Health Report 2007, Tables A-20 and A-21,* Canberra, 2007.

46 McKay R, McDonald R, Coombs T, *Benchmarking older persons mental health organizations,* Australasian Psychiatry, 19(1), 45–48, 2011.

47 McKay R, Draper B, *Is it too late to prevent a decline in mental health care for older*

*Australians?* Medical Journal of Australia, 197(2), 87–88, 2012.

48  Department of Health, *The Fifth National Mental Health and Suicide Prevention Plan,* Canberra, Commonwealth of Australia, 2017.

49  Andrews G, Henderson S, Hall W, *Prevalence, comorbidity, disability and service utilisation: Overview of the Australian National Mental Health Survey,* British Journal of Psychiatry, 178, 145–153, 2001.

50  Slade T, Johnston A, Teeson M, et al., *The Mental Health of Australians 2: Report on the 2007 National Survey of Mental Health and Wellbeing,* Canberra, Department of Health and Ageing, 2009.

51  Snowdon J, Draper B, Chiu E, Ames D, Brodaty H, *Surveys of mental health and wellbeing: Critical comments,* Australasian Psychiatry, 6, 246–247, 1998.

52  O'Connor DW, Parslow RA, *Different responses to K-10 and CIDI suggest that complex structured psychiatric interviews underestimate rates of mental disorder in older people,* Psychological Medicine, 39, 1527–1531, 2009.

53  O'Connor DW, Parslow RA, *Differences in older people's responses to CIDI's depression screening and diagnostic questions may point to age-related bias,* Journal of Affective Disorders, 125 (1–3), 361–364, 2010.

54  O'Connor DW, Jackson K, Lie D, McGowan H, McKay R, *Survey of aged psychiatry services' support of older Australians with very severe, persistent behavioural symptoms of dementia,* Australasian Journal on Ageing, 37(4), E133-E138, 2018.

55  Reisberg B, *About the 1991 Awards,* IPA Bulletin, 8 (2), 10, 1991.

56  Over R, *Interest patterns of Australian psychologists,* Australian Psychologist, 26, 49–53, 1991.

57  Koder DA, Helmes E, *The current status of clinical geropsychology in Australia: A survey of practising psychologists,* Australian Psychologist, 43(1), 22–26, 2008.

58  Koder DA, Helmes E, *Predictors of working with older adults in an Australian psychologist sample: revisiting the influence of contact,* Professional Psychology: Research and Practice, 39(3), 276–282, 2008.

59  Pachana N, Emery E, Konnert C, Woodhead E, Edelstein B, *Geropsychology content in clinical training programs: a comparison of Australian, Canadian and US data,* International Psychogeriatrics, 22, 909–918, 2010.

60  Pachana N, Helmes E, Koder D, *Guidelines for the provision of psychological services for older adults,* Australian Psychologist, 41, 15–22, 2006.

61  Australian Institute of Health and Welfare, *Mental Health Services in Australia, Medicare-subsidised mental health-specific services 2018–2019,* March 2021.

62  Department of Health, *Psychological treatment services for persons with mental illness in residential aged care facilities,* Canberra, Commonwealth of Australia, 2018.

63  Queensland Centre for Mental Health Research, *National Mental Health Service*

*Planning Framework Reports,* National Mental Health Service Planning Framework Reports – qcmhr (accessed 28 April 2021).

## 14 The Development of Older People's Mental Health Services in Victoria and NSW 1980–2020

1    Chiu E, Ames D, Hassett A, *Old Age Psychiatry in the Department,* In Chiu E & Preston J (eds) The Department of Psychiatry at the University of Melbourne 1964–2009: personal reminiscences. University of Melbourne, 180–184, 2010.

2    Harrison AW, Kernutt GJ, Piperoglou MV, *A survey of patients in a regional geriatric psychiatry inpatient unit,* Australian and New Zealand Journal of Psychiatry, 22, 412–417, 1988.

3    Bonwick R, *The Older Veteran's Psychiatry Program (OVPP), Melbourne* FPOA News, June, 9, 1999.

4    O'Bryan RJ, *Developing a community responsive psycho-geriatric service,* Australian Journal on Ageing, 6(4), 15–18, 1987.

5    Office of Psychiatric Services, Health Department of Victoria, *Psychiatric services for older people in Victoria,* Melbourne, Office of Psychiatric Services, May 1988.

6    Ibid. p. 7.

7    Ibid. 5, although the policy statement mainly used the term 'geriatric psychiatry', in places such as with the community assessment teams, the term 'psychogeriatric' was used.

8    Loi S, Hassett A, *Evolution of aged persons mental health services in Victoria: the history behind their development.* Australasian Journal on Ageing, 30(4), 226–230, 2011.

9    Ibid. 1.

10   The information covered here is distilled from personal communications and a podcast interview I did with Daniel O'Connor in 2019. The interview can be accessed from the RANZCP website History of psychiatry of old age podcast | RANZCP.

11   Duke M, *Spotlight on one institution in Australia,* IPA Bulletin, 11(2), 20, 1994.

12   Snowdon J, Ames D, Chiu E, Wattis J, *A survey of psychiatric services for elderly people in Australia,* Australian and New Zealand Journal of Psychiatry, 29, 207–214, 1995.

13   Auditor General of Victoria, *Building Better Cities: a joint government approach to urban development, Special Report No. 45,* Melbourne, Victorian Government Printer, 1996.

14   Hall K, *Mainstreaming aged psychiatric services: the Caulfield experience,* unpublished lecture, 2005.

15   Ibid. 8.

16   Victoria Psychiatric Services Division, *Victoria's mental health service: the framework for service delivery: aged persons services,* Melbourne, Department of Health and

Community Services, April 1996.

17 Victoria Aged, Community and Mental Health Division, *Victoria's mental health service: generic brief for a psychogeriatric assessment and admissions unit – 20 bed,* Melbourne, Aged, Community and Mental Health Division, Department of Human Services, 1997.

18 Victoria Aged, Community and Mental Health Division, *Victoria's mental health service: generic brief for a psychogeriatric nursing home – 30 bed,* Melbourne, Aged, Community and Mental Health Division, Department of Human Services, 1997.

19 Ibid. 1.

20 Ibid. 8.

21 O'Connor D, Stafrace S, *From Victoria,* FPOA News, September, 8, 2001.

22 Hunter C, Doyle C, *Dementia policy in Australia and the 'social construction' of infirm old age,* Health and History, 16(2), 44–62, 2014.

23 Hall K, *Memory clinics in Victoria,* IPA Bulletin, 16(4), 12–14, 1999.

24 O'Connor D, Melding P, *A survey of publicly funded aged psychiatry services in Australia and New Zealand,* Australian and New Zealand Journal of Psychiatry, 40, 368–373, 2006.

25 George K, Giri S, *An Intensive Community Team in aged persons mental health,* Australasian Psychiatry, 19(1), 56–58, 2011.

26 Ibid. 8.

27 Ibid. 1.

28 Department of Human Services, *Specialist mental health service components,* State Government Victoria, April 2005.

29 Bonwick R, *Service development in the private sector in Victoria,* FPOA News, 12, April 2011.

30 O'Connor DW, Jackson K, Lie D, McGowan H, McKay R, *Survey of aged psychiatry services' support of older Australians with very severe, persistent behavioural symptoms of dementia,* Australasian Journal on Ageing, 37(4), E133–E138, 2018.

31 Ibid. 24.

32 Royal Commission into Victoria's Mental Health System, *Final Report, Summary and Recommendations,* Melbourne, Victorian Government Printer, February 2021.

33 Commissioner for Senior Victorians, *Submission Royal Commission into Victoria's Mental Health System,* Melbourne, Victorian Government Printer, 2019.

34 COTA Victoria, *Submission Royal Commission into Victoria's Mental Health System,* Melbourne, COTA, July 2019.

35 NSW Branch RANZCP, *Submission to Inquiry into Health Services for the Psychiatrically Ill and Developmentally Disabled,* RANZCP, October 1982. I have retained the terms used in the submission which used 'geriatric psychiatry' and 'psychogeriatric' in

different sections.

36 The information covered here is distilled from personal communications and a podcast interview I did with Sid Williams in 2019. The interview can be accessed from the RANZCP website History of psychiatry of old age podcast | RANZCP.

37 Richmond D (Chair), *Inquiry into Health Services for the Psychiatrically Ill and Developmentally Disabled,* NSW State Health, March 1983.

38 Aftercare, *Aftercare: our journey 1907–2017,* Sydney, Australia, 2017 www.aftercare.com.au (accessed 8 April 2019).

39 Ibid. 37, Part 4.

40 Ibid. 37, Part 4, p. 3.

41 Ibid. 37, Part 4, p. 13.

42 Ibid. 37, Part 4, p. 10.

43 Ibid. 37.

44 Williams S, Sammut A, *Submission to the NSW Consultative Committee on Ageing re psychogeriatric care,* 1983.

45 Shea P, *Defining Madness,* Leichhardt, Hawkins Press, 1999, pp. 103–112.

46 Ibid. pp. 113–129.

47 Draper B, *Correspondence with Dr Noel Wilton NSW Director of Mental Health,* 14 March 1995.

48 The information covered here is distilled from personal communications and a podcast interview I did with Richard Fleming in November 2019. The interview can be accessed from the RANZCP website History of psychiatry of old age podcast | RANZCP.

49 Fleming R, Bowles J, *Units for the confused and disturbed elderly: development, design, programming, and evaluation,* Australian Journal on Ageing, 6(4), 25–28, 1987.

50 Bird M, Anderson K, Blair A, MacPherson S, *Evaluation of the T-BASIS Unit Initiative and Model of Care,* Sydney, NSW Department of Health, August 2011.

51 O'Neill TJ, *Correspondence with Sid Williams, Working Party on Geriatric Psychiatry in NSW,* 29 August 1988.

52 Ibid. 49.

53 Williams S, *Correspondence with Peter Anderson, NSW Minister for Health,* 17 December 1986.

54 The information about service developments in Newcastle are from personal communication by email with Stephen Ticehurst 2 August 2021.

55 Ibid.

56 Russell B, *Correspondence with Sid Williams, Working Party on Geriatric Psychiatry in NSW,* 31 August 1988.

57 NSW Institute of Psychiatry 'Psychiatry of Old Age Course 1989', RANZCP

Archives, May 1989.

58   Russell RJ, *Psychogeriatric services in Australia*, IPA Bulletin, 9(1), 20, May 1992.

59   Snowdon J, *Psychiatric services for the elderly*, Australian and New Zealand Journal of Psychiatry, 21, 131–136, 1987.

60   Psychogeriatrics Working Party, Ministerial Implementation Committee on Mental Health and Developmental Disability (Chair WA Barclay). *Report to the Minister for Health, Volume Three*. Sydney, NSW Minister for Health, November 1988.

61   Balaraman CS, *Correspondence with Sid Williams, Working Party on Geriatric Psychiatry in NSW*, 8 September 1988.

62   Sammut A, Williams S, *Submission to the NSW Consultative Committee on Ageing re Psychogeriatric Care*, Circa 1993.

63   Brodaty H, *The need for distinctive psychogeriatric services*, RANZCP News and Notes, 24, 27–28, February 1991.

64   Draper B, Meares S, McIntosh H, *A Psychogeriatric Outreach Service to Nursing Homes in Sydney*, Australasian Journal on Ageing 17, 184–186, 1998.

65   Personal communication with Judy Raymond who provided psychiatric consultations to Kenmore Hospital, 28 June 2021.

66   Andrews G, *Reply to Snowdon re Health Services Research into the Future of Australian Psychiatry*, Australian and New Zealand Journal of Psychiatry, 24, 435–436, 1990.

67   Snowdon J, *Letter to the Editor, Health Services Research into the Future of Australian Psychiatry*, Australian and New Zealand Journal of Psychiatry, 24, 435, 1990.

68   Snowdon J, *Bed requirements for an area psychogeriatric service*, Australian and New Zealand Journal of Psychiatry, 25, 56–62, 1991.

69   NSW Ministerial Taskforce on Psychotropic Medication Use in Nursing Homes, *Discussion Paper*, NSW Health, May 1997.

70   Russell R, *NSW news*, FPOA News, 1, 8, June 1999.

71   NSW Health Department, *Caring for Older People's Mental Health: a Strategy for the Delivery of Mental Health Care for Older People in NSW*, State Health Publication No. *(CMH) 990009*, Gladesville, NSW Department of Health, January 1999.

72   Ibid. 69.

73   Draper B, Jochelson T, Kitching D, Snowdon J, Brodaty H, Russell B, *Mental health service delivery to older people in NSW: perceptions of aged care, adult mental health and mental health services for older people*, Australian and New Zealand Journal of Psychiatry, 37, 735–740, 2003.

74   Ibid. 24.

75   Chiu A, Nguyen HV, Reutens S, et al., *Clinical outcomes and length of stay of a co-located psychogeriatric and geriatric unit*, Archives of Gerontology and Geriatrics, 49, 233–236, 2009.

76  NSW Department of Health, *Summary Report: The management and accommodation of older people with severely and persistently challenging behaviours in residential care,* Gladesville, NSW Department of Health, 2006.

77  Brodaty H, Draper B, Low L-F, *Behavioural and Psychological Symptoms of Dementia – a 7 tiered Model of Service Delivery,* Medical Journal of Australia, 178, 231–234, 2003.

78  Personal communication from Kate Jackson, Director Older Persons Mental Health Policy Unit, 21 May 2021.

79  NSW Department of Health, *NSW Service Plan for Specialist Mental Health Services for Older people (SMHSOP) 2005–2015,* Gladesville, NSW Department of Health, 2006.

80  Ibid. 77.

81  In 2005 I chaired a review of the training of psychiatrists for the NSW Institute of Medical Education and Training (IMET) while Morris Iemma was Minister for Health. As reported to me by the Clinical Director of IMET, Mark Brown, Iemma had a very favourable attitude towards funding enhancements for training in mental health. When Iemma became Premier in August 2005, he also took on the role of Treasurer and so still had a strong input into budget expenditure. His replacement as Minister for Health, John Hatzigeros, did not undo any of the funding promises made by Iemma, but of note in the area of medical training, subsequent training reviews in other medical specialties did not receive the same level of funding enhancements.

82  Group Report, *Community Mental Health Care,* unpublished report involving Kate Jackson for Executive Masters of Public Administration, Sydney University – cites sections of Morris Iemma's National Press Club address from the 1 June 2006. The quote comes from page 4 of the National Press Club transcript, December 2007.

83  NSW Department of Health, *NSW: a new direction for Mental Health,* North Sydney, NSW Department of Health, 2006.

84  Health Policy Analysis, *Evaluation of NSW Service Plan for Specialist Mental Health Services for Older People – Final report Volume 1 (Summary),* NSW Ministry of Health, Sydney, p. 5–6, 2011.

85  NSW Department of Health, *The NSW Dementia Services Framework, 2010–2015,* North Sydney, NSW Department of Health, 2010.

86  Draper B, Hudson C, Peut A, Karmel R, Chan C, Gibson D, *Hospital Dementia Services Project: Aged care and dementia services in NSW hospitals,* Australasian Journal on Ageing, 33(4), 237–243, 2014.

87  Stewart J, O'Connor D, Cameron I, Kurrle S, *Final Report: Review of Confused And Disturbed Elderly (CADE) units in New South Wales.* Sydney, NSW Department of

Health, 2006.

88 Anderson K, Bird M, Blair A, MacPherson S, *Development and effectiveness of an integrated inpatient and community service for challenging behaviour in late life: from Confused and Disturbed Elderly to Transitional Behavioural Assessment and Intervention Service*, Dementia, 15(6), 1340–57, 2016.

89 Ibid. 49.

90 NSW Department of Health, *Evaluation of the Mental Health Aged Care Partnership Initiative*, Sydney, NSW Department of Health, December 2009.

91 NSW Ministry of Health, *NSW Older People's Mental Health Services, Service Plan 2017–2027*, North Sydney, NSW Ministry of Health, 2017, Appendix 2.

92 Ibid. 83, p. 4.

93 Ibid. 83, p. 14.

94 Ibid. 30.

95 NSW Ministry of Health, *Specialist Mental Health Services for Older People (SMHSOP) Acute Inpatient Unit Model of Care Project Report*, Sydney, NSW Health, 2012.

96 Ibid. 90.

97 Ibid. 90, iv–v.

98 NSW Ministry of Health, *SMHSOP Acute Inpatient Unit Model of Care Guideline*, Mental Health & Drug and Alcohol Office, Ministry of Health North Sydney, 23 June 2016.

99 Dobrohotoff JT, Llewellyn-Jones RH, *Psychogeriatric inpatient unit design: a literature review*, International Psychogeriatrics, 23(2), 174–189, 2011.

100 Jackson K, Roberts R, McKay R, *Older people's mental health in rural areas: Converting policy into service development, service access, and sustainable workforce*, Australian Journal of Rural Health, 27 (4), 358–365, 2019.

101 NSW Ministry of Health, *NSW Older People's Mental Health Community Services: Key Features of the Model of Care*, North Sydney, NSW Ministry of Health, 2020.

102 Ibid. 90.

## 15 The Development of Older People's Mental Health Services in Other States and Territories 1980–2020

1 Hills NF, *Promise and practice: WA psychiatry for the elderly*, Australasian Psychiatry, 3(4), 260–262, 1995.

2 Hills N, *Asylum to Mainstream. The Closure and Replacement of Swanbourne Hospital 1979–1985*, Unpublished 2nd edition, 2019.

3 Much of this section was provided by Neville Hills to me by way of personal communications in emails in 2020 and 2021.

4 Ibid. 2, 55–56.

5   Ibid. 2, 68–70.

6   Ibid. 2, 82–86.

7   Ibid. 2, 71–80.

8   Ibid. 1.

9   Snowdon J, Ames D, Chiu E, Wattis J, *A survey of psychiatric services for elderly people in Australia,* Australian and New Zealand Journal of Psychiatry, 29, 207–214, 1995.

10  Ibid. 2, p. 146.

11  Information obtained in my personal records of psychiatry of old age advanced training for that period.

12  O'Connor M, *Western Australia Update,* FPOA News, 9, September 2001.

13  O'Connor M, *Report from Western Australia*, FPOA News, 8, April 2002.

14  Restifo S, *Branch Report from Western Australia*, FPOA News, 10, October 2003.

15  O'Connor D, Melding P, *A survey of publicly funded aged psychiatry services in Australia and New Zealand,* Australian and New Zealand Journal of Psychiatry, 40, 368–373, 2006.

16  Personal communication email from Helen McGowan who is co-lead of the Older Adult Mental Health Sub-network.

17  Personal communication with Leon Flicker, 25 June 2021.

18  Department of Health Western Australia, *Dementia Model of Care,* Perth, Aged Care Network, Department of Health, Western Australia, 2011.

19  O'Connor DW, Jackson K, Lie D, McGowan H, McKay R, *Survey of aged psychiatry services' support of older Australians with very severe, persistent behavioural symptoms of dementia,* Australasian Journal on Ageing, 37(4), E133–E138, 2018.

20  Ibid. 16.

21  Western Australian Department of Health, *Older Adult Mental Health Sub Network Establishment Report,* Perth, Health Networks, Western Australian Department of Health, 2016.

22  Mental Health Commission, *Draft Western Australian Mental Health, Alcohol and Other Drug Services Plan 2015 2025 (Plan) Update 2018*, Mental Health Commission, Government of Western Australia, 2019.

23  Department of Health, *The North Metropolitan Older Adult Mental Health Program Model of Care,* North Metropolitan Health Service Mental Health, WA Department of Health, 2014.

24  Ibid. 16.

25  Dibden W, *A biography of psychiatry: The story of events and the people involved in the development of services for the psychiatrically ill in South Australia 1939–1989.* Adelaide, University of Adelaide Library, 2001, p. 243.

26  Groves A, Thomson D, McKellar D, Procter N, *The Oakden Report.* Adelaide, South

Australia, SA Health, Department for Health and Ageing, 2017, p. 23.

27  Ibid. 9.

28  Ibid. 26, p. 14.

29  McLean S, *News from South Australia,* SPOA Newsletter, 5, Winter 1997.

30  Ibid. 26, p. 24.

31  Ibid. 29.

32  Ibid. 15.

33  Ibid. 26.

34  Rischbieth S, *Letter from South Australia,* FPOA Newsletter, 11, April 2011.

35  Ibid. 26.

36  South Australian Social Inclusion Board, *Stepping Up: A Social Inclusion Action Plan for Mental Health Reform 2007–2012,* South Australia, Social Inclusion Board, January 2007, p. 70.

37  Ibid. 26, p. 16.

38  Ibid. 34.

39  Rischbieth S, *Letter from South Australia,* FPOA Newsletter, 11, September 2011.

40  Rischbieth S, *Letter from South Australia,* FPOA Newsletter, 7, April 2012.

41  Ibid. 26, p. 16.

42  Ibid. 19.

43  Personal communication with Duncan Mackellar, Clinical Advisor Old Age Mental Health, South Australia, 25 June 2021.

44  Ibid. 26.

45  Ibid. 26, p. 100.

46  Ibid. 26.

47  South Australian Government, *The 'Oakden Report' Response,* South Australia Health, June 2018.

48  Ibid. 43.

49  Personal communication from Dr Eddie Tan who worked at Toowoomba in the 1970s and early 1980s and again from 1999 to 2018, 31 May 2021.

50  Personal communication from Dr John McIntyre who worked at Toowoomba from 1982, 11 June 2021.

51  Thompson J, *Obituary Joan Metcalf Ridley,* Psychiatric Bulletin, 18, 525–526, 1994.

52  Queensland Government, Chapter 8, *Health* in 'Queensland Past and Present: 100 years of statistics 1896–1996, pp. 246–254. State of Queensland, 2009.

53  The information covered here is distilled from personal communications and a podcast interview I did with Gerard Byrne in January 2020. The interview can be accessed from the RANZCP website History of psychiatry of old age podcast | RANZCP.

54 Ibid. 9.

55 Personal communication with David Lie, 26 May 2021.

56 Ibid. 53.

57 Queensland Government, *Mental Health Services for Older People,* State of Queensland, 1996.

58 Leong M, *News from Queensland,* SPOA Newsletter, 5, Winter 1997.

59 Lie D, *Queensland update,* FPOA News, 8, May 2001.

60 Ibid. 53.

61 Ibid. 15.

62 Lie D, *Aged Care Mental Health Service, Princess Alexandra Hospital, Brisbane,* FPOA News, 6, April 2003.

63 Queensland Health, *Queensland Health's Directions for Aged Care 2004 – 2011,* Brisbane, Queensland Health, 2004.

64 Mental Health Branch, Queensland Health, *The Queensland Plan for Mental Health 2007–2017,* The State of Queensland, Queensland Health, June 2008.

65 Lie D, *Public psychogeriatric services in Queensland,* FPOA News, 5, July 2008.

66 Ibid. 19.

67 Ibid. 55.

68 Personal Communication with Dr Shirlony Morgan, Chair of the Queensland Older Persons Mental Health Network, 31 May 2021.

69 Kerr A, *David William Kilbourne Kay,* Royal College of Physicians Inspiring Physicians, David William Kilbourne Kay | RCP Museum (rcplondon.ac.uk) (accessed 26 May 2021).

70 Henderson AS, Scott R, Kay DWK, *The elderly who live alone: their mental health and social relationships,* Australian and New Zealand Journal of Psychiatry, 20, 202–209, 1986.

71 Kay DWK, Holding TA, Jones B, Littler S, *Psychiatric morbidity in Hobart's dependent aged,* Australian and New Zealand Journal of Psychiatry, 21, 463–475, 1987.

72 Draper B, *Correspondence with Sharon Brownie, CEO RANZCP, nominating John Tooth for a College Citation,* 27 November 2007.

73 Blackwood M, *1384.6 – Statistics – Tasmania, 2002 Feature Article – Mental health services* Released 13/09/2002, 1384.6 – Statistics – Tasmania, 2002 (abs.gov.au) (accessed 1 February 2021).

74 Ibid. 72.

75 Cohen-Mansfield J, Bester A, *Flexibility as a management principle in dementia care: the ADARDS example,* The Gerontologist, 46(4), 540–544, 2006.

76 Fleming R, Zeisel J, Bennett K, *World Alzheimer Report 2020 Design Dignity Dementia: dementia-related design and the built environment Volume 1.* London,

England, Alzheimer's Disease International, 2020.

77   Tooth JSH, *Submission to Senate Enquiry into 'Care and management of younger and older people with dementia and behavioural and psychological symptoms of dementia,* 15 April 2013 Submissions – Parliament of Australia (aph.gov.au) (accessed 26 May 2021).

78   Budget Estimates Committee, Tasmania, *Uncorrected proof issue of minutes 24 June 2009.* Microsoft Word – cestawed2.doc (parliament.tas.gov.au) (accessed 26 May 2021).

79   Ibid. 9.

80   Herst L, *Other news from around Australia – Tasmania,* FPOA News, Issue 1, 8, June 1999.

81   Herst L, *Report from Tasmania,* FPOA News, Issue 3, 7, December 2000.

82   Herst L, *Report from Tasmania,* FPOA News, Issue 5, 7, September 2001.

83   Ibid. 15.

84   Personal communication with Martin Morrissey, 13 May 2021.

85   Ibid. 19.

86   Ibid. 84.

87   Tasmanian Government, *Rethink 2020: a state plan for mental health in Tasmania 2020–2025,* Tasmanian Government, November 2020.

88   Primary Health Tasmania, *Suicide prevention,* Suicide prevention – Primary Health Tasmania (accessed 27 May 2021).

89   Personal communication with Judy Raymond, 28 June 2021.

90   Ibid.

91   Raymond J, Kirkwood H, Looi J, *Commitment and collaboration for excellence in older persons' mental health: the ACT experience,* Australasian Psychiatry, 12(2), 130–133, 2004.

92   Personal communication Jeff Looi, 19 July 2021.

93   Ibid. 89.

94   Ibid. 15.

95   ACT Health, *Agreed requirements for ACT Plan under Subacute Care Component of National Partnership Agreement,* ACT Health 30 April 2009.

96   Ibid. 89.

97   Personal communication with Julia Lane, old age psychiatrist, ACT, 4 June 2021.

98   Capital Health Network, *Australian Capital Territory Mental Health and Suicide Prevention Plan for 2019–2024,* Canberra, ACT Primary Health Network, 2019.

99   Pettigrew J, *What is happening in the Northern Territory,* FPOA News, 6–7, January 2008.

100 Personal communication with Jill Pettigrew old age psychiatrist NT, 2 June 2021.

101 Personal communication with Judy Ratajec and Mary Ingrame, 16 June 2021.

102 Ibid.

## 16 Services for Aboriginal and Torres Strait Islander Peoples after the Second World War

1   Daniels D, *Social security payments for the aged, people with disabilities and carers 1901 to 2010*, Canberra, Parliament of Australia, 2011.

2   Australian Institute of Health and Welfare, *Older Aboriginal and Torres Strait Islander People*, Canberra, AIHW, May 2011.

3   Tatz C, *The Social and Political contexts,* In Tatz C, Aboriginal Suicide is Different: A Portrait of Life and Self-destruction, Aboriginal Studies Press, p. 1–17, 2001.

4   Ibid. 2.

5   Australian Bureau of Statistics, *Life Tables for Aboriginal and Torres Strait Islander Australians, 2015–2017, 3302.0.55.003*, ABS, 28 November 2018.

6   Department of the Prime Minister and Cabinet, *Closing the Gap Report 2020*, Canberra, Commonwealth of Australia, 2020.

7   Cotter PR, Condon JR, Barnes T, Anderson IPS, Smith LR, Cunningham T, *Do Indigenous Australians age prematurely? The implications of life expectancy and health conditions of older Indigenous people for health and aged care policy.* Australian Health Review, 36, 68–74, 2012.

8   Arkles R, Jackson Pulver L, Robertson H, et al., *Ageing, Cognition and Dementia in Australian Aboriginal and Torres Strait Islander Peoples: A life Cycle Approach,* Neuroscience Research Australia and Muru Marri Indigenous Health Unit, University of New South Wales, June 2010.

9   Ibid. 2.

10  Australian Institute of Health and Welfare, *Australian Burden of Disease Study: Impact and causes of illness and death in Aboriginal and Torres Strait Islander people 2011,* Canberra, AIHW, 2016.

11  Ibid. 2.

12  Australian Bureau of Statistics, *Census of Population and Housing: Reflecting Australia – Stories from the Census, 2016. Aboriginal and Torres Strait Islander population, 2016.* ABS cat.no. 2071.0. Canberra, ABS, 2017.

13  Temple JB, Wilson T, Taylor A, Kelaher M, Eades S, (2020). *Ageing of the Aboriginal and Torres Strait Islander population: numerical, structural, timing, and spatial aspects,* Australian and New Zealand Journal of Public Health, 44, 271–278, 2020.

14  Cawte J, *Ethnopsychiatry in Central Australia: I. Traditional illnesses in the Eastern Aranda People,* British Journal of Psychiatry, 111, 1069–1077, 1965.

15  Cawte J, Kidson MA, *Ethnopsychiatry in Central Australia: II. The evolution of illness in a Walbiri lineage,* British Journal of Psychiatry, 111, 1079–1085, 1965.

16  Berndt RM, Berndt CH. *The World of the First Australians*, Ure Smith, Sydney, 1964, p. 210.

17  Elkin AP, *The Australian Aborigines*, Angus & Robertson, Australia, 1974, p. 114.

18  Pollitt PA, *The problem of dementia in Australian Aboriginal and Torres Strait Islander communities: an overview*, International Journal of Geriatric Psychiatry, 12, 155–163, 1997.

19  Fraser J, *The Aborigines of New South Wales*, Royal Society of NSW, 1882–83, p. 228.

20  Ibid. 16.

21  Kidson MA, *Psychiatric disorders in the Walbiri, Central Australia*, Australian and New Zealand Journal of Psychiatry, 1, 14–22, 1967.

22  Coolican RE, In: Cawte J, *Medicine is the Law*, Honolulu, University Press of Hawaii, 21–22, 1974.

23  Harper C, *Wernicke's encephalopathy in Western Australia: a common preventable disease*, Australian Alcohol Drug Review, 2(1), 71–73, 1983.

24  Ridley N, Draper B, Withall A, *Alcohol-related Dementia: an update of the evidence*, Alzheimer's Research & Therapy, 5: 3. http://alzres.com/content/5/1/3, 2013.

25  Ibid. 23.

26  Zann S, *Identification of Support, Education and Training Needs of Rural/Remote Health Care Service Providers Involved in Dementia Care. Rural Health, Support, Education and Training (RHSET) Project Progress Report*, Northern Regional Health Authority, Queensland, 1994.

27  Alzheimer's Australia South Australia, *Dementia Learning Resource for Aboriginal and Torres Strait Islander Communities*, Commonwealth of Australia, 2007.

28  Calabria B, Doran CM, Vos T, Shakeshaft AP, Hall W, *Epidemiology of alcohol-related burden of disease among Indigenous Australians*, Australian and New Zealand Journal of Public Health, 34(S1), S47–S51, 2010.

29  Wilson M, Stearne A, Gray D, Sherry S, *The harmful use of alcohol amongst Indigenous Australians*, Australian Indigenous HealthInfoNet, 2010 http://www.healthinfonet. ecu.edu.au/alcoholuse_review (accessed 31 July 2013).

30  Australian Institute of Health and Welfare, *Dementia in Australia*, Cat No Age 70, Canberra, AIHW, 38, Table 3.7, 2012.

31  LoGiudice D, Smith K, Thomas J, et al., *Kimberley Indigenous Cognitive Assessment tool (KICA): Development of a cognitive assessment tool for older Indigenous Australians*, International Psychogeriatrics, 18, 269–280, 2006.

32  Personal communication with Leon Flicker, 25 June 2021.

33  Smith K, Flicker L, Lautenschlager NT, et al., *High prevalence of dementia and cognitive impairment in Indigenous Australians*, Neurology 71(19), 1470–3, 2008.

34  Smith K, Flicker L, Dwyer A, et al., *Factors associated with dementia in Aboriginal Australians,* Australian and New Zealand Journal of Psychiatry, 44, 888–893, 2010.

35  LoGiudice D, *The health of older Aboriginal and Torres Strait Islander peoples,* Australasian Journal on Ageing, 35(2), 82–85, 2016.

36  The information covered here is distilled from personal communications and a podcast interview I did with Tony Broe in 2020. The interview can be accessed from the RANZCP website History of psychiatry of old age podcast | RANZCP.

37  Radford K, Mack HA, Draper B, et al., *Prevalence of dementia and cognitive impairment in urban and regional Aboriginal Australians,* Alzheimer's & Dementia, 11, 271–279, 2015.

38  Radford K, Lavrencic LM, Delbaere K, et al., *Factors associated with the high prevalence of dementia in older Aboriginal Australians,* Journal of Alzheimer's Disease 70(s1), 1–11, 2018.

39  Radford K, Delbaere K, Draper B, et al., *Childhood stress and adversity is associated with late-life dementia in Aboriginal Australians,* American Journal of Geriatric Psychiatry, 25(10), 1097–1106, 2017.

40  Radford K, Mack HA, Draper B, et al., *Comparison of three cognitive tools for dementia screening in urban and regional aboriginal Australians,* Dementia and Geriatric Cognitive Disorders, 40, 22–32, 2015.

41  Li SQ, Guthridge SL, Aratchige PE, et al., *Dementia prevalence and incidence among the Indigenous and non-Indigenous populations of the Northern Territory,* Medical Journal of Australia, 200(8), 465–469, 2014.

42  Russell SG, Quigley R, Thompson F, et al., *Prevalence of dementia in the Torres Strait,* Australasian Journal on Ageing, 40 (2). e125–e132, 2021.

43  Gubhaju L, McNamara BJ, Banks E, et al., *The overall health and risk factor profile of Australian Aboriginal and Torres Strait Islander participants from the 45 and up study,* BMC Public Health, 13, 661, 2013.

44  Almeida OP, Flicker L, Fenner S, et al., *The Kimberley Assessment of Depression of Older Indigenous Australians: Prevalence of depressive disorders, risk factors and validation of the KICA-dep Scale,* PLoS ONE, 9, e94983, 2014.

45  Shen Y, Radford K, Daylight G, Cumming R, Broe T, Draper B, *Depression, Suicidal Behaviour and Mental Disorders in Older Aboriginal Australians,* The International Journal of Environmental Research and Public Health 15(3), 447, 2018.

46  AIHW: Kreisfeld R, Harrison JE, *Indigenous injury deaths: 2011–12 to 2015–16. Injury research and statistics series no. 130. Cat. no. INJCAT 210.* Canberra, AIHW, 2020.

47  Hunter E, *Aboriginal communities and suicide,* Australasian Psychiatry, 4(4), 195–199, 1996.

48  National Aboriginal and Torres Strait Islander Health Council, *National Strategic Framework for Aboriginal and Torres Strait Islander Health: Context,* National Aboriginal and Torres Strait Islander Health Council, Canberra, July 2003.

49  Department of Health and Family Services, *Mid-plan report of the National Action Plan for Dementia Care,* Canberra, Australian Government Publishing Service, 1996.

50  Australian Bureau of Statistics, *The Health and Welfare of Australia's Aboriginal and Torres Strait Islander Peoples 2008,* Commonwealth of Australia, Canberra, 2008.

51  Access Economics, *The Dementia Epidemic: Economic impact and positive solutions for Australia,* Canberra, Alzheimer's Australia, March 2003.

52  Department of Health and Ageing, *Report to the Minister for Ageing on Residential Care and People with Psychogeriatric Disorders,* Canberra, Australian Government Publishing Service, 2008.

53  Ibid. 2.

54  Health Policy Analysis, *Evaluation of NSW Service Plan for Specialist Mental Health Services for Older People – Final report Volume 1 (Summary),* NSW Ministry of Health, Sydney, 2011.

55  Aged Care Sector Committee Diversity Sub-group, *Aged Care Diversity Framework,* Canberra, Commonwealth of Australia, 2017.

56  National Advisory Group for Aboriginal and Torres Strait Islander Aged Care, *Submission to the Royal Commission into Aged Care Quality and Safety,* September 2019.

57  Department of Health, *Actions to support older Aboriginal and Torres Strait Islander people – a Guide for Aged Care Providers,* Canberra, Commonwealth of Australia, February 2019.

58  Department of Health, *Actions to support older Aboriginal and Torres Strait Islander people – a Guide for Consumers,* Canberra, Commonwealth of Australia, February 2019.

59  NSW Department of Community Services, *Working with Aboriginal people and communities,* Ashfield, NSW Department of Community Services, February 2009.

60  Ibid. 56.

61  Garvey G, Simmonds D, Clements V, et al., *Understanding Dementia amongst Indigenous Australians,* Aboriginal and Islander Health Worker Journal, 35 (2), 16–18, 2011.

62  Ibid. 8.

63  Commonwealth of Australia, *National Strategic Framework for Aboriginal and Torres Strait Islander Peoples' Mental Health and Social and Emotional Wellbeing,* Canberra, Department of the Prime Minister and Cabinet, 2017.

64  NSW MHDAO Older People's Mental Health Policy Unit, *Aboriginal Older People's*

*Mental Health: Resources for Local Health District SMHSOP Services,* Orange, Older People's Mental Health Policy Unit, 2015.

## 17 The Impact of the Ageing Culturally and Linguistically Diverse Population on Service Development

1  Australian Institute of Health and Welfare, *Older Australia at a glance* Cat No AGE 87, Canberra, AIHW, 2018.

2  Wand APF, Pourmand D, Draper B, *Using interpreters with culturally and linguistically diverse older adults: what do we need to know?* Australasian Journal on Ageing, 39 (3): 175–177, 2020.

3  Department of Health, *Review of the Culturally and Linguistically Diverse (CALD) Ageing and Aged Care Strategy. Publication Number: 12060* Canberra, Commonwealth of Australia, 2017.

4  Federation of Ethnic Communities' Councils of Australia, *Review of Australian Research on Older People from Culturally and Linguistically Diverse Backgrounds,* Curtin ACT, FECCA, 2015.

5  Kratiuk S, Young J, Rawson G, Williams S, *A Double Jeopardy: A Report on Dementia Clients of Non-English Speaking Backgrounds,* South Western Area Health Services, Sydney, 1992.

6  Department of Health and Family Services, *Mid-plan report of the National Action Plan for Dementia Care,* Canberra, Australian Government Publishing Service, 1996.

7  LoGiudice D, Hassett A, Cook R, Flicker L, Ames D, *Equity of Access to a Memory Clinic in Melbourne? Non-English Speaking Background Attenders Are More Severely Demented and Have Increased Rates of Psychiatric Disorders,* International Journal of Geriatric Psychiatry, 16(3), 327–34, 2001.

8  Alzheimer's Australia, *National Cross Cultural Dementia Network,* Alzheimer's Australia, 2010 Microsoft Word – NCCDN_background_paper_100719_final.doc (dementia.org.au) (accessed 30 June 2021).

9  Access Economics, *The Dementia Epidemic: Economic impact and positive solutions for Australia,* Canberra, Alzheimer's Australia, March 2003.

10  Low LF, Draper B, Cheng A, et al., *Future Research on Dementia Relating to Culturally and Linguistically Diverse Communities,* Australasian Journal on Ageing, 28(3), 144–148, 2009.

11  Access Economics, *Keeping dementia front of mind: incidence and prevalence 2009–2050,* Alzheimer's Australia, August 2009.

12  Australian Institute of Health and Welfare, *Dementia in Australia,* Cat No Age 70, Canberra, AIHW, 2012.

13  Australian Institute of Health and Welfare, *Dementia among Aged Care Residents: First Information from the Aged Care Funding Instrument,* AIHW, Canberra, 2011.

14  Low LF, Anstey KJ, Lackersteen SM, et al., *Recognition, Attitudes and Causal Beliefs Regarding Dementia in Italian, Greek and Chinese Australians,* Dementia and Geriatric Cognitive Disorders, 30(6), 499–508, 2010.

15  Cultural and Indigenous Research Centre Australia, *CALD Dementia Strategic Model,* Sydney, Office for Ageing, 2008.

16  Alzheimer's Australia Victoria, *Perceptions of dementia in ethnic communities,* Hawthorn, Alzheimer's Australia Victoria, 2008.

17  Low LF, Harrison F, Kochan NA, et al., *Can Mild Cognitive impairment be accurately diagnosed in English speakers from ethnic minorities? Results from the Sydney Memory and Ageing Study,* American Journal of Geriatric Psychiatry, 20(10), 845–853, 2012.

18  Rowland JT, Basic D, Storey JE, Conforti DA, *The Rowland Universal Dementia Assessment Scale (RUDAS) and the Folstein MMSE in a Multicultural Cohort of Elderly Persons,* International Psychogeriatrics, 18(01), 111–120, 2006.

19  Wand A, Draper B, Pourmand D, *Working with interpreters in the psychiatric assessment of older adults from culturally and linguistically diverse backgrounds,* International Psychogeriatrics, 32 (1), 11–16, 2020.

20  Ibid. 2.

21  NHMRC National Institute for Dementia Research, *Culturally and Linguistically Diverse (CALD) Dementia Research Action Plan,* Canberra, NNIDR, 2020.

22  Department of Health and Ageing, *Report to the Minister for Ageing on Residential Care and People with Psychogeriatric Disorders,* Canberra, Australian Government Publishing Service, 2008.

23  Ibid. 16.

24  Productivity Commission, *Caring for Older Australians, Inquiry Report No 53,* Canberra, Australian Government, 2011.

25  Department of Health, *Review of the Culturally and Linguistically Diverse Ageing and Aged Care Strategy,* Canberra, Commonwealth of Australia (Department of Health), 2017.

26  Ibid. 4.

27  Ibid. 15.

28  Radermacher H, Feldman S, Browning C, *Review of Literature Concerning the Delivery of Community Aged care Services to Ethnic Groups – Mainstream Versus Ethno-Specific Services: It's Not an 'Either Or',* Ethnic Communities' Council of Victoria and Partners, 2008.

29  Xiao LD, De Bellis A, Kyriazopoulos H, Draper B, Ullah S, *The effect of a personalized dementia care intervention for caregivers from minority groups,* American Journal of Alzheimer's Disease and Other Dementias, 31 (1), 57–67, 2016.

30  Ibid. 16.

31 Runci SJ, Eppingstall BJ, van der Ploeg ES, O'Connor DW, *Comparison of family satisfaction in Australian ethno-specific and mainstream aged care facilities,* Journal of Gerontological Nursing, 40(4), 54–63, 2014.

32 Runci SJ, Eppingstall BJ, O'Connor DW, *A comparison of verbal communication and psychiatric medication use by Greek and Italian residents with dementia in Australian ethno-specific and mainstream aged care facilities,* International Psychogeriatrics, 24(5), 733–741, 2012.

33 Runci SJ, Eppingstall BJ, van der Ploeg ES, Graham G, O'Connor DW, *The language needs of residents from linguistically diverse backgrounds in Victorian aged care facilities,* Australasian Journal on Ageing, 34(3), 195–198, 2015.

34 Ibid.

35 Department of Health, *Review of the Culturally and Linguistically Diverse Ageing and Aged Care Strategy,* Canberra, Commonwealth of Australia (Department of Health), 2017.

36 Ibid. 4.

37 Tang GWG, Dennis S, Comino E, *Anxiety and Depression in Chinese Patients Attending an Australian GP Clinic,* Australian Family Physician, 38(7), 552–555, 2009.

38 Ibid. 4.

39 Hassett A, George K, Harrigan S, *Admissions of elderly patients from English-speaking and non-English-speaking backgrounds to an inpatient psychogeriatric unit,* Australian and New Zealand Journal of Psychiatry, 33, 576–582, 1999.

40 Hassett A, George K, *Access to a community aged psychiatry service by elderly from non-English speaking backgrounds,* International Journal of Geriatric Psychiatry, 17, 623–28, 2002.

41 Health Policy Analysis, *Evaluation of NSW Service Plan for Specialist Mental Health Services for Older People – Final report Volume 3 (Appendices),* NSW Ministry of Health, Sydney, 2011.

42 Health Policy Analysis, *Evaluation of NSW Service Plan for Specialist Mental Health Services for Older People – Final report Volume 2 (Main Report),* NSW Ministry of Health, Sydney, 2011.

43 Australian Government, *Diversity Action Plan,* Commonwealth of Australia (Department of Health), 2019.

## 18 Concluding Observations and Future Prospects

1 Australian Institute of Health and Welfare, *Older Australia at a glance*, Cat. No. AGE 87, Canberra, AIHW, 2018.

2 Australian Bureau of Statistics, *Life Tables 2017–2019*, ABS, 4 November 2020.

3 Australian Bureau of Statistics, *Life Tables, States, Territories and Australia, 2016–*

*2018 3302.0.55.001,* ABS, 30 October 2019.

4    Australian Bureau of Statistics, *National, State and Territory Population,* ABS, December 2020.

5    National Seniors Productive Ageing Centre, *Ageing Baby Boomers in Australia: Informing actions for better retirement,* ACT, National Seniors Productive Ageing Centre, August 2012.

6    Ibid. 1.

7    Australian Institute of Health and Welfare, *National Drug Strategy Household Survey 2019,* Canberra, AIHW, 2020.

8    NSW Ministry of Health, *Older People's Drug and Alcohol project,* North Sydney, NSW Ministry of Health, 2015.

9    Mi9, *Australian Baby Boomers,* February 2013 02282_fuel_mi9_Baby-Boomers-2564x1200px_v07_11.jpg (763×1632) (marketing.com.au) (accessed 7 July 2021).

10   Ibid. 1.

11   Australian Human Rights Commission, *National prevalence survey of age discrimination in the workplace – 2015,* Australian Human Rights Commission, 2015.

12   Healy J, Williams R, *Are Australians ageist?* Centre for Workplace Leadership, University of Melbourne, 2016.

13   Council of Attorneys General, *National Plan to Respond to the Abuse of Older Australians (Elder Abuse) 2019–2023,* Canberra, Commonwealth of Australia, 2019, https://www.ag.gov.au/ElderAbuseNationalPlan (accessed 1 June 2020).

14   Ibid. 5.

15   Hamilton M, Hamilton C, *Baby boomers and retirement: Dreams, fears and anxieties,* ACT, The Australia Institute, September 2006.

16   Ibid. 1.

17   Dementia Australia, *Dementia Key Facts and Statistics – updated January 2021,* Dementia statistics | Dementia Australia (accessed 14 July 2021).

18   Ibid. 5.

19   Royal Commission into Aged Care Quality and Safety, *Final Report: Care, Dignity and Respect Volume 1,* Canberra, Commonwealth of Australia, 2021.

20   Department of Health, *Australian Government response to the Final Report of the Royal Commission into Aged Care Quality and Safety,* Commonwealth of Australia (Department of Health), 2021.

21   Ibid. 19.

22   Ibid. 20, pp. 4–12.

23   Ibid. 19, p. 220.

24   Ibid. 20, pp. 14–15.

25  Dementia Australia, *A Roadmap for Quality Dementia Care,* Dementia Australia, March 2021 A roadmap for quality dementia care (accessed 8 July 2021).

26  Ibid. 19, p. 220.

27  Ibid. 19, pp. 221 & 252.

28  Pharmaceutical Benefit Advisory Committee, PBAC Meeting Outcomes, November 2021 meeting, pbac-web-outcomes-11-2021.pdf (pbs.gov.au) (accessed 12 May 2022).

29  Ibid. 20, pp. 15–17 & 44–45.

30  Aged Care Quality and Safety Commission, *regulation of restrictive practices and the role of the Senior Practitioner, Restrictive Practices,* Regulatory Bulletin RB 2021–13, 28 June 2021.

31  Ibid. 19, p. 249.

32  Ibid. 20, p. 42.

33  Ibid. 25.

34  Ibid. 19, pp. 239–240 & pp. 258–262.

35  Ibid. 20, pp. 33–34 & 49–56.

36  Department of Health, *Diversity Action Plan,* Australian Government (Department of Health), 2019.

37  Ibid. 19, pp. 240–244.

38  Ibid. 20, pp. 35–38.

39  Ibid. 19, pp. 256–57.

40  Cations M, Day S, Laver K, Withall A, Draper B, *Post-diagnosis young-onset dementia care in the National Disability Insurance Scheme.* Australian and New Zealand Journal of Psychiatry, 56 (3), 270–280, 2022 doi.org/10.1177/00048674211011699.

41  Australian Government, *Budget 2021–22,* Commonwealth of Australia 2021, Budget 2021-22 – Overview (accessed 12 July 2021).

42  Richardson D, Stanford J, *Funding High Quality Aged Care Services,* The Australia Institute, May 7 2021, Funding High-Quality Aged Care Services | The Australia Institute (accessed 12 July 2021).

43  NHMRC, *NHMRC National Institute for Dementia Research,* NHMRC, NHMRC National Institute for Dementia Research | NHMRC (accessed 13 July 2021).

44  NHMRC National Institute for Dementia Research, *Strategic Roadmap for Dementia Research and Translation,* NHMRC 2019, NHMRC National Institute for Dementia Research | NHMRC (accessed 13 July 2021).

45  Australian Dementia Network, Home – Australian Dementia Network (accessed 13 July 2021).

46  Ibid. 44.

47  Alzheimer's Disease International and the Global Coalition on Aging, *Dementia*

*Innovation Readiness Index 2020: 30 Global Cities,* ADI & GCOA, October 2020.

48    Ibid. 19, pp. 170–173.

49    Bhome R, Huntley J, Dalton-Locke C, et al., *Impact of the COVID-19 pandemic on older adults mental health services: A mixed-methods study,* International Journal of Geriatric Psychiatry, 1–11, 2021, https://doi.org/10.1002/gps.5596.

50    Alzheimer's Disease International, *WHO 73rd World Health Assembly Statement on COVID-19,* ADI, May 2020.

51    Howard R, Burns A, *COVID-19 and dementia: a deadly combination,* International Journal of Geriatric Psychiatry, 36, 1120–1121, 2021.

52    Ibid. 49.

53    Australian Dementia Network, *Managing memory clinics during the COVID-19 pandemic: initial perspectives from the Australian Dementia Network Memory Clinics network,* Australian Dementia Network, April 2020.

54    Liu KY, Howard R, Banerjee S, et al., *Dementia well-being and COVID-19: Review and expert consensus on current research and knowledge gaps,* International Journal of Geriatric Psychiatry, 1–43, 2021, https://doi.org/10.1002/gps.5567.

55    Sorinmade OA, Kossoff L, Peisah C, *COVID-19 and Telehealth in older adult psychiatry – opportunities for now and the future,* International Journal of Geriatric Psychiatry, 35, 1427–30, 2020.

56    Macquarie University, *Stepped Care Effectiveness Trial for Ageing Adults,* Macquarie University – Stepped Care Effectiveness Trial for Ageing Adults (mq.edu.au) (accessed 14 July 2021).

57    Personal communication with Duncan Mackellar, Clinical Advisor Old Age Mental Health, South Australia, 25 June 2021.

58    Draper B, Low LF, *What is the effectiveness of old age mental health services?* World Health Organization Regional Office for Europe Health Evidence Network, Copenhagen, Denmark, 2004.

59    Dobrohotoff J, Llewellyn-Jones R, *Psychogeriatric inpatient unit design: a literature review,* International Psychogeriatrics, 23(2), 174–189, 2011.

60    Futeran S, Draper B, *An examination of the needs of older patients with chronic mental illness in public mental health services,* Aging & Mental Health, 16, 327–334, 2012.

61    Lintzeris N, Rivas G, Monds L, Leung S, Withall A, Draper B, *Substance use, health status and service utilisation of older clients attending specialist D&A services,* Drug and Alcohol Review, 35 (2), 223–231, 2016.

62    McKay R, McDonald R, Lie D, McGowan H, *Reclaiming the best of the biopsychosocial model of mental health care and 'recovery' for older people through a person-centred approach,* Australasian Psychiatry, 20(6), 492–495, 2012.

63    SMHSOP Recovery-oriented Practice Improvement Project, *Communique 1,* NSW

Mental Health Drug and Alcohol Older People's Mental Health Policy Unit, 15 May 2015.

64   Grey F, O'Hagan M, *The effectiveness of services led or run by consumers in mental health: rapid review of evidence for recovery-oriented outcomes: an Evidence Check rapid review brokered by the Sax Institute for the Mental Health Commission of New South Wales,* Sax Institute, August 2015.

65   Brodaty H, Draper B, Low L-F, *Behavioural and Psychological Symptoms of Dementia – a 7 tiered Model of Service Delivery,* Medical Journal of Australia, 178, 231–234, 2003.

66   Draper B, Brodaty H, Low LF, *A tiered model of mental health service delivery for older persons: an evidence-based approach,* International Journal of Geriatric Psychiatry, 21, 645–653, 2006.

# Bibliography

## Primary Sources

### Archived Materials

*NSW State Archives and Records*
Medical Casebooks from Gladesville Hospital (NRS5031) and Callan Park Hospital (NRS4994), the Consolidated Indexes to Medical Casebooks (NRS5032), Index to Admission Registers Gladesville (NRS5037), Letters Concerning Patients Callan Park (NRS5002), and Liverpool State Hospital Surgeon Superintendent's Weekly Reports (NRS4951) and Medical Registers (NRS4952).
Report on Care of the Aged (Health Advisory Council) (NRS5170)

*State Library of NSW*
Frederic Norton Manning – report on Lunatic Asylums, Thomas Richards, Governor Printer, Sydney, 1868; Annual Reports of the Inspector General of the Insane (1881–1917), Inspector General of Mental Hospitals (1918 – 1957/58), and Director of State Psychiatric Services (1958/59 – 1970/71); NSW Government Asylums Inquiry Board Report, Charles Potter, Government Printer, Sydney May 1887; Report on Hospitals for the Insane in South Australia 1886; Report of Royal Commission on Charitable Institutions Victoria 1895; Report of the Callan Park Mental Hospital Royal Commission Sydney, Government Printer, 1961

*Libraries Tasmania*
Archives Series – *Hospital for the Insane, Cascades, Case Book HSD54, Royal Derwent Hospital, TA465*

*State Records Office of Western Australia*
Register of Patients Fremantle Asylum (S4507 Cons1120 25), Inspector General of the Insane A/Report 1919/1920 (S675 Cons752 1920/2115), Annual Report Inspector General of Insane 31.12.1932 (S675 Cons752 1933/0564), Report Inspector General of Insane 31 December 1940 (S4410 Cons1067 1941/114)

*Queensland State Archives*
Annual Reports of the Inspector of Hospitals for the Insane 1937–1963

*Public Records Office of Victoria*
VPRS 7680 P1 Register of Patients (VA2840), Kew 1871–1919, Units 1–4

*State Library of Victoria*
Annual Reports of the Inspector of Asylums on the Hospitals for the Insane (1868–69), Inspector of Lunatic Asylums on the Hospitals for the Insane (1870–1904), Inspector-General of the Insane on the Hospitals for the Insane (1905, 1907), Report of the Mental Hygiene Authority (1954–1975).
Office of Psychiatric Services Health Department Victoria – Psychiatric Services for Older People in Victoria 1988

*RANZCP Archives*
Correspondence from G Vernon Davies, Herbert Bower, Ed Chiu, David Ames, John Snowdon, Brian Draper to various RANZCP officers.
Correspondence from RANZCP officers to SPOA and FPOA Executive members
Copies of Australasian Psychiatric Bulletin 1960–1964
Media releases of the Australian National Association for Mental Health, 1988
Copy of NSW Institute of Psychiatry 'Psychiatry of Old Age Course, 1989'

*NSW Association for Mental Health*
Governing Council minutes, Correspondence and Annual Reports pertinent to the founding of ADARDS, 1981–1988

## Newspapers

These were accessed through Trove and the National Library of Australia
*Adelaide Advertiser, Adelaide Mail, Adelaide News, Adelaide Observer, Adelaide Register, Adelaide Times, Australian Town and Country Journal, Ballarat Star, Braidwood Dispatch and Mining Journal, Brisbane Telegraph, Brisbane Week, Camperdown Chronicle, Catholic Weekly* (Sydney), *Colonial Times* (Hobart), *Clarence and Richmond Examiner, Courier-Mail* (Brisbane), *Cumberland Argus and Fruitgrowers Advocate, Daily Herald* (Adelaide), *Daily News* (Perth), *Daily Standard* (Brisbane), *Daily Telegraph* (Sydney), *Don Dorrigo Gazette and Guy Fawkes Advocate, Evening Journal* (Adelaide), *Evening News* (Sydney), *Freeman's Journal, Geelong Advertiser, Gympie Times and Mary River Mining Gazette, Hobart Mercury, Inquirer and Commercial News* (Perth), *Kalgoorlie Western Argus, Launceston Advertiser, Launceston Daily Telegraph, Mount Alexander Mail, Northern Star* (Lismore), *Ovens and Murray Advertiser, Queanbeyan Observer, Queensland Times, Ipswich Herald and General*

*Advertiser, South Australian Advertiser, South Australian Chronicle and Weekly Mail, South Australian Register, South Australian Weekly Chronicle, Sydney Gazette and New South Wales Advertiser, Sydney Mail, Sydney Monitor and Commercial Advertiser, Sydney Morning Herald, Tasmanian News, The Age, The Argus* (Melbourne), *The Banner* (Melbourne), *The Express and Telegraph* (Adelaide), *The Herald* (Melbourne), *Warragul Guardian and Buln Buln and Narracan Shire Advocate, Weekly Herald* (Adelaide), *Weekly Times* (Melbourne), *West Australian, West Australian Sunday Times, Western Mail* (Perth), *Wodonga and Towong Sentinel*

Annual Reports of the Inspector General of the Insane (or equivalent) from each of the Colonies/States were often reported in newspapers either in full or excerpts. These were used to supplement the reports accessed in the various State Libraries and Archives and were particularly useful for the reports from South Australia (for both the lunatic and destitute asylums), Western Australia, Queensland and Tasmania.

## Government, Agency and Non-Government Organisation Reports

Access Economics, *The Dementia Epidemic: Economic impact and positive solutions for Australia,* Canberra, Alzheimer's Australia, March 2003

Access Economics, *Keeping dementia front of mind: incidence and prevalence 2009–2050,* Alzheimer's Australia, August 2009

Access Economics, *Caring Places: planning for aged care and dementia 2010–2050,* Canberra, Access Economics, July 2010

ACT Health, *Agreed requirements for ACT Plan under Subacute Care Component of National Partnership Agreement,* ACT Health 30 April 2009 Hospital and Health workforce Reform – Subacute Care – ACT (federalfinancialrelations.gov.au) (accessed 31 May 2021)

Aged Care Quality and Safety Commission, *regulation of restrictive practices and the role of the Senior Practitioner, Restrictive Practices,* Regulatory Bulletin RB 2021–13, 28 June 2021

Aged Care Sector Committee Diversity Sub-group, *Aged Care Diversity Framework,* Canberra, Commonwealth of Australia, 2017

Alzheimer's Australia Victoria, *Perceptions of dementia in ethnic communities,* Hawthorn, Alzheimer's Australia Victoria, 2008

Alzheimer's Disease International, *WHO 73rd World Health Assembly Statement on COVID-19,* ADI, May 2020

Alzheimer's Disease International and the Global Coalition on Aging, *Dementia Innovation Readiness Index 2020: 30 Global Cities,* ADI & GCOA, October 2020

Auditor General of Victoria, *Building Better Cities: a joint government approach to urban development, Special Report No. 45,* Melbourne, Victorian Government Printer, 1996

Australian Bureau of Statistics, *Australian Historical Population Statistics, Cat No 3105.0.65.001* Canberra, Commonwealth of Australia, 2006

Australian Bureau of Statistics, *Census of Population and Housing: Reflecting Australia – Stories from the Census, 2016. Aboriginal and Torres Strait Islander population, 2016.* ABS cat.no. 2071.0. Canberra: ABS, 2017

Australian Bureau of Statistics, *Life Tables for Aboriginal and Torres Strait Islander Australians, 2015–2017, 3302.0.55.003,* ABS, 28/11/2018

Australian Bureau of Statistics, *The Health and Welfare of Australia's Aboriginal and Torres Strait Islander Peoples 2008,* Commonwealth of Australia, Canberra, 2008

Australian Government Department of Health, *Diversity Action Plan,* Commonwealth of Australia (Department of Health), 2019

Australian Government Department of Health. *Psychological Treatment Services for people with mental illness in Residential Aged Care Facilities.* Canberra, Australian Government Department of Health; 2018.

Australian Human Rights Commission, *National prevalence survey of age discrimination in the workplace – 2015,* Australian Human Rights Commission, 2015

Australian Institute of Health and Welfare, *Dementia in Aged Care Residents 2011, AIHW Aged Care Series Statistics No 32,* Canberra, AIHW, 2011

Australian Institute of Health and Welfare, *Older Aboriginal and Torres Strait Islander People*, Canberra, AIHW, May 2011

Australian Institute of Health and Welfare, *Dementia among Aged Care Residents: First Information from the Aged Care Funding Instrument,* AIHW, Canberra, 2011

Australian Institute of Health and Welfare, *Dementia in Australia*, Cat No Age 70, Canberra, AIHW, 2012

Australian Institute of Health and Welfare, *Australian Burden of Disease Study: Impact and causes of illness and death in Aboriginal and Torres Strait Islander people 2011,* Canberra, AIHW, 2016

AIHW: Kreisfeld R, Harrison JE, *Indigenous injury deaths: 2011–12 to 2015–16. Injury research and statistics series no. 130. Cat. no. INJCAT 210.* Canberra, AIHW, 2020

Australian Institute of Health and Welfare, *Older Australia at a Glance*, Cat. No. AGE 87, Canberra, AIHW, 2018

Australian Institute of Health and Welfare, *Older Australia at a Glance,* Canberra, Australian Government Publishing Service, 1997

Australian Institute of Health and Welfare, *Australia's Welfare,* Canberra, AIHW, 2007

Australian Institute of Health and Welfare, *National Drug Strategy Household Survey 2019,* Canberra, AIHW, 2020

Beveridge W, *Social insurance and allied services – a report*, London, HM Stationery Office, November 1942

Bird M, Anderson K, Blair A, MacPherson S, *Evaluation of the T-BASIS Unit Initiative and Model of Care,* Aged Care Evaluation Unit, NSW Greater Southern Area Health Service, August 2011

Capital Health Network, *Australian Capital Territory Mental Health and Suicide Prevention Plan for 2019–2024,* Canberra, ACT Primary Health Network, 2019

Clinical Epidemiology and Health Service Evaluation Unit, Melbourne Health, *Clinical Practice Guidelines for the Management of Delirium in Older People,* Melbourne, Victorian Government Department of Human Services, October 2006

Commissioner for Senior Victorians, *Submission Royal Commission into Victoria's Mental Health System,* Melbourne, Victorian Government Printer, 2019

Commonwealth of Australia, *National Strategic Framework for Aboriginal and Torres Strait Islander Peoples' Mental Health and Social and Emotional Wellbeing,* Canberra, Department of the Prime Minister and Cabinet, 2017

COTA Victoria, *Submission Royal Commission into Victoria's Mental Health System,* Melbourne, COTA, July 2019

Cultural and Indigenous Research Centre Australia, *CALD Dementia Strategic Model,* Sydney, Office for Ageing, 2008

Dementia Australia, *A Roadmap for Quality Dementia Care,* Dementia Australia, March 2021

Department of Community Services and Health, *Nursing Home and Hostels Review.* Canberra, Australian Government Publishing Service, 1986

Department of Community Services and Health, *Living in a Nursing Home. Outcome Standards for Australian Nursing Homes.* Canberra, Australian Government Publishing Service, 1987

Department of Health, *The North Metropolitan Older Adult Mental Health Program Model of Care,* North Metropolitan Health Service Mental Health, WA Department of Health, 2014

Department of Health, *Review of the Culturally and Linguistically Diverse Ageing and Aged Care Strategy,* Canberra, Commonwealth of Australia (Department of Health), 2017

Department of Health, *Diversity Action Plan,* Australian Government (Department of Health), 2019

Department of Health and Ageing, *A New Strategy for Community Care: The Way Forward,* Canberra, August 2004

Department of Health and Ageing, *National Mental Health Report 2005, Table A-9,* Canberra, 2005

Department of Health and Ageing, *National Mental Health Report 2007, Tables A-20 and A-21,* Canberra, 2007

Department of Health and Ageing, *Community Packaged Care Guidelines,* Canberra, Australian Government Publishing Service, 2007

Department of Health and Ageing, *Report to the Minister for Ageing on Residential Care and People with Psychogeriatric Disorders.* Canberra, Australian Government Publishing Service, 2008

Department of Health and Ageing, *Review of the Aged Care Funding Instrument,* Canberra, DOHA, 2011

Department of Health and Ageing, *The Dementia and Veterans' Supplements in Aged Care, Consultation Paper,* Canberra, DOHA, April 2013

Department of Health and Family Services, *Mid-plan report of the National Action Plan for Dementia Care,* Canberra, Australian Government Publishing Service, 1996

Department of Health, Housing, and Community Services, *Mid-term Review of the Aged Care Reform Strategy Report, A*ustralian Government Publishing Service, Canberra, 1991

Department of Health, Housing, and Community Services, *Putting the Pieces Together: a National Action Plan for Dementia Care.* Canberra, Australian Government Publishing Service, 1992

Department of Health, *Geriatric Medicine 2016 Fact Sheet.* Canberra, Commonwealth of Australia, 2017

Department of Health, *The Fifth National Mental Health and Suicide Prevention Plan,* Canberra, Commonwealth of Australia, 2017

Department of Health, *Review of the Culturally and Linguistically Diverse (CALD) Ageing and Aged Care Strategy. Publication Number: 12060,* Canberra, Commonwealth of Australia, 2017

Department of Health, *Specialist Dementia Care Program Framework,* Canberra, Department of Health, December 2018

Department of Health, *2017–18 Report on the Operation of the Aged Care Act 1997,* Canberra, Commonwealth of Australia, 2018

Department of Health, *2018–19 Report on the Operation of the Aged Care Act 1997.* Online ISBN: 978-1-76007-413-5, Canberra, Commonwealth of Australia, 2019, p. 7

Department of Health, *Actions to support older Aboriginal and Torres Strait Islander people – a Guide for Aged Care Providers,* Canberra, Commonwealth of Australia, February 2019

Department of Health, *Actions to support older Aboriginal and Torres Strait Islander people – a Guide for Consumers,* Canberra, Commonwealth of Australia, February 2019

Department of Health, *Australian Government response to the Final Report of the Royal Commission into Aged Care Quality and Safety,* Commonwealth of Australia (Department of Health), 2021

Department of Health Western Australia, *Dementia Model of Care,* Perth, Aged Care Network, Department of Health, Western Australia, 2011

Department of Human Services, *Specialist mental health service components,* State Government Victoria, April 2005

Department of the Prime Minister and Cabinet, *Closing the Gap Report 2020,* Canberra, Commonwealth of Australia, 2020

Department of Social Services, *Phase one – Severe Behaviour Response Teams Operational Guidelines,* Canberra, DSS, May 2015

Draper B, Low LF, *What is the effectiveness of old age mental health services?* World Health Organization Regional Office for Europe Health Evidence Network, Copenhagen, Denmark, 2004

Fleming R, Zeisel J, Bennett K, *World Alzheimer Report 2020 Design Dignity Dementia: dementia-related design and the built environment Volume 1.* London, England, Alzheimer's Disease International, 2020

Gray L, *Two year review of aged care reforms,* Canberra, Commonwealth of Australia, 2001

Groves A, Thomson D, McKellar D, Procter N, *The Oakden Report,* Adelaide, South Australia, SA Health, Department for Health and Ageing, 2017

Health Policy Analysis, *Evaluation of NSW Service Plan for Specialist Mental Health Services for Older People – Final report Volume 1 (Summary), Volume 2 (Main Report), Volume 3 (Appendices),* NSW Ministry of Health, Sydney, 2011

Hicks J, Allen G, *A Century of Change: Trends in UK statistics since 1900,* Research Paper 99/111, Social and General Statistics Section, House of Commons Library, 21 December 1999

Human Rights and Equal Opportunities Commission, *Human Rights and Mental Illness: Report of the National Inquiry into the Human Rights of People with Mental Illness – Part III.* Canberra, Australian Government Publishing Service, 1993

Hutchinson B, *Old People in a Modern Australian Community: A social Survey,* Carlton, MUP, 1954

KPMG, *Dementia services pathways – an essential guide to effective service planning,* KPMG, February 2011

Kratiuk S, Young J, Rawson G, Williams S, *A Double Jeopardy: A Report on Dementia Clients of Non-English Speaking Backgrounds,* South Western Area Health Services, Sydney, 1992

Masso M, Duncan C, Grootematt P, et al., *Specialist dementia care units: an Evidence Check rapid review* brokered by the Sax Institute (www.saxinstitute.org.au) for the

Commonwealth Department of Health, 2017.

Mental Health Branch, Queensland Health, *The Queensland Plan for Mental Health 2007–2017*, The State of Queensland, Queensland Health, June 2008

Mental Health Commission, *Draft Western Australian Mental Health, Alcohol and Other Drug Services Plan 2015 2025 (Plan) Update 2018*, Mental Health Commission, Government of Western Australia, 2019

Ministerial Conference on Ageing, *Communique,* 15 December 2010

Myer Foundation, *2020: a vision for aged care in Australia.* Melbourne, Myer Foundation, 2002

National Aboriginal and Torres Strait Islander Health Council, *National Strategic Framework for Aboriginal and Torres Strait Islander Health: Context,* National Aboriginal and Torres Strait Islander Health Council, Canberra, July 2003

National Advisory Group for Aboriginal and Torres Strait Islander Aged Care, *Submission to the Royal Commission into Aged Care Quality and Safety,* September 2019

National Institute for Health and Care Excellence, *Donepezil, galantamine, rivastigmine and memantine for the treatment of Alzheimer's disease. (TA217)* National Institute for Health and Care Excellence, Published 23 March 2011, last updated 20 June 2018

NHMRC National Institute for Dementia Research, *Culturally and Linguistically Diverse (CALD) Dementia Research Action Plan,* Canberra, NNIDR, 2020

NSW Department of Community Services, *Working with Aboriginal people and communities,* Ashfield, NSW Department of Community Services, February 2009

NSW Department of Health, *NSW: a new direction for Mental Health,* North Sydney, NSW Department of Health, 2006

NSW Department of Health, *Summary Report: The management and accommodation of older people with severely and persistently challenging behaviours in residential care,* Gladesville, NSW Department of Health, 2006

NSW Department of Health, *NSW Service Plan for Specialist Mental Health Services for Older people (SMHSOP) 2005–2015,* Gladesville, NSW Department of Health, 2006

NSW Department of Health, *Evaluation of the Mental Health Aged Care Partnership Initiative,* Sydney, NSW Department of Health, December 2009

NSW Department of Health, *The NSW Dementia Services Framework, 2010–2015,* North Sydney, NSW Department of Health, 2010

NSW Health Department, *Caring for Older People's Mental Health: a Strategy for the Delivery of Mental Health Care for Older People in NSW,* State Health Publication No. (CMH) 990009, Gladesville, NSW Department of Health, January 1999

NSW MHDAO Older People's Mental Health Policy Unit, *Aboriginal Older People's*

*Mental Health: Resources for Local Health District SMHSOP Services,* Orange, Older People's Mental Health Policy Unit, 2015

NSW Ministerial Taskforce on Psychotropic Medication Use in Nursing Homes, *Discussion Paper,* NSW Health, May 1997

NSW Ministry of Health and the Royal Australian and New Zealand College of Psychiatrists, *Assessment and Management of People with Behavioural and Psychological Symptoms of Dementia (BPSD),* North Sydney, NSW Ministry of Health, May 2013

NSW Ministry of Health, *Older People's Drug and Alcohol project,* North Sydney, NSW Ministry of Health, 2015

NSW Ministry of Health, *NSW Older People's Mental Health Services, Service Plan 2017–2027,* North Sydney, NSW Ministry of Health, 2017, Appendix 2

NSW Ministry of Health, *Specialist Mental Health Services for Older People (SMHSOP) Acute Inpatient Unit Model of Care Project Report,* Sydney, NSW Health, 2012

NSW Ministry of Health, *SMHSOP Acute Inpatient Unit Model of Care Guideline,* Mental Health & Drug and Alcohol Office, Ministry of Health North Sydney, 23 June 2016

NSW Ministry of Health, *NSW Older People's Mental Health Community Services: Key Features of the Model of Care,* North Sydney, NSW Ministry of Health, 2020

Parliament of Australia, *In a home or at home? Home care and accommodation for the aged.* Report of the House of Representatives Standing Committee on Expenditure. Chair: LB McLeay, Canberra, Australian Government Publishing Service, 1981

Parliament of Australia, *Private Nursing Homes in Australia: Their Conduct, Administration and Ownership. Report by the Senate Select Committee on Private Hospitals and Nursing Homes,* Canberra, Australian Government Publishing Service, 1985, p. 61

Parliament of Australia, *Residential care for the aged: an overview of Government policy from 1962 to 1993,* Social Policy Group, Department of the Parliamentary Library, Canberra, Commonwealth of Australia, 1993

Prince M, Wimo A, Guerchet M, Ali GC, Wu YT, Prina M, *World Alzheimer Report 2015: the Global Impact of Dementia: An analysis of prevalence, incidence, costs and trends.* London, Alzheimer's Disease International, August 2015

Productivity Commission, *Caring for Older Australians, Inquiry Report No 53,* Canberra, Australian Government, 2011

Psychogeriatrics Working Party, Ministerial Implementation Committee on Mental Health and Developmental Disability (Chair WA Barclay), *Report to the Minister for Health, Volume Three.* Sydney, NSW Minister for Health, November 1988

Queensland Government, *Mental Health Services for Older People,* State of Queensland, 1996

Queensland Government, Chapter 8, *Health* in 'Queensland Past and Present: 100 years of statistics 1896–1996, pp. 246–254. State of Queensland, 2009

Queensland Health. *The Road to Recovery – a history of mental health services in Queensland 1859–2009.* Queensland Government, 2013

Queensland Health, *Queensland Health's Directions for Aged Care 2004 – 2011,* Brisbane, Queensland Health, 2004

RANZCP Position Statement 22, *Psychiatric Services for the Elderly.* RANZCP Archives, May 1987

RANZCP Position Statement 29, *Relationships between Geriatric and Psychogeriatric Services.* RANZCP Archives, May 1990

RANZCP Position Statement 81, *Use of antidepressants to treat depression in dementia,* RANZCP Archives, January 2015

Rosewarne R, Opie J, Bruce A, et al., *Care Needs of People with Dementia and Challenging Behaviour Living in Residential Facilities,* Canberra, Australian Government Publishing Service, 1997

Richmond D (Chair), *Inquiry into Health Services for the Psychiatrically Ill and Developmentally Disabled,* NSW State Health, March 1983

Royal Commission into Aged Care Quality and Safety, *Interim Report: Neglect.* Canberra, Commonwealth of Australia, 2019

Royal Commission into Aged Care Quality and Safety, *Final Report: Care, Dignity and Respect Volume 1,* Canberra, Commonwealth of Australia, 2021

Royal Commission into Victoria's Mental Health System, *Final Report, Summary and Recommendations,* Melbourne, Victorian Government Printer, February 2021

Sainty MR, Johnson KA (eds), *Census of New South Wales – November 1828,* Sydney, Public Library of Australian History, 1980

Sax S, *Report for the Consultative Committee for the Care of the Aged,* NSW Department of Public Health, August 1965

Slade T, Johnston A, Teeson M, et al., *The Mental Health of Australians 2: Report on the 2007 National Survey of Mental Health and Wellbeing,* Canberra, Department of Health and Ageing, 2009

SMHSOP Recovery-oriented Practice Improvement Project, *Communique 1,* NSW Mental Health Drug and Alcohol Older People's Mental Health Policy Unit, 15 May 2015

South Australian Government, *The 'Oakden Report' Response,* South Australia Health, June 2018

South Australian Social Inclusion Board, *Stepping Up: A Social Inclusion Action Plan for Mental Health Reform 2007–2012,* South Australia, Social Inclusion Board, January 2007

Stewart J, O'Connor D, Cameron I, Kurrle S, *Final Report: Review of Confused And Disturbed Elderly (CADE) units in New South Wales*, Sydney, NSW Department of Health, 2006

Stoller A, Arscott KW, *Report on Mental Health Facilities and Needs of Australia*, Canberra, Commonwealth of Australia, 1955

Tasmanian Government, *Rethink 2020: a state plan for mental health in Tasmania 2020–2025*, Tasmanian Government, November 2020

The Lunacy Statute, 1867. Victorian Government Gazette, Supplement, 10 September 1867

United Nations Department of Economic and Social Affairs, *Report on the World Social Situation 2003. Social Vulnerability: Sources and Challenges*, New York, United Nations, 2003

US Bureau of the Census, *65+ in the United States*. Current Population Reports, Special Studies, p. 23–190, Washington DC, US Government Printing Office, 1996

Victoria Aged, Community and Mental Health Division, *Victoria's mental health service: generic brief for a psychogeriatric assessment and admissions unit – 20 bed*, Melbourne: Aged, Community and Mental Health Division, Department of Human Services, 1997

Victoria Aged, Community and Mental Health Division, *Victoria's mental health service: generic brief for a psychogeriatric nursing home – 30 bed*, Melbourne : Aged, Community and Mental Health Division, Department of Human Services, 1997

Victoria Psychiatric Services Division, *Victoria's mental health service: the framework for service delivery: aged persons services*, Melbourne, Department of Health and Community Services, April 1996

Western Australian Department of Health, *Older Adult Mental Health Sub Network Establishment Report*, Perth, Health Networks, Western Australian Department of Health, 2016

World Health Organisation, *Mental Health Problems of Aging and the Aged*. Geneva: WHO, 1959

World Health Organisation, *Psychogeriatrics*, Geneva, WHO, 1972

World Health Organization, *A glossary of terms for community health care and services for older persons*, Geneva, WHO, 2004

## Unpublished Correspondence, submissions, lectures

NSW Branch RANZCP, *Submission to Inquiry into Health Services for the Psychiatrically Ill and Developmentally Disabled*, RANZCP, October 1982

Australian National Association for Mental Health, *Annual Report 1982–83*. ANAMH, Melbourne, 1983

Balaraman CS, *Correspondence with Sid Williams, Working Party on Geriatric Psychiatry in NSW,* 8 September 1988

Hall K, *Mainstreaming aged psychiatric services: the Caulfield experience,* unpublished lecture notes, 2005

Merlin M, *The development of a psychogeriatric service at Parramatta.* Unpublished lecture notes, Clinicians Conference, Sydney, 19 June 1981

O'Neill TJ, *Correspondence with Sid Williams, Working Party on Geriatric Psychiatry in NSW,* 29 August 1988

Russell B, *Correspondence with Sid Williams, Working Party on Geriatric Psychiatry in NSW,* 31 August 1988

Sammut A, Williams S, *Submission to the NSW Consultative Committee on Ageing re Psychogeriatric Care,* Circa 1993

Williams S, *What is psychogeriatrics in NSW?* Unpublished lecture notes, Clinicians Conference, Sydney, 19 June 1981

Williams S, *Correspondence with Peter Anderson, NSW Minister for Health,* 17 December 1986

Williams S, Sammut A, *Submission to the NSW Consultative Committee on Ageing re psychogeriatric care,* 1983

## Journal articles

Almeida OP, Flicker L, Fenner S, et al., *The Kimberley Assessment of Depression of Older Indigenous Australians: Prevalence of depressive disorders, risk factors and validation of the KICA-dep Scale,* PLoS ONE, 9, e94983, 2014

Ames D, Flicker L, Helme R, *A memory clinic at a geriatric hospital: rationale, routine and results from the first 100 patients,* Medical Journal of Australia, 156, 618–622, 1992

Ames D, *Edmond Chiu installed as President of IPA,* IPA Bulletin, 16 (3), 1, 1999

Anderson K, Bird M, Blair A, MacPherson S, *Development and effectiveness of an integrated inpatient and community service for challenging behaviour in late life: from Confused and Disturbed Elderly to Transitional Behavioural Assessment and Intervention Service,* Dementia, 15(6), 1340–57, 2016

Andrews G, *Reply to Snowdon re health Services Research into the Future of Australian Psychiatry,* Australian and New Zealand Journal of Psychiatry, 24, 435–436, 1990

Andrews G, Henderson S, Hall W, *Prevalence, comorbidity, disability and service utilisation: Overview of the Australian National Mental Health Survey,* British Journal of Psychiatry, 178, 145–153, 2001

Anonymous, *Report of the Thirty-Seventh Annual Meeting of the Medico-Psychological Association,* Journal of Mental Science, 28, 460, 1882

Anonymous, *Bower praised as Australian doyen*, IPA Bulletin, Winter 1995 – Spring 1996, p. 12

Bhome R, Huntley J, Dalton-Locke C, et al., *Impact of the COVID-19 pandemic on older adults mental health services: A mixed-methods study*, International Journal of Geriatric Psychiatry, 1–11, 2021, https://doi.org/10.1002/gps.5596

Bonwick R, *The Older Veteran's Psychiatry Program (OVPP), Melbourne* FPOA News, June, 9, 1999

Bonwick R, *Service development in the private sector in Victoria*, FPOA News, 12, April 2011

Bower HM, *Sensory stimulation and the treatment of senile dementia*, Medical Journal of Australia, i(22), 1113–1119, 1967

Bower HM, *The first psychogeriatric day-centre in Victoria*, Medical Journal of Australia, I (May 17), 1047–1050, 1969

Bower H, *Dr Herbert Bower – Psychiatrist 19/12/1914 – 29/8/2004*, Australasian Psychiatry, 12(4), 430–432, 2004

Brodaty H, *The need for distinctive psychogeriatric services*, RANZCP News and Notes, 24, 27–28 February 1991

Brodaty H, *Low diagnostic yield in a memory disorders clinic*, International Psychogeriatrics, 2(2), 149–159, 1990

Brodaty H, Ames D, Snowdon J, et al., *A randomized placebo-controlled trial of risperidone for the treatment of aggression, agitation and psychosis of dementia*, Journal of Clinical Psychiatry, 64, 134–143, 2003

Brodaty H, Draper B, Low L-F, *Behavioural and Psychological Symptoms of Dementia – a 7 tiered Model of Service Delivery*, Medical Journal of Australia, 178, 231–234, 2003

Brodaty H, Draper B, Miller J, et al., *Randomised controlled trial of different models of care for nursing home residents with dementia complicated by psychosis or depression*, Journal of Clinical Psychiatry, 64, 63–72, 2003

Brodaty H, Gresham M, *Effect of a training programme to reduce stress in carers of patients with dementia*, British Medical Journal, 2;299(6712), 1375–9, 1989

Brodaty H, Gresham M, Luscombe G, *The Prince Henry Hospital dementia caregivers' training programme*, International Journal of Geriatric Psychiatry, 12(2), 183–92, 1997

Burvill P, *Psychiatric population of nursing homes*, Australian and New Zealand Journal of Psychiatry, 3, 75–79, 1969

Calabria B, Doran CM, Vos T, Shakeshaft AP, Hall W, *Epidemiology of alcohol-related burden of disease among Indigenous Australians*, Australian and New Zealand Journal of Public Health, 34(S1), S47–S51, 2010

Carter J, *States of confusion: Australian policies and the elderly confused*, Social Welfare

Research Centre Report Proceedings, No. 4, University of New South Wales, Sydney, 1981

Cations M, Withall A, White F, et al., *Why aren't people with young onset dementia and their caregivers using formal services? Results from the INSPIRED study.* PLOS ONE, 12(7): e0180935, 2017

Cations M, Day S, Laver K, Withall A, Draper B, *Experiences and satisfaction with post-diagnosis young onset dementia care in the National Disability Insurance Scheme.* Australian and New Zealand Journal of Psychiatry, doi. org/10.1177/00048674211011699 published online 13 May 2021

Cawte J, *Ethnopsychiatry in Central Australia: I. Traditional illnesses in the Eastern Aranda People,* British Journal of Psychiatry, 111, 1069–1077, 1965

Cawte J, Kidson MA, *Ethnopsychiatry in Central Australia: II. The evolution of illness in a Walbiri lineage,* British Journal of Psychiatry, 111, 1079–1085, 1965

Chester TE, *The Guillebaud Report,* Public Administration, 34 (2), 199–210, June 1956

Chiu A, Nguyen HV, Reutens S, et al., *Clinical outcomes and length of stay of a co-located psychogeriatric and geriatric unit,* Archives of Gerontology and Geriatrics, 49, 233–236, 2009

Chiu E, *Spirit in Ageing, 7th Congress Chairman's Report,* IPA Bulletin, 12 (2), 10, Winter 1995 – Spring 1996

Chiu E, *Cane toads, jacarandas, headstones and the MCG – a very fortunate journey.* FPOA News, March, 11–13, 2005

Clifford W, Marjoram J, *Suicide in South Australia,* Australian Institute of Criminology, 1979

Cohen-Mansfield J, Bester A, *Flexibility as a management principle in dementia care: the ADARDS example,* The Gerontologist, 46(4), 540–544, 2006

Cook L, Dax E, Maclay W, *The geriatric problem in mental hospitals,* Lancet, 259, 377–382, 1952

Daniel R, *A two-year study of geriatric admissions in a Queensland mental hospital,* The Medical Journal of Australia, i: 1034–1039, 1968

Davies V, *Clinical advances in geriatric psychiatry,* The Medical Journal of Australia, ii, 43–46, 1959

Davies GV, *The relation of physical and mental disease in later life,* The Medical Journal of Australia, July 22, 48(2), 152–154, 1961

Davies GV, *The geriatric population of a mental hospital,* The Medical Journal of Australia, I, 181–184, 1965

Davies GV, *Female geriatric admissions to a mental hospital,* The Medical Journal of Australia, ii, 309–312, 1965

Davies GV, *Family relationships of elderly mental hospital patients,* Australian and New

Zealand Journal of Psychiatry, 2, 264–271, 1968

Davies GV, Teltscher B, Davies B, *Senile and arteriosclerotic dementia – a study of personal, social and family data*, Australian and New Zealand Journal of Psychiatry, 3, 398–400, 1969

Dobbie JA, *A survey of older admissions to psychiatric hospitals in Sydney*, Australian and New Zealand Journal of Psychiatry, 1, 80–85, 1967

Draper B, *Psychogeriatric training in Australia and New Zealand: a survey of psychiatry trainees and training program coordinators*, Australian and New Zealand Journal of Psychiatry, 28, 121–128, 1994

Draper B, *Psychogeriatric services in Australia*, IPA Bulletin, 11(2), 19–20, Winter 1994

Draper B, *Older people in hospitals for the insane in New South Wales, Australia, 1849–1905*, History of Psychiatry, 2021, doi.org/10.1177/0957154X211029479

Draper B, *Dementia in nineteenth-century Australia*, Health and History, 23(1), 38–60, 2021

Draper B, *G Vernon Davies: Unsung pioneer of old age psychiatry in Victoria*, Australasian Psychiatry, 30(2), 203–205, 2022

Draper B, Brodaty H, Low L-F, et al., *Use of psychotropic drugs in Sydney nursing homes: Associations with depression, psychosis and behavioural disturbances*, International Psychogeriatrics, 13(1), 107–120, 2001

Draper B, Brodaty H, Low LF, *A tiered model of mental health service delivery for older persons: an evidence-based approach*, International Journal of Geriatric Psychiatry, 21, 645–653, 2006

Draper B, Hudson C, Peut A, Karmel R, Chan C, Gibson D, *Hospital Dementia Services Project: Aged care and dementia services in NSW hospitals*, Australasian Journal on Ageing, 33(4), 237–243, 2014

Draper B, Jochelson T, Kitching D, Snowdon J, Brodaty H, Russell B, *Mental health service delivery to older people in NSW: perceptions of aged care, adult mental health and mental health services for older people*, Australian and New Zealand Journal of Psychiatry, 37, 735–740, 2003

Draper B, Low L-F, *Psychiatric services for the 'old' old*, International Psychogeriatrics, 22, 582–588, 2010

Draper B, Meares S, McIntosh H, *A Psychogeriatric Outreach Service to Nursing Homes in Sydney*, Australasian Journal on Ageing 17, 184–186, 1998

Draper B, Reutens S, Subau D, *Workforce and advanced training survey of the RANZCP Faculty of Psychiatry of Old Age: issues and challenges for the field.* Australasian Psychiatry, 18, 142–145, 2010

Draper B, Snowdon J, *Psychiatry of old age: from Section to Faculty*, Australian and New Zealand Journal of Psychiatry, 33, 785–788, 1999

Duke M, *Spotlight on one institution in Australia*, IPA Bulletin, 11(2), 20, 1994

Fejer I, *From Robin Hood to the Pharaohs – History of the Forming Phase of IPA,* The International Psychogeriatric Association Newsletter, 8(1), 24–28, 1991

Fleming R, Bowles J, *Units for the confused and disturbed elderly: development, design, programming, and evaluation,* Australian Journal on Ageing, 6(4), 25–28, 1987

Folstein ME, Folstein SE, McHugh PR, *Mini-Mental State: a practical method for grading the state of patients for the clinician,* Journal of Psychiatric Research, 12, 189–198, 1975

Futeran S, Draper B, *An examination of the needs of older patients with chronic mental illness in public mental health services,* Aging & Mental Health, 16, 327–334, 2012

Garvey G, Simmonds D, Clements V, et al., *Understanding Dementia amongst Indigenous Australians.* Aboriginal and Islander Health Worker Journal, 35 (2), 16–18, 2011

George K, Giri S, *An Intensive Community Team in aged persons mental health,* Australasian Psychiatry, 19(1), 56–58, 2011

Gubhaju L, McNamara BJ, Banks E, et al., *The overall health and risk factor profile of Australian Aboriginal and Torres Strait Islander participants from the 45 and up study,* BMC Public Health, 13, 661, 2013

Hall K, *Memory Clinics in Victoria.* IPA Bulletin, 16(4), 12–14, 1999

Harper C, *Wernicke's encephalopathy in Western Australia: a common preventable disease,* Australian Alcohol Drug Review, 2(1), 71–73, 1983

Harrison AW, *Assessment and accommodation of demented patients in the community,* Australian and New Zealand Journal of Psychiatry, 15, 53–55, 1981

Harrison AW, Kernutt GJ, Piperoglou MV, *A survey of patients in a regional geriatric psychiatry inpatient unit,* Australian and New Zealand Journal of Psychiatry, 22, 412–417, 1988

Hassett A, George K, Harrigan S, *Admissions of elderly patients from English-speaking and non-English-speaking backgrounds to an inpatient psychogeriatric unit,* Australian and New Zealand Journal of Psychiatry, 33, 576–582, 1999

Hassett A, George K, *Access to a community aged psychiatry service by elderly from non-English speaking backgrounds,* International Journal of Geriatric Psychiatry, 17, 623–28, 2002

Henderson AS, Scott R, Kay DWK, *The elderly who live alone: their mental health and social relationships,* Australian and New Zealand Journal of Psychiatry, 20, 202–209, 1986

Herst L, *Other news from around Australia – Tasmania,* FPOA News, Issue 1, 8, June 1999

Herst L, *Report from Tasmania,* FPOA News, Issue 3, 7, December 2000

Herst L, *Report from Tasmania,* FPOA News, Issue 5, 7, September 2001

Howard R, Burns A, *COVID-19 and dementia: a deadly combination,* International Journal of Geriatric Psychiatry, 36, 1120–1121, 2021

Jorm AF, Mackinnon AJ, Henderson AS, et al., *The Psychogeriatric Assessment Scales: a multidimensional alternative to categorical diagnoses of dementia and depression in the elderly,* Psychological Medicine, 25, 447–460, 1995

Kay DWK, Beamish P, Roth M, *Old age mental disorders in Newcastle upon Tyne Part 1: A study of prevalence,* British Journal of Psychiatry, 110, 146–158, 1964

Kay DWK, Beamish P, Roth M, *Old age mental disorders in Newcastle upon Tyne Part 2: A study of possible social and medical causes,* British Journal of Psychiatry, 110, 668–682, 1964

Kay DWK, Holding TA, Jones B, Littler S, *Psychiatric morbidity in Hobart's dependent aged,* Australian and New Zealand Journal of Psychiatry, 21, 463–475, 1987

Kidson MA, *Psychiatric disorders in the Walbiri, Central Australia,* Australian and New Zealand Journal of Psychiatry, 1, 14–22, 1967

Kiloh LG, *Pseudo-dementia,* Acta Psychiatrica Scandinavica, 37, 336–351, 1961

Koder DA, Helmes E, *The current status of clinical geropsychology in Australia: A survey of practising psychologists,* Australian Psychologist, 43(1), 22–26, 2008

Koder DA, Helmes E, *Predictors of working with older adults in an Australian psychologist sample: revisiting the influence of contact,* Professional Psychology: Research and Practice, 39(3), 276–282, 2008

Laver K, Cumming R, Dyer S, et al., *Clinical Practice Guidelines for Dementia in Australia,* Medical Journal of Australia, 204(5), 191–193, 2016

Lefroy RB, *Permanent Care of Elderly People in Institutions,* Medical Journal of Australia, 707–12, 4 October 1969

Leong M, *News from Queensland,* SPOA Newsletter, 5, Winter 1997

Levy R, *President's Report. A Precedent-setting success: Congress brings 1300 to Sydney,* IPA Bulletin, 12 (2), 1–2, Winter 1995 – Spring 1996

Li SQ, Guthridge SL, Aratchige PE, et al., *Dementia prevalence and incidence among the Indigenous and non-Indigenous populations of the Northern Territory,* Medical Journal of Australia, 200(8), 465–469, 2014

Lintzeris N, Rivas G, Monds L, Leung S, Withall A, Draper B, *Substance use, health status and service utilisation of older clients attending specialist D&A services,* Drug and Alcohol Review, 35 (2), 223–231, 2016

Liu KY, Howard R, Banerjee S, et al., *Dementia well-being and COVID-19: Review and expert consensus on current research and knowledge gaps,* International Journal of Geriatric Psychiatry, 1–43, 2021, https://doi.org/10.1002/gps.5567

Lie D, *Queensland update,* FPOA News, 8, May 2001

Lie D, *Aged Care Mental Health Service, Princess Alexandra Hospital, Brisbane,* FPOA News, 6, April 2003

Lie D, *Public psychogeriatric services in Queensland,* FPOA News, 5, July 2008

LoGiudice D, Hassett A, Cook R, Flicker L, Ames D, *Equity of Access to a Memory Clinic in Melbourne? Non-English Speaking Background Attenders Are More Severely Demented and Have Increased Rates of Psychiatric Disorders.* International Journal of Geriatric Psychiatry, 16(3), 327–34, 2001

LoGiudice D, Smith K, Thomas J, et al., *Kimberley Indigenous Cognitive Assessment tool (KICA): Development of a cognitive assessment tool for older Indigenous Australians,* International Psychogeriatrics, 18, 269–280, 2006

LoGiudice D, Strivens E, Smith K, et al., *The KICA Screen: the psychometric properties of a shortened version of the KICA (Kimberley Indigenous Cognitive Assessment),* Australasian Journal on Ageing, 30(4), 215–219, 2011

Low LF, Anstey KJ, Lackersteen SM, et al., *Recognition, Attitudes and Causal Beliefs Regarding Dementia in Italian, Greek and Chinese Australians,* Dementia and Geriatric Cognitive Disorders, 30(6), 499–508, 2010

Low LF, Harrison F, Kochan NA, et al., *Can Mild Cognitive impairment be accurately diagnosed in English speakers from ethnic minorities? Results from the Sydney Memory and Ageing Study,* American Journal of Geriatric Psychiatry, 20(10), 845–853, 2012

Manning FN, *Insanity in Australian Aborigines with a brief analysis of 32 cases,* Intercolonial Medical Congress of Australasia, 4, 857–860, 1889

Mayer-Gross W, *Electric convulsion treatment in patients over 60,* Journal of Mental Science, 91, 101–103, 1945

McKay R, *From the Chair,* Faculty of Psychiatry of Old Age Newsletter, 2–3 April 2013

McKhann G, Drachman D, Folstein M, Katzman R, Price D, Stadlan EM, *Clinical diagnosis of Alzheimer's disease: report of the NINCDS-ADRDA Work Group under the auspices of the Department of Health and Human Services Task Force on Alzheimer's disease,* Neurology, 34(7): 939–944, 1984

McKhann GM, Knopman DS, Chertkow H, et al., *The diagnosis of dementia due to Alzheimer's disease: recommendations from the National Institute on Aging-Alzheimer's Association workgroups on diagnostic guidelines for Alzheimer's disease.* Alzheimer's and Dementia, 7(3), 263–269, 2011

Nascher I, *Geriatrics,* New York Medical Journal, 90, 358–359, 1909

O'Bryan RJ, *Developing a community responsive psycho-geriatric service,* Australian Journal on Ageing, 6(4), 15–18, 1987

O'Connor DW, Parslow RA, *Different responses to K-10 and CIDI suggest that complex structured psychiatric interviews underestimate rates of mental disorder in older people,* Psychological Medicine, 39, 1527–1531, 2009

O'Connor DW, Parslow RA, *Differences in older people's responses to CIDI's depression screening and diagnostic questions may point to age-related bias,* Journal of Affective Disorders, 125 (1–3), 361–364, 2010

O'Connor DW, Jackson K, Lie D, McGowan H, McKay R, *Survey of aged psychiatry services' support of older Australians with very severe, persistent behavioural symptoms of dementia,* Australasian Journal on Ageing, 37(4), E133–E138, 2018

O'Connor D, Melding P, *A survey of publicly funded aged psychiatry services in Australia and New Zealand,* Australian and New Zealand Journal of Psychiatry, 40, 368–373, 2006

O'Connor D, Stafrace S, *From Victoria,* FPOA News, September, 8, 2001

O'Connor M, *Western Australia Update,* FPOA News, 9, September 2001

O'Connor M, *Report from Western Australia,* FPOA News, 8, April 2002

Over R, *Interest patterns of Australian psychologists,* Australian Psychologist, 26, 49–53, 1991

Pachana N, Emery E, Konnert C, Woodhead E, Edelstein B, *Geropsychology content in clinical training programs: a comparison of Australian, Canadian and US data,* International Psychogeriatrics, 22, 909–918, 2010

Pachana N, Helmes E, Koder D, *Guidelines for the provision of psychological services for older adults,* Australian Psychologist, 41, 15–22, 2006

Peterson BH, *The Age of Ageing,* Australian and New Zealand Journal of Psychiatry, 7, 9–15, 1973

Pettigrew J, *What is happening in the Northern Territory,* FPOA News, 6–7 January 2008

Prince M, Ali GC, Guerchet M, Prina AM, Albanese E, Wu YT, *Recent global trends in the prevalence and incidence of dementia, and survival with dementia,* Alzheimer's Research & Therapy, 8, 23, 2016, DOI 10.1186/s13195-016-0188-8

Pritchard RJ, *Psychogeriatric nursing in Victoria, Australia,* IPA Bulletin, 8(1), 19–20, 1991

Radford K, Mack HA, Draper B, et al., *Prevalence of dementia and cognitive impairment in urban and regional Aboriginal Australians,* Alzheimer's & Dementia, 11, 271–279, 2015

Radford K, Lavrencic LM, Delbaere K, et al., *Factors associated with the high prevalence of dementia in older Aboriginal Australians,* Journal of Alzheimer's Disease 70(s1), 1–11, 2018

Radford K, Mack HA, Draper B, et al., *Comparison of three cognitive tools for dementia screening in urban and regional aboriginal Australians,* Dementia and Geriatric Cognitive Disorders, 40, 22–32, 2015

Radford K, Delbaere K, Draper B, et al., *Childhood stress and adversity is associated with late-life dementia in Aboriginal Australians,* American Journal of Geriatric Psychiatry,

25(10):, 1097–1106, 2017

Reisberg B, *About the 1991 Awards,* IPA Bulletin, 8 (2), 10, 1991

Restifo S, *Branch Report from Western Australia,* FPOA News, 10 October 2003

Rischbieth S, *Letter from South Australia,* FPOA Newsletter, 11 April 2011

Rischbieth S, *Letter from South Australia,* FPOA Newsletter, 11 September 2011

Rischbieth S, *Letter from South Australia,* FPOA Newsletter, 7 April 2012

Robinson RA, *The Evolution of Geriatric Psychiatry,* Medical History, 16(2), 184–193, 1972

Roth M, *The natural history of mental disorders in old age,* Journal of Mental Science, 101, 281–301, 1955

Rowland JT, Basic D, Storey JE, Conforti DA, *The Rowland Universal Dementia Assessment Scale (RUDAS) and the Folstein MMSE in a Multicultural Cohort of Elderly Persons,* International Psychogeriatrics, 18(01), 111–120, 2006

Runci SJ, Eppingstall BJ, O'Connor DW, *A comparison of verbal communication and psychiatric medication use by Greek and Italian residents with dementia in Australian ethno-specific and mainstream aged care facilities,* International Psychogeriatrics, 24(5), 733–741, 2012

Runci SJ, Eppingstall BJ, van der Ploeg ES, O'Connor DW, *Comparison of family satisfaction in Australian ethno-specific and mainstream aged care facilities,* Journal of Gerontological Nursing, 40(4), 54–63, 2014

Runci SJ, Eppingstall BJ, van der Ploeg ES, Graham G, O'Connor DW, *The language needs of residents from linguistically diverse backgrounds in Victorian aged care facilities,* Australasian Journal on Ageing, 34(3), 195–198, 2015

Russell RJ, *Psychogeriatric services in Australia,* IPA Bulletin, 9(1), 20, May 1992

Russell R, *NSW news,* FPOA News, 1, 8, June 1999

Schneider LS, Tariot PN, Dagerman KS, et al., *Effectiveness of atypical antipsychotic drugs in patients with Alzheimer's disease,* New England Journal of Medicine, 355(15), 1525–38, 2006

Shen Y, Radford K, Daylight G, Cumming R, Broe T, Draper B, *Depression, Suicidal Behaviour and Mental Disorders in Older Aboriginal Australians,* The International Journal of Environmental Research and Public Health 15(3), 447, 2018

Smith K, Flicker L, Lautenschlager NT, et al., *High prevalence of dementia and cognitive impairment in Indigenous Australians.* Neurology 71(19), 1470–3, 2008

Smith K, Flicker L, Dwyer A, et al., *Factors associated with dementia in Aboriginal Australians,* Australian and New Zealand Journal of Psychiatry, 44, 888–893, 2010

Snowdon J, *Letter to the Editor, Health Services Research into the Future of Australian Psychiatry,* Australian and New Zealand Journal of Psychiatry, 24, 435, 1990

Snowdon J, *Medication use by elderly persons in Sydney,* Australian Journal on Ageing,

12(2), 14–21, 1993

Snowdon J, *Bed requirements for an area psychogeriatric service,* Australian and New Zealand Journal of Psychiatry, 25, 56–62, 1991

Snowdon J, *A follow-up survey of psychotropic drug use in Sydney nursing homes,* Medical Journal of Australia, 170, 293–294, 1999

Snowdon J, Ames D, Chiu E, Wattis J, *A survey of psychiatric services for elderly people in Australia,* Australian and New Zealand Journal of Psychiatry, 29, 207–214, 1995

Snowdon J, Vaughan R, Miller R, Burgess E, Tremlett P, *Psychotropic drug use in Sydney nursing homes,* Medical Journal of Australia, 163, 70–72, 1995

Tang GWG, Dennis S, Comino E, *Anxiety and Depression in Chinese Patients Attending an Australian GP Clinic,* Australian Family Physician, 38(7), 552–555, 2009

Teltscher B, *Misreferral of patients to a geriatric hospital,* The Medical Journal of Australia, i: 218–219, 1968

Thompson J, *Obituary Joan Metcalf Ridley,* Psychiatric Bulletin, 18, 525–526, 1994

Turner J, *Letter to the Editor,* PGNA Newsletter, 8–9 November 2020

Wattis J, Wattis L, Arie T, *Psychogeriatrics: A National Survey of a New Branch of Psychiatry,* British Medical Journal, 282, 1529–33, 1981

Wilson K, Mottram P, Sivanranthan A, Nightingale A, *Antidepressants versus placebo for the depressed elderly,* Cochrane Database of Systematic Reviews 2001, Issue 1, CD000561. DOI: 10.1002/14651858.CD000561.

Woodward MC, Woodward E, *A national survey of memory clinics in Australia,* International Psychogeriatrics, 21(4), 696–702, 2009

World Health Organisation and GPWorldPA, *Organisation of care in psychiatry of the elderly – a technical consensus statement,* Aging and Mental Health, 2, 246–252, 1998

Xiao LD, De Bellis A, Kyriazopoulos H, Draper B, Ullah S, *The effect of a personalized dementia care intervention for caregivers from minority groups,* American Journal of Alzheimer's Disease and Other Dementias, 31 (1), 57–67, 2016

## Books and Chapters

American Psychiatric Association, *Diagnostic and Statistical Manual of Mental Disorders. Third Edition,* Washington DC, American Psychiatric Association, 1980

American Psychiatric Association, *Diagnostic and Statistical Manual of Mental Disorders. Fifth Edition,* Arlington, VA, American Psychiatric Association, 2013

Chiu E, Ames D, Hassett A, *Old Age Psychiatry in the Department,* In Chiu E & Preston J (eds) The Department of Psychiatry at the University of Melbourne 1964–2009: personal reminiscences. University of Melbourne, 180–184, 2010

Collins D, *An Account of the English Colony in New South Wales – Volume 1,* London,

Cadell & Davies, 1798, Project Gutenberg 2004

Dax EC, *Asylum to Community: The Development of the Mental Hygiene Service in Victoria, Australia,* Melbourne, FW Cheshire, 1961

Mace N, Rabins P, *The 36-Hour Day: A family guide to caring for persons with Alzheimer's disease, related dementing illnesses, and memory loss in later life,* 1st ed, Baltimore, Johns Hopkins University Press, 1981

Prichard JC, *A Treatise on Insanity and other disorders affecting the mind,* London, Sherwood, Gilbert and Piper, 1835

Sweetser W, *Mental hygiene, or, an examination of the intellect and passions,* New York, J & HG Langley, 1843

Tench W, *A Complete Account of the Settlement at Port Jackson.* London, 1793. Project Gutenberg, http://gutenberg.net.au/ebooks/e00084.html#13 (accessed 28 May 2020)

Thomas J, *The Vagabond papers: Sketches of Melbourne Life in Light and.....* Melbourne, George Robertson, 1877

Trollope A, *Trollope's Australia,* edited by Hugh Dow. Melbourne, Thomas Nelson, 1966

## Internet Pages

ABC Four Corners, *Who Cares?* Posted 17 September 2018, Who Cares? – Four Corners (abc.net.au) (accessed 15 April 2021)

Australian Bureau of Statistics. *Causes of Death, Australia 2018.* https://www.abs.gov.au/statistics/health/causes-death/causes-death-australia/2018 (accessed 23 September 2020)

Australian Bureau of Statistics. *Australian Demographic Statistics, June 2020.* National, state and territory population, June 2020 | Australian Bureau of Statistics (abs.gov.au) (accessed 4 February 2021)

Australian Bureau of Statistics, *Life Tables, States, Territories and Australia, 2016–2018 3302.0.55.001.* ABS, 30/10/2019 https://www.abs.gov.au/ausstats/abs@.nsf/mf/3302.0.55.001 (accessed 29 May 2020)

Australian Bureau of Statistics, *Life Tables 2017–2019,* Life tables, 2017–2019 | Australian Bureau of Statistics (abs.gov.au) ABS (accessed 5 July 2021)

Australian Bureau of Statistics, *National, State and Territory Population,* December 2020, National, state and territory population, December 2020 | Australian Bureau of Statistics (abs.gov.au) (accessed 6 July 2021)

Australian Government, *Budget 2021–22,* Commonwealth of Australia 2021, Budget 2021–22 – Overview (accessed 12 July 2021)

Australian Institute of Health and Welfare, *Mental Health Services in Australia, Medicare-subsidised mental health-specific services 2018–2019,* March 2021, Mental health services in Australia, Medicare-subsidised mental health-specific services – Australian Institute of Health and Welfare (aihw.gov.au) (accessed 26 April 2021)

Budget Estimates Committee, Tasmania, *Uncorrected proof issue of minutes 24 June 2009*. Microsoft Word – cestawed2.doc (parliament.tas.gov.au) (accessed 26 May 2021)

Council of Attorneys General, *National Plan to Respond to the Abuse of Older Australians (Elder Abuse) 2019–2023*. Canberra, Commonwealth of Australia, 2019, https://www.ag.gov.au/ElderAbuseNationalPlan (accessed 1 June 2020)

Department of Health, *Specialist Dementia Care Program,* Specialist Dementia Care Program (SDCP) | Australian Government Department of Health (accessed 15 April 2021*)*

Department of Health, *Psychological treatment services for persons with mental illness in residential aged care facilities,* Canberra, Commonwealth of Australia, 2018 11PHN Guidance – Psychological treatment services in Residential Aged Care.pdf (health. gov.au) (accessed 26 April 2021)

First Fleet OnLine. http://firstfleet.uow.edu.au/objectv.html (accessed 23 January 2020)

Histpop – the online historical population reports website. *Census of England and Wales, 1861* http://www.histpop.org/ohpr/servlet/Show?page=Home (accessed 17 June 2020)

InflationTool, *Value of 1955 Australian dollars today.* Value of 1955 Australian Dollars today – Inflation calculator (inflationtool.com) (accessed 4 February 2021)

Joint Commissioning Panel for Mental Health. *Guidance for commissioners of older people's mental health services* May 2013 http://www.jcpmh.info/wp-content/uploads/jcpmh-olderpeople-guide.pdf (accessed 19 January 2021)

Lunacy Act 1847. South Australia Parliament. https://dspace.flinders.edu.au/xmlui/handle/2328/2048 (accessed 20 July 2020)

Macquarie University, *Stepped Care Effectiveness Trial for Ageing Adults,* Macquarie University – Stepped Care Effectiveness Trial for Ageing Adults (mq.edu.au) (accessed 14 July 2021)

NHMRC, *NHMRC National Institute for Dementia Research,* NHMRC, NHMRC National Institute for Dementia Research | NHMRC (accessed 13 July 2021)

NHMRC National Institute for Dementia Research, *Strategic Roadmap for Dementia Research and Translation,* NHMRC 2019, NHMRC National Institute for Dementia Research | NHMRC (accessed 13 July 2021)

Office for National Statistics. *Living longer: is age 70 the new age 65?* November 2019 https://www.ons.gov.uk/peoplepopulationandcommunity/birthsdeathsandmarriages/ageing/articles/livinglongerisage70thenewage65/2019-11-19 (accessed 21 May 2020)

Primary Health Tasmania, *Suicide prevention,* Suicide prevention – Primary Health Tasmania (accessed 27 May 2021)

Queensland Centre for Mental Health Research, *National Mental Health Service Planning Framework Reports,* National Mental Health Service Planning Framework Reports – qcmhr (accessed 28 April 2021)

Report of the Mid Staffordshire NHS Foundation Trust Public Inquiry. London: The Stationery Office, 2013. www.midstaffspublicinquiry.com (accessed 20 March 2017)

Richardson D, Stanford J, *Funding High Quality Aged Care Services,* The Australia Institute, May 7 2021, Funding High-Quality Aged Care Services | The Australia Institute (accessed 12 July 2021)

States Records Office of WA. https://archive.sro.wa.gov.au/index.php/various-records-mental-health-hospitals-au-wa-s4867 (accessed 3 November 2019)

State Records Office of WA. *Claremont Mental Hospital.* AU WA A543 – CLAREMONT MENTAL HOSPITAL – State Records Office of WA (sro.wa.gov.au) (accessed 19 February 2021)

State Records Office of WA. *Sunset Hospital, Nedlands.* AU WA A810 – SUNSET HOSPITAL, NEDLANDS – State Records Office of WA (sro.wa.gov.au) (accessed 1 March 2021)

The Lunatics Act 1864. South Australia Parliament. https://dspace.flinders.edu.au/xmlui/handle/2328/2485 (accessed 20 July 2020)

Tooth JSH, *Submission to Senate Enquiry into 'Care and management of younger and older people with dementia and behavioural and psychological symptoms of dementia,* April 15 2013 Submissions – Parliament of Australia (aph.gov.au) (accessed 26 May 2021)

Wood P, *Restrictions on dementia drugs dropped*, Australian Doctor, 24 April 2013, www.australiandoctor.com.au/news/latest-news/restrictions-on-dementia-drugs-dropped (accessed 25 April 2013)

## Personal communications by interviews and emails

David Ames, Elizabeth Beattie, Richard Bonwick, Henry Brodaty, Tony Broe, Gerard Byrne, Ed Chiu, Marianne Cummins, Colleen Doyle, Richard Fleming, Leon Flicker, Meredith Gresham, Neville Hills, Mary Ingrames, Kathy Hall, Kate Jackson, Deborah Koder, Julia Lane, David Lie, Jeff Looi, Helen McGowan, John McIntyre, Duncan McKellar, Rod McKay, Martin Morrissey, Bob Moss, Daniel O'Connor, Jill Pettigrew, Judy Ratajec, Judy Raymond, Wayne Reid, John Snowdon, Richard Steel, Janine Stevenson, Eddie Tan, Stephen Ticehurst, Sid Williams

# Secondary Sources

## Government, Agency and Non-Government Organisation Reports

Arkles R, Jackson Pulver L, Robertson H, Draper B, Chalkley S, Broe GA (Tony), *Ageing, Cognition and Dementia in Australian Aboriginal and Torres Strait Islander Peoples: A life Cycle Approach,* Neuroscience Research Australia and Muru Marri Indigenous Health Unit, University of New South Wales, June 2010

Cummins CJ, *The Development of the Benevolent (Sydney) Asylum 1788–1855,* Sydney, Department of Health, 1971

Cummins CJ, *A History of Medical Administration in NSW 1788–1973,* 2nd edition, Sydney, NSW Department of Health, 2003

Federation of Ethnic Communities' Councils of Australia, *Review of Australian Research on Older People from Culturally and Linguistically Diverse Backgrounds,* Curtin ACT, FECCA, 2015

Grey F, O'Hagan M, *The effectiveness of services led or run by consumers in mental health: rapid review of evidence for recovery-oriented outcomes: an Evidence Check rapid review brokered by the Sax Institute for the Mental Health Commission of New South Wales,* Sax Institute, August 2015

Hamilton M, Hamilton C, *Baby boomers and retirement: Dreams, fears and anxieties,* ACT, The Australia Institute, September 2006

Henderson AS, Jorm AF. *Dementia in Australia. Aged and Community Care Service Development and Evaluation Reports, Number 35.* Canberra, Australian Government Publishing Service, 1998.

National Seniors Productive Ageing Centre, *Ageing Baby Boomers in Australia: Informing actions for better retirement,* ACT, National Seniors Productive Ageing Centre, August 2012

Norman LG, *Historical notes on Newtown,* Sydney, Council of the City of Sydney, 1963

Radermacher H, Feldman S, Browning C, *Review of Literature Concerning the Delivery of Community Aged care Services to Ethnic Groups – Mainstream Versus Ethno-Specific Services: It's Not an 'Either Or',* Ethnic Communities' Council of Victoria and Partners, 2008

Royal Commission into Aged Care Quality and Safety, *Background Paper 1. Navigating the maze: an overview of Australia's current aged care system,* Canberra, Commonwealth of Australia, February 2019

Royal Commission into Aged Care Quality and Safety, *Medium- and long-term pressures on the system: the changing demographics and dynamics of aged care. Background Paper 2.* Commonwealth of Australia, 2019

# Journal Articles

Andrews ES, *Institutionalising senile dementia in 19th century Britain,* Sociology of Health & Illness, 39 (2), 244–257, 2017 doi: 10.1111/1467-9566.12452

Anonymous, *The Mental Hospital Services,* Medical Journal of Australia, June 20 1925, 678–680

Anonymous, *The Mental Hospital Services,* Medical Journal of Australia, November 20, 1926, 705–706

Anonymous, *The Mental Hospital Services,* Medical Journal of Australia, November 26, 1927, 755–758

Bell M. *From the 1870s to the 1970s: the changing face of public psychiatry in South Australia,* Australasian Psychiatry, 11(1), 79–86, 2003

Berrios GE, *Delirium and confusion in the nineteenth century: a conceptual history,* British Journal of Psychiatry, 139, 439–449, 1981

Berrios GE, *'Depressive pseudodementia' or 'melancholic dementia': a nineteenth century view,* Journal of Neurology, Neurosurgery, and Psychiatry, 48, 393–400, 1985

Berrios GE, *Dementia during the seventeenth and eighteenth centuries: a conceptual history,* Psychological Medicine, 17, 829–837, 1987

Berrios GE, *Historical aspects of psychoses: 19th century issues,* British Medical Bulletin, 43(3), 484–498, 1987

Berrios GE, *Melancholia and depression during the nineteenth century: a conceptual history,* British Journal of Psychiatry, 153, 298–304, 1988

Berrios GE, *J.C. Prichard and the concept of 'moral insanity',* History of Psychiatry, 10(37), 111–126, 1999

Berrios GE, *The insanities of the third age: a conceptual history of paraphrenia,* Journal of Nutrition, Health & Ageing, 7 (6), 394–399, 2003

Blashfield RK, *Pre-Kraepelin names for mental disorders,* Journal of Nervous and Mental Disease, 207, 726–730, 2019

Bower HM, T*he Beattie-Smith Lectures – Part 1. Old Age in Western Society,* Medical Journal of Australia, II (8), 285–292, 1964

Bower HM, *The Beattie-Smith Lectures – Part 2. Old Age in Western Society,* Medical Journal of Australia, II (9), 325–332, 1964

Brewer GJ, *Copper-2 ingestion, plus increased meat eating leading to increased copper absorption, are major factors behind the current epidemic of Alzheimer's disease,* Nutrients, 7, 10053–10064, 2015

Brodaty H, Ames D, Boundy KL, et al., *Pharmacological treatment of cognitive deficits in Alzheimer's disease,* Medical Journal of Australia, 175, 324–329, 2001

Brodaty H, Cumming A, *Dementia services in Australia,* International Journal of Geriatric Psychiatry, 25, 887–895, 2010

Brunton W, 'At variance with the most elementary principles': the state of British colonial lunatic asylums in 1863, History of Psychiatry, 26 (2), 147–165, 2015

Burnham JC, The Royal Derwent Hospital in Tasmania: historical perspectives on the meaning of community psychiatry, Australian and New Zealand Journal of Psychiatry, 9, 163–167, 1975

Coleborne C, The 'scientific management' of the insane and the problem of 'difference' in the asylum in Victoria 1870s–1880s, Australasian Victorian Studies Journal, 2 (1), 126–137, 1996

Coleman W, Six problems in the biography of Alfred Deakin, Agenda, 25, number 1, ANU Press, Canberra 2018

Cotter PR, Condon JR, Barnes T, Anderson IPS, Smith LR, Cunningham T, Do Indigenous Australians age prematurely? The implications of life expectancy and health conditions of older Indigenous people for health and aged care policy. Australian Health Review, 36, 68–74, 2012

Cuijpers P, Karyotaki E, Pot AM, Park M, Reynolds III, CF, Managing depression in older age: Psychological interventions, Maturitas, 79, 160-169, 2014

Davis G, The most deadly disease of asylumdom: general paralysis of the insane and Scottish psychiatry c1840-1940, Journal of the Royal College of Physicians of Edinburgh, 42, 266-273, 2012

Dax EC, The first 200 years of Australian psychiatry, Australian and New Zealand Journal of Psychiatry, 23, 103-110, 1989

Dax EC, The evolution of community psychiatry, Australian and New Zealand Journal of Psychiatry, 26, 295-301, 1992

Dobrohotoff J, Llewellyn-Jones R, Psychogeriatric inpatient unit design: a literature review, International Psychogeriatrics, 23(2), 174-189, 2011

Draper B, Richard Mahony: the Misfortunes of Younger Onset Dementia, Medical Journal of Australia, 190, 94–95, 2009

Draper B, Suicidal behaviour and suicide prevention in later life, Maturitas, 79(2), 179–183, 2014

Draper B, Withall A, Young onset dementia. Internal Medicine Journal, 46(7): 779–786, 2016

Dunk J, Work, paperwork and the imaginary Tarban Creek Lunatic Asylum, 1846, Rethinking History, 22(3), 326–355, 2018

Earnshaw B, The lame, the blind, the mad, the malingerers: sick and disabled convicts within the colonial community, Journal of the Royal Australian Historical Society, 81, part 1, 1995

Edwards GA, Restraint in the treatment of the mentally ill in the late 19th century, Australian and New Zealand Journal of Psychiatry, 4, 201–205, 1970

Ellis AS, *Early Psychiatry in Western Australia: Dr Nicholas Langley – a born loser*, Australian and New Zealand Journal of Psychiatry, 12, 283–286, 1978

Ford AH, *Neuropsychiatric aspects of dementia*, Maturitas, 79, 209–215, 2014

Förstl H, Howard R, Burns A, Levy R, *'The strange mental state of an old man who thought he would be slaughtered' – an early report of dementia with delusion (1785)*, Journal of the Royal Society of Medicine, 84, 432–434, 1991

Fox P, *From senility to Alzheimer's disease: The rise of the Alzheimer's disease movement*, The Milbank Quarterly, 67, (1), 58–102, 1989

Fraser J, *The Aborigines of New South Wales*, Royal Society of NSW, 1882–83

Gilleard C, *The other Victorians: age, sickness and poverty in 19th-century Ireland*, Ageing & Society, 36, 1157–1184, 2016

Goedert M, *Oskar Fischer and the study of dementia*, Brain, 132, 1102–1111, 2009

Goldney R, *Lessons from history: the first 25 years of psychiatric hospitals in South Australia*, Australasian Psychiatry, 15 (5), 368–371, 2007

Grimshaw P, Willett G, *Family Structure in colonial Australia*, Australia 1888, No. 4, 5–27, May 1980

Gurwitz JH, Bonner A, Berwick DM, *Reducing excessive use of antipsychotic agents in nursing homes*, JAMA, 318(2), 118–119, 2017

Harris J, *Hiding the bodies: the myth of the humane colonisation of Aboriginal Australia*, Aboriginal History, 27, 79–104, 2003

Henderson AS, *The Coming Epidemic of Dementia*, Australian and New Zealand Journal of Psychiatry, 17, 117–127, 1983

Hendricks S, Peetoom K, Bakker C, et al., *Global prevalence of young-onset dementia. A systematic review and meta-analysis*, JAMA Neurology, doi:10.1001/jamaneurol.2021.2161, published online 19 July 2021

Hills NF, *Promise and practice: WA psychiatry for the elderly*, Australasian Psychiatry, 3(4), 260–262, 1995

Hilton C, *Joint geriatric and old-age psychiatric wards in the UK, 1940s to early 1990s: a historical study*, International Journal of Geriatric Psychiatry, 29, 1071–1078, 2014

Hilton C, *Psychogeriatrics in England in the 1950s: greater knowledge with little impact on the provision of services*, History of Psychiatry, 27(10), 3–20, 2016

Hilton C, *Psychogeriatrics in England: Its route to recognition by the government as a distinct medical specialty c.1970–89*, Medical History, 60(2), 206–228, 2016

Howe AL, *From states of confusion to a national action plan for dementia care: the development of policies for dementia care in Australia*, International Journal of Geriatric Psychiatry, 12, 165–171, 1997

Hunter C, *Nursing and care for the aged in Victoria: 1950s to 1970s*, Nursing Inquiry, 12, 278–286, 2005

Hunter C, Doyle C, *Dementia policy in Australia and the 'social construction' of infirm old age*, Health and History, 16(2), 44–62, 2014

Hunter E, *Aboriginal communities and suicide*, Australasian Psychiatry, 4(4), 195–199, 1996

Jackson K, Roberts R, McKay R, *Older people's mental health in rural areas: Converting policy into service development, service access, and sustainable workforce*, Australian Journal of Rural Health, 27 (4), 358–365, 2019

Jervis J, *The Mental Hospital, Parramatta*, Royal Australian Historical Society Journal and Proceedings, 19, 191–196, 1933

Kelly BD, *Dr William Saunders Halloran and psychiatric practice in nineteenth century Ireland*, Irish Journal of Medical Science, 177, 79–84, 2008

Kirkby KC, *History of Psychiatry in Australia, pre-1960*, History of Psychiatry, x, 191–204, 1999

Knopman DS, Petersen RC, Jack Jr CR, *A brief history of 'Alzheimer's disease': Multiple meanings separated by a common name*, Neurology, 92(22), 1053–1059, 2019

Kosky R, *From morality to madness: a reappraisal of the asylum movement in psychiatry, 1800–1940*, Australian and New Zealand Journal of Psychiatry, 20,180–187, 1986

Lawrence J, *A Century of Psychiatry in Queensland*, Australasian Psychiatry, 10 (2), 155–161, 2002

Lefroy RB, *The development of geriatric medicine in Australia*, Medical Journal of Australia, 161, 18–20, 1994

LoGiudice D, *The health of older Aboriginal and Torres Strait Islander peoples*, Australasian Journal on Ageing, 35(2), 82–85, 2016

Loi S, Hassett A, *Evolution of aged persons mental health services in Victoria: the history behind their development.* Australasian Journal on Ageing, 30(4), 226–230, 2011

Low LF, Draper B, Cheng A, et al., *Future Research on Dementia Relating to Culturally and Linguistically Diverse Communities*, Australasian Journal on Ageing, 28(3), 144–148, 2009

Massoud F, Gauthier S, *Update on the pharmacological treatment of Alzheimer's disease*, Current Neuropharmacology, 8, 69–80, 2010

Maurer K, Volk S, Gerbaldo H, *Auguste D and Alzheimer's disease*, The Lancet, 349, May 24, 1546–1549, 1997

Maynard J, *Australian history – Lifting Haze or Descending Fog?* Aboriginal History, 27, 139–145, 2003

McDonald DI, *Gladesville Hospital: the formative years 1838–1850*, Journal Royal Australian Historical Society, 51, 273–295, 1965

McDonald DI, *Dr Francis Campbell & the Tarban Creek Asylum*, Journal Royal Australian Historical Society, 53, 222–255, 1967

McDonald DI, *Frederic Norton Manning, 1839–1903*, Journal Royal Australian Historical Society, 58, 190–201, 1972

McKay R, Draper B, *Is it too late to prevent a decline in mental health care for older Australians?* Medical Journal of Australia, 197(2), 87–88, 2012

McKay R, McDonald R, Coombs T, *Benchmarking older persons mental health organizations,* Australasian Psychiatry, 19(1), 45–48, 2011

McKay R, McDonald R, Lie D, McGowan H, *Reclaiming the best of the biopsychosocial model of mental health care and 'recovery' for older people through a person-centred approach,* Australasian Psychiatry, 20(6), 492–495, 2012

McSherry W, *Dignity in care: meanings, myths and the reality of making it work in practice,* Nursing Times, 106(40), 20–23, 2010

Miller MD, Mark D, *Using Psychoanalytically Oriented Psychotherapy with the Elderly,* Jefferson Journal of Psychiatry, 4 (1), 13–21, 1986

Nitrini R, *A cure of one of the most frequent types of dementia: a historical parallel.* Alzheimer's Disease and Associated Disorders, 19, 156–158, 2005

Noble HN, *The Management of the Elderly Mentally Frail,* Australasian Psychiatric Bulletin, 2(2), 23–24, 1961

Nusteling HPH, *The population of England, 1539–1873: an issue of demographic homeostasis,* Histoire & Mesure, VIII–1/2, 59–92, 1993

O'Shane P, *The Psychological Impact of White Colonialism on Aboriginal People,* Australasian Psychiatry, 3 (3), 149–153, 1995

Parkinson JP, *The Castle Hill Lunatic Asylum (1811–1826) and the Origins of Eclectic Pragmatism in Australian Psychiatry,* Australian and New Zealand Journal of Psychiatry, 15, 319–322, 1981

Patrick R, *The Case of Dr Jonathan Labatt.* John Oxley Journal: a bulletin for historical research in Queensland, 1 (6), 7–15, 1980

Peisah C, Burns K, Edmonds S, Brodaty H, *Rendering visible the previously invisible in health care: the ageing LGBTI communities.* Medical Journal of Australia, 209(3), 106–108, 2018

Peters T, *King George III and the porphyria myth – causes, consequences and re-evaluation of his mental illness with computer diagnostics,* Clinical Medicine, 15 (2), 168–172, 2015

Piddock S, *Convicts and the free: nineteenth century lunatic asylums in South Australia and Tasmania (1830–1883),* Australasian Historical Archaeology, 19, 84–96, 2001

Piddock S, *Possibilities and realities: South Australia's asylums in the 19th Century,* Australasian Psychiatry, 12 (2), 172–175, 2004

Piper A, *Admission to charitable institutions in colonial Tasmania: from individual failing to social problem,* Tasmanian Historical Studies, 9, 43–62, 2004

Pollitt PA, *The problem of dementia in Australian Aboriginal and Torres Strait Islander communities: an overview,* International Journal of Geriatric Psychiatry, 12, 155–163, 1997

Raeburn T, Liston C, Hickmott J, Cleary M, *Liverpool 'lunatic asylum': a forgotten chapter in the history of Australian health care,* Collegian, 25, 347–353, 2018

Raeburn T, Liston C, Hickmott J, Cleary M, *Colonial surgeon Patrick Hill (1794–1852): unacknowledged pioneer of Australian mental health care,* History of Psychiatry, 30 (1), 90–103, 2019

Ratcliffe E, Kirkby K, *Psychiatry in Tasmania: from old cobwebs to new brooms,* Australasian Psychiatry, 9, (2), 128–132, 2001

Raymond J, Kirkwood H, Looi J, *Commitment and collaboration for excellence in older persons' mental health: the ACT experience,* Australasian Psychiatry, 12(2), 130–133, 2004

Reynolds H, *That hated stain: the aftermath of transportation in Tasmania,* Historical Studies, 14: 19, 1969

Ridley N, Draper B, Withall A, *Alcohol-related Dementia: an update of the evidence,* Alzheimer's Research & Therapy, 5: 3. doi:10.1186/alzrt157, 2013

Robson B, *From mental hygiene to community mental health: psychiatrists and Victorian public administration from the 1940s to 1990s,* Provenance: The Journal of Public Record Office Victoria, issue 7, 2008, ISSN 1832–2522

Russell SG, Quigley R, Thompson F, et al., *Prevalence of dementia in the Torres Strait,* Australasian Journal on Ageing, published online 10 November 2020, https://doi.org/10.1111/ajag.12878

Rybakowski JK, *120th anniversary of the Kraepelinian dichotomy of psychiatric disorders,* Current Psychiatry Reports, 21, 65, 2019

Sax S, *How it all began – geriatric medicine in Australia,* Australian Journal on Ageing, 13, (1), 5–7, 1994

Schwartz MF, Stark JA, *The distinction between Alzheimer's disease and senile dementia: Historical Considerations,* Journal of the History of the Neurosciences, 1, 3, 169–187, 2009

Shlomowitz E, Garton S, '*How much more generally applicable are remedial words than medicines': Care of the Mentally Ill in South Australia, 1858–1884,* Journal of Australian Colonial History, 4(1), 81–103, 2002

Skerritt P, Ellis A, Prendergast F, Harrold C, Blackmore H, Derham B, *Psychiatry in Western Australia since Federation: an eloquent testimony,* Australasian Psychiatry, 9 (3), 226–228, 2001

Snowdon J, *Psychiatric services for the elderly,* Australian and New Zealand Journal of Psychiatry, 21, 131–136, 1987

Snowdon J, *Psychiatry of Old Age*, Australasian Psychiatry, 3(6), 431–435, 1995

Snowdon J, *The early days of old age psychiatry in New South Wales*, PGNA Newsletter, 4–5, November 2020

Snowdon J, Draper B, *The Faculty of Psychiatry of Old Age*, Australasian Psychiatry, 7(1), 30–32, 1999

Snowdon J, Draper B, Chiu E, Ames D, Brodaty H, *Surveys of mental health and wellbeing: Critical comments*, Australasian Psychiatry, 6, 246–247, 1998

Sorinmade OA, Kossoff L, Peisah C, *COVID-19 and Telehealth in older adult psychiatry – opportunities for now and the future*, International Journal of Geriatric Psychiatry, 35, 1427–30, 2020

Stewart M, Debattista J, Fitzgerald L, Williams O, *Syphilis, General Paralysis of the Insane, and Queensland asylums*, Health and History, 19 (1), 60–79, 2017

Temple JB, Wilson T, Taylor A, Kelaher M, Eades S, *Ageing of the Aboriginal and Torres Strait Islander population: numerical, structural, timing, and spatial aspects*, Australian and New Zealand Journal of Public Health, 44, 271–278, 2020

Thane P, 'Social Histories of Old Age and Aging', *Journal of Social History*, 37, (1), Special Issue, 93–111, 2003

Toole JF, *Dementia in world leaders and its effects upon international events: the examples of Franklin D Roosevelt and T Woodrow Wilson*, European Journal of Neurology, 6, 115–119, 1999

Virtue R, *Lunacy and Social Reform in Western Australia 1886–1903*, Studies in Western Australia History, 1, 29–65, 1977

Vreugdenhil A, '*Incoherent and violent if crossed': The admission of older people to the New Norfolk Lunatic Asylum in the nineteenth century*, Health and History, 14 (2), 91–111, 2012

Wand APF, Pourmand D, Draper B, *Using interpreters with culturally and linguistically diverse older adults: what do we need to know?* Australasian Journal on Ageing, 39 (3), 175–177, 2020

Wand A, Draper B, Pourmand D, *Working with interpreters in the psychiatric assessment of older adults from culturally and linguistically diverse backgrounds*, International Psychogeriatrics, 32 (1), 11–16, 2020

Warne R, *Issues in the development of geriatric medicine in Britain and Australia*, Medical Journal of Australia, 146, 139–141, 1987

Whitlock FA, *Prichard and the concept of 'moral insanity'*, Australian and New Zealand Journal of Psychiatry, 1, 72–79, 1967

Willis E, … *of 'unsound mind'*, Historic Environment, 14, (2), 33–38, 1999

Willmuth LR, *Medical views of depression in the elderly: historical notes*, Journal of the American Geriatrics Society, 27 (2), 495–499, 1979

Wilson D, *Quantifying the quiet epidemic: Diagnosing dementia in late 20th Century Britain,* History of the Human Sciences, 27(5), 126–146, 2014

Yorston G, Haw C, *Old and mad in Victorian Oxford: a study of patients aged 60 and over admitted to the Warneford and Littlemore Asylums in the nineteenth century,* History of Psychiatry, 16(4), 395–421, 2005

## Books and Book Chapters

Barnard M, *A History of Australia,* 2nd edition, Sydney, Angus & Robertson, 1963

Berndt RM, Berndt CH, *The World of the First Australians,* Sydney, Ure Smith, 1964

Bostock J, *The Dawn of Australian Psychiatry 1788–1850,* Sydney, Australasian Medical Publishing Company, 1968

Brothers CRD, *Early Victorian Psychiatry,* Government Printer, Melbourne, 1962

Brown JC, *'Poverty is not a Crime'. The development of social services in Tasmania, 1803–1900,* Hobart, Tasmanian Historical Research Association, 1972

Butlin NG, *Our original aggression: Aboriginal populations of southeastern Australia, 1788–1850,* Sydney, Allen and Unwin, 1983

Cawte J, *Medicine is the Law,* Honolulu, University Press of Hawaii, 21–22, 1974

Cobley J, *Sydney Cove 1788,* Sydney, Angus & Robertson, 1980

Cobley J, *The Crimes of the First Fleet convicts,* Sydney, Angus & Robertson, 1989

Cooke S, *'Terminal old age': Ageing and suicide in Victoria 1841–1921,* In: Walker D & Garton S (eds) Ageing, Australian Cultural History 14, Geelong, Deakin University, 76–91, 1995

Craig DA, *The Lion of Beechworth,* Beechworth, Victoria, 2000

Crowther A, *Administration and the Asylum,* In: Coleborne, C. & MacKinnon, D. (eds), 'Madness' in Australia: histories, heritage, and the asylum. St Lucia, Queensland, Queensland University Press, 93–95, 2003

Davison G, *'Our youth is spent and our backs are bent': The origins of Australian ageism,* In: Walker D & Garton S (eds) Ageing, Australian Cultural History 14, Geelong, Deakin University, 40–62, 1995

Dickey B, *No Charity There: a short history of social welfare in Australia,* Sydney, Allen & Unwin, 1980

Draper B, *Understanding Alzheimer's and Other Dementias.* Sydney, Longueville Media, 2011

Dunk J, *Bedlam at Botany Bay,* Sydney, NewSouth Publishing, 2019

Elkin AP, *The Australian Aborigines,* Australia, Angus & Robertson, 1974

Ellis AS, *Eloquent Testimony,* Perth, UWA Press, 1983

Ellis MH, *John Macarthur,* Penrith, Discovery Press, 1972

Finnane M, *Wolston Park Hospital, 1865–2001: a Retrospect,* Queensland Review, 15

(2),39–58, 2008

Flenley R, Spencer R, *Modern German History*, 4th edition, London, JM Dent & Sons, 1968

Flynn M, *The Second Fleet – Britain's Grim Convict Armada of 1790*, Sydney, Library of Australian History, 2001

Ford R, *Sexuality and 'Madness': regulating women's gender deviance through the asylum, the Orange Asylum in the 1930s*, In: Coleborne, C. & MacKinnon, D. (eds), 'Madness' in Australia: histories, heritage, and the asylum. St Lucia, Queensland, Queensland University Press, 109–119, 2003

Garton S, *Medicine and Madness: a Social history of insanity in New South Wales, 1880–1940*, New South Wales University Press, Kensington, 1988

Garton S, *Out of Luck: Poor Australians and Social Welfare 1788–1988*, Sydney, Allen & Unwin, 1990

Gillen M, *The Founders of Australia: a biographical dictionary of the First Fleet*, Sydney, Library of Australian History, 1989

Gowlland RW, *Troubled asylum: the history of…the Royal Derwent Hospital*, New Norfolk, Tasmania, 1981

Hall J, *'May they rest in peace': The History and Ghosts of the Fremantle Lunatic Asylum*, Hesperian Press, Carlisle WA, 2013

Healy J, *Community services: long term care at home?* In: Kendig HL, McCallum J (eds) Grey Policy: Australian policies for an ageing society, Sydney, Allen & Unwin, 127–149, 1990

Hetherington P, *Paupers, Poor Relief & Poor Houses in Western Australia 1829–1910*, Crawley, UWA Publishing, 2009

Hilton C, Arie T, *The Development of Old Age Psychiatry in the UK*, In: Abou-Saleh Mohammed T, Katona Cornelius, and Kumar Anand (Eds) Principles and Practice of Geriatric Psychiatry, 3rd ed, John Wiley, 7–11, 2011

Historical Records of Australia, Series 1, vol xiii

Holt AG, *Hillcrest Hospital: the first 50 years*, Victoria, the Hillcrest Hospital Heritage Committee, 1999

Hughes M, *Providing responsive services to LGBT individuals with dementia*, In S. Westwood & E. Price (Eds.), Lesbian, gay, bisexual and trans individuals living with dementia: Concepts, practice and rights. London, England: Routledge New York, 2016

Hughes R, *The Fatal Shore. A History of the Transportation of Convicts to Australia 1787–1868*, London, Vintage, 2003

Irish P, *Hidden in Plain View. The Aboriginal people of coastal Sydney*, NewSouth, Sydney, 2017

Jalland P, *Old Age in Australia: a History*, Melbourne, Melbourne University Press, 2015

Karskens G, *Declining life: on the Rocks in early Sydney,* In: Walker D & Garton S (eds) Ageing, Australian Cultural History 14, Geelong, Deakin University, 63–75, 1995

Karskens G, *The Colony: a history of early Sydney,* Sydney, Allen & Unwin, 2009

Kay HT, *1870–1970. Commemorating the Centenary of Glenside Hospital,* Netley, SA: Griffin Press, 1970

Kehoe M, *The Melbourne Benevolent Asylum, Hotham's Premier Building,* Hotham History Project, 1998

Lewis M, *Managing Madness: Psychiatry and Society in Australia, 1788–1980,* Canberra, Australian Government Publishing Service, 1988

Lewis M, Garton S, *Mental Health in Australia, 1788–2015: A History of Responses to Cultural and Social Challenges,* In: Minas H, Lewis M (eds) Mental Health in Asia and the Pacific. Historical and Cultural Perspectives, New York, Springer Nature, 289–313, 2017

Luke S, *Callan Park: Hospital for the Insane,* Sydney, Australian Scholarly Publishing Pty Ltd, 2018

Moyle H, *Tasmania in the 19th and early 20th centuries,* In 'Australia's Fertility Transition', 41–62, ANU Press, 2020

Neil WD, *The lunatic asylum at Castle Hill: Australia's first psychiatric hospital 1811–1826,* Sydney, Dryas, 1992

O'Brien A, *Poverty's Prison. The poor in NSW 1880–1918,* Carlton, Victoria, Melbourne University Press, 1988

Ottaway SR, *The Decline of Life: Old Age in Eighteenth-Century England,* Cambridge University Press, Cambridge, 2004

Peace SM, *The development of residential and nursing home care in the United Kingdom,* In: Katz, Jeanne Samson and Peace, Sheila M. eds. End of Life in Care Homes: a Palliative Approach. Oxford, Oxford University Press, 15–42, 2003

Pybus C, *Truganini – Journey through the apocalypse,* Allen & Unwin, Sydney, 2020

Rathbone R, *A very present help – caring for Australians since 1813. The History of the Benevolent Society of NSW,* Sydney, State Library of NSW Press, 1994

Richards J, *Going up the Line to Goodna – a History of Woogaroo Lunatic Asylum, Goodna Mental Hospital, and Wolston Park Hospital 1865–2015,* Queensland Government, 2017

Robson L, *The Convict Settlers of Australia,* Melbourne, Melbourne University Press, 1973

Rollett C, Parker J, *Population and Family,* In: Halsey, A.H. (ed) Trends in British Society since 1900, UK, Palgrave MacMillan, 20–63, 1972

Rowley CD, *Outcasts in White Australia, Melbourne,* Pelican Books, 1973

Rubinstein WD, Rubinstein HL, *Menders of the Mind. A History of the Royal Australian* and New Zealand College of Psychiatrists, 1946–1996, Oxford, Oxford University Press, 1996

Rumsey HJ, *The Pioneers of Sydney Cove*, Sydney, Sunnybrook Press, 1937

Saggers S, Gray D, *Explanations of Indigenous alcohol use,* In: Gray, D. & Saggers, S. (eds) Indigenous Australian alcohol and other drug issues: Research from the National Drug Research Institute, Perth, Curtin University of Technology, 68–88, 2002

Seitz D, Lawlor B, *Module 6 – Pharmacological management.* In: Draper, B., Brodaty, H., Finkel, S. (eds) The IPA Complete Guides to Behavioral and Psychological Symptoms of Dementia (BPSD), Chicago, International Psychogeriatric Association, 2015

Shea P, *Defining Madness*, Leichhardt, Hawkins Press, 1999

Stoller A, *Growing Old – Problems of Old Age in the Australian Community*, Melbourne, Cheshires, 1960

Tampke J, *The Germans in Australia*, Melbourne, Cambridge University Press, 2006

Thane P, *The Cultural History of Old Age,* In: Walker D & Garton S (eds) Ageing, Australian Cultural History 14, Geelong, Deakin University, 1995

Thane P, *Old Age in English History. Past Experiences, Present Issues,* Oxford, Oxford University Press, 2000

Vreugdenhil AJ, *Out of Sight, out of Mind. Senile dementia in nineteenth century Launceston,* In: Effecting a Cure: Aspects of Health and Medicine in Launceston, P.A.C. Richards, B. Valentine, T. Dunning (eds), Launceston, Myola House of Publishing, 74–87, 2006

Webster C, *The elderly and the early National Health Service,* In: Life and Death and the Elderly ed. Margaret Pelling, Richard Smith. London: Routledge, 165–193, 1991

Whyntie A, *The History of Sunset Hospital*, Perth, B&S Printing, 1999

## Australian Dictionary of Biography

Conway J, *Blaxland, Gregory (1778–1852)*, Australian Dictionary of Biography, National Centre of Biography, Australian National University, http://adb.anu.edu.au/biography/blaxland-gregory-1795/text2031, published first in hardcopy 1966 (accessed 14 September 2019)

Dowd BT, *Alt, Augustus Theodore (1731–1815)*, Australian Dictionary of Biography, National Centre of Biography, Australian National University, http://adb.anu.edu.au/biography/alt-augustus-theodore-1702/text1845, published first in hardcopy 1966 (accessed 18 January 2020)

Fletcher BH, *Phillip, Arthur (1738–1814)*, Australian Dictionary of Biography, National Centre of Biography, Australian National University, http://adb.anu.

edu.au/biography/phillip-arthur-2549/text3471, published first in hardcopy 1967 (accessed 1 June 2020)

Gray AJ, *Brewer, Henry (1739–1796),* Australian Dictionary of Biography, National Centre of Biography, Australian National University, http://adb.anu.edu.au/ biography/brewer-henry-1825/text2095, published first in hardcopy 1966 (accessed 9 January 2020)

Gunson N, *Oakes, Francis (1770–1844),* Australian Dictionary of Biography, National Centre of Biography, Australian National University, http://adb.anu.edu.au/ biography/oakes-francis-2513/text3397 published first in hardcopy 1967 (accessed 14 September 2019)

Hone JA, *Chirnside, Thomas (1815–1887),* Australian Dictionary of Biography, National Centre of Biography, Australian National University, http://adb.anu.edu. au/biography/chirnside-thomas-3203/text4815, published first in hardcopy 1969 (accessed 15 September 2019)

Hume SH, *Hume, Hamilton (1797–1873),* Australian Dictionary of Biography, National Centre of Biography, Australian National University, http://adb.anu.edu. au/biography/hume-hamilton-2211/text2869, published first in hardcopy 1966 (accessed 15 September 2019)

McDonald DI, *Campbell, Francis Rawdon (1798–1877),* Australian Dictionary of Biography, National Centre of Biography, Australian National University, http:// adb.anu.edu.au/biography/campbell-francis-rawdon-3156/text4715 published first in hardcopy 1969 (accessed 3 June 2020)

Norris R, *Deakin, Alfred (1856–1919),* Australian Dictionary of Biography, National Centre of Biography, Australian National University, http://adb.anu.edu.au/ biography/deakin-alfred-5927/text10099, published first in hard copy 1981 (accessed 10 October 2019)

Piggin S, *Abbott, William Edward (Wingen) (1844–1924),* Australian Dictionary of Biography, National Centre of Biography, Australian National University, http:// adb.anu.edu.au/biography/abbott-william-edward-wingen-6/text8233, published first in hardcopy 1979 (accessed 25 September 2019)

Shepherd M, *Lewis, Sir Aubrey Julian (1900–1975),* Australian Dictionary of Biography, National Centre of Biography, Australian National University, http:/adb.anu.edu. au/biography/lewis-sir-aubrey-julian-10823/text19201, published first in hardcopy 2000 (accessed 13 January 2021)

Steven M, *Birnie, James (1762–1844),* Australian Dictionary of Biography, National Centre of Biography, Australian National University, http://adb.anu.edu.au/ biography/birnie-james-1783/text2007 published first in hardcopy 1966 (accessed 14 September 2019)

Steven M, *Macarthur, John (1767–1834)*, Australian Dictionary of Biography, National Centre of Biography, Australian National University, http://adb.anu.edu.au/biography/macarthur-john-2390/text3153 published first in hardcopy 1967 (accessed 17 September 2019)

Tamblyn M, *'Johns, Joseph Bolitho (1827–1900)'*, Australian Dictionary of Biography, National Centre of Biography, Australian National University, http://adb.edu.au/biography/johns-joseph-bolitho-3859/text6139, published first in hardcopy 1972 (accessed 15 September 2019)

Van der Poorten HM, *Darrell, George Frederick Price (1851–1921)*, Australian Dictionary of Biography, National Centre of Biography, Australian National University, http://adb.anu.edu.au/biography/darrell-george-frederick-price-3369/text5089, published first in hardcopy 1972 (accessed 10 October 2019)

Walsh GP, *Divine, Nicholas (1769–1830)*, Australian Dictionary of Biography, National Centre of Biography, Australian National University, http://adb.anu.edu.au/biography/divine-nicholas-1979/text2399, published first in hardcopy 1966 (accessed 15 September 2019)

Walter J, *Davies, Alan Fraser (1924–1987)*, Australian Dictionary of Biography, National Centre of Biography, Australian National University, https://adb.anu.edu.au/biography/davies-alan-fraser-12406/text22303 published first in hardcopy 2007 (accessed 2 February 2021)

## Theses

Andrews ES, *Senility before Alzheimer: Old age in British psychiatry, c1835–1912*, Doctoral thesis, University of Warwick, April 2014

Atkinson M, *From 'barbarous relics' to an 'emphasis on cure'? Suicide in Tasmania 1868–1943*, Doctoral thesis, University of Tasmania, March 2019

Bonwick R, *The history of Yarra Bend Lunatic Asylum, Melbourne*, Master's thesis, University of Melbourne, Melbourne, November 1995

Day C, *Magnificence, misery, and madness. A history of the Kew Asylum 1872–1915*, Doctoral thesis, University of Melbourne, 1998

Evans RL, *Charitable Institutions of the Queensland Government to 1919*, Master's Thesis, University of Queensland, 1969

Goodall JB, *Whom nobody owns: The Dunwich Benevolent Asylum, an Institutional biography 1866–1946*, Doctoral thesis, Department of History, University of Queensland, 1992

Hargrave J, *A pauper establishment is not a jail: old crawlers in Tasmania 1856–1895*, Master's thesis, University of Tasmania, 1993

Hilton C, *The development of psychogeriatric services in England from circa 1940 until*

*1989*, Doctoral thesis, King's College, London, 2014

Hunter CE, *Doctoring old age. A social history of geriatric medicine in Victoria*, Doctoral thesis, University of Melbourne, February 2003

Kippen R, *Death in Tasmania: using civil death registers to measure nineteenth century cause-specific mortality*, Doctoral thesis, Australian National University, 2002

Piddock S, *A Space of their Own: Nineteenth century lunatic asylums in England, South Australia and Tasmania*, Doctoral thesis, Flinders University of South Australia, 2003

Piper A, *Beyond the convict system: the aged poor and institutionalisation in colonial Tasmania*, Doctoral thesis, University of Tasmania, 2003

Roth DT, *Life, Death and Deliverance at Callan Park Hospital for the Insane 1877–1923*, Doctoral thesis, Australian National University, May 2020

Smith TG, '*With tact, intelligence and a special acquaintance with the insane'. A history of the development of mental health care (nursing) in NSW Australia, from colonisation to federation, 1788–1901*, Doctoral thesis, University of Western Sydney, 2005

## Unpublished lectures, papers, letters

Dibden W, *A biography of psychiatry: The story of events and the people involved in the development of services for the psychiatrically ill in South Australia 1939–1989*. Adelaide, University of Adelaide Library, 2001

Group Report, *Community Mental Health Care*, unpublished report involving Kate Jackson for Executive Masters of Public Administration, Sydney University – cites sections of Morris Iemma's National Press Club address from 1 June 2006. The quote comes from page 4 of the National Press Club transcript, December 2007

Hills N, *Asylum to Mainstream. The Closure and Replacement of Swanbourne Hospital 1979–1985*. Unpublished 2nd edition, 2019

## Internet Pages

Age UK. *Our history.* https://www.ageuk.org.uk/about-us/people/our-history/ (accessed 28 May 2020)

Alfred Deakin Prime Ministerial Library. *Alfred Deakin.* https://www.deakin.edu.au/library/special-collections/alfred (accessed 17 November 2020)

Alzheimer's Australia, *National Cross Cultural Dementia Network,* Alzheimer's Australia, 2010 Microsoft Word – NCCDN_background_paper_100719_final.doc (dementia.org.au) (accessed 30 June 2021)

Alzheimer's Disease International, *About Us.* https://www.alzint.org/about-us/ (accessed 18 January 2021)

Aftercare. *Aftercare: Our Journey 1907–2017*. Sydney, Australia. www.aftercare.com.au (accessed 8 April 2019)

Australian Association of Gerontology. *Our History.* Our History – Australian Association of Gerontology (aag.asn.au) (accessed 4 February 2021)

Australian Dementia Network, Home – Australian Dementia Network (accessed 13 July 2021)

Australian Dementia Network, *Managing memory clinics during the COVID-19 pandemic: initial perspectives from the Australian Dementia Network Memory Clinics network,* Australian Dementia Network, April 2020, Home – Australian Dementia Network (accessed 13 July 2021)

Blackwood M, 1384.6 – Statistics – Tasmania, 2002 Feature Article – Mental health services Released 13/09/2002, 1384.6 – Statistics – Tasmania, 2002 (abs.gov.au) (accessed 1 February 2021)

Blaxland Wine Group. *Gregory Blaxland.* https://blaxwine.com.au/gregory-blaxland/ (accessed 21 September 2020)

Darebin Heritage, Yarra Bend Lunatic Asylum. Darebin Libraries, http://heritage. darebinlibraries.vic.gov.au/article/631 (accessed 6 July 2020)

Dementia Australia, *Dementia Key Facts and Statistics – updated January 2021,* Dementia statistics | Dementia Australia (accessed 14 July 2021)

Denham, Michael. *A Brief History of the Care of the Elderly.* British Geriatrics Society, June 2016 https://www.bgs.org.uk/resources/a-brief-history-of-the-care-of-the-elderly (accessed 6 May 2020)

Healy J, Williams R, *Are Australians ageist?* Centre for Workplace Leadership, University of Melbourne, 2016 https://fbe.unimelb.edu.au/__data/assets/pdf_file/0007/2729140/Research-Snapshot.pdf (accessed 1 June 2020)

Kerr A, *David William Kilbourne Kay,* Royal College of Physicians Inspiring Physicians, David William Kilbourne Kay | RCP Museum (rcplondon.ac.uk) (accessed 26 May 2021)

Martyr P, *Claremont Hospital for the Insane has a Shadowy Past,* MeDeFacts, University of Western Australia, 12–13, September 2010

Mary Marshall eFestchrift, Personal Social Services Unit, University of Manchester, 2005. Microsoft Word – marymarshall eFestschrift booklet web.doc (pssru.ac.uk) (accessed 18 January 2021)

Mi9, *Australian Baby Boomers,* February 2013 02282_fuel_mi9_Baby-Boomers-2564x1200px_v07_11.jpg (763×1632) (marketing.com.au) (accessed 7 July 2021)

Murphy, Matt. *Newtown Ejectment Case.* https://www.newtownproject.com.au/portfolio-items/newtown-ejectment-case/ (accessed 9 November 2020)

National Archives of Australia. *Alfred Deakin: after office.* https://www.naa.gov.au/

explore-collection/australias-prime-ministers/alfred-deakin/after-office (accessed 17 November 2020)

NSW Office of Environment and Heritage. Rydalmere Hospital Precinct (former). https://www.environment.nsw.gov.au/heritageapp/ViewHeritageItemDetails. aspx?id=5000658 (accessed 1 September 2020)

Reynolds, Emma. *Madman on the money: How Australian pioneer John Macarthur died in obscurity after being declared a lunatic.* Finance, News.com.au, 27 January 2015. https://www.news.com.au/finance/money/madman-on-the-money-how-australian-pioneer-john-macarthur-died-in-obscurity-after-being-declared-a-lunatic/news-story /5c5745846b66e309e79f694206bbac42 (accessed 30 September 2020)

Sanders A, *Dax, Eric Cunningham (1908–2008)*, Obituaries Australia, National Centre of Biography, Australian National University, http://oa.anu.edu.au/obituary/dax-eric-cunningham-13941/text24835 (accessed 13 January 2021)

Thane P, *History of Social Care in England* Memorandum submitted to the House of Commons' Health Committee Inquiry: Social Care, October 2009. https:// publications.parliament.uk/pa/cm200809/cmselect/cmhealth/1021/1021we49.htm (accessed 28 May 2020)

The History of Parliament Trust, *Mills, George Galway (1765–1828),* History of Parliament online, https://www.historyofparliamentonline.org/volume/1790-1820/ member/mills-george-galway-1765-1828 (accessed 9 November 2020)

The Prince Charles Hospital, *TPCH History: Home.* Home TPCH History LibGuides at The Prince Charles Hospital (accessed 18 February 2021)

Williams S, *Support for the elderly during the 'crisis of the Old Poor Law", c.1790–1834.* Population, economy, and welfare, 1200–2000. Cambridge, September 2011 https://www.campop.geog.cam.ac.uk/events/richardsmithconference/papers.html (accessed 27 May 2020)

Wilson M, Stearne A, Gray D, Sherry S, *The harmful use of alcohol amongst Indigenous Australians,* Australian Indigenous HealthInfoNet, 2010, http://www.healthinfonet. ecu.edu.au/alcoholuse_review (accessed 31 July 2013)

# Index

Aged Care Funding Instrument (ACFI) (see Residential Aged Care Facilities)

Aged Care Quality and Safety Commission 283, 285

Aged Care Reform Strategy 172, 175, 181, 219, 223

Aged Care Reforms (1997) 180–181

Aged Care Program 175–176, 184, 223, 266–267, 277, 283, 286

Aged Care Standards and Accreditation Agency 180

Aged Persons Mental Health Services (Victoria) (see also older people's mental health services) 214–217, 291, 293

Ageing
    and general health 15–16, 58–64, 71–73, 85, 93–95, 99–100, 103–104, 127–128, 139–141, 152–153, 158, 164–165, 192, 258
    and mental disorders 9, 11–13, 33–35, 46–55, 67–71, 73–74, 78–83, 87–89, 92–96, 99–100, 102, 107–118, 129–136, 141–145, 149–150, 155–164, 206–207, 211, 245, 264–265, 277
    population 1, 9–12, 32–41, 52, 64, 72, 75, 83, 99, 102, 105–106, 126–134, 137–139, 171, 253, 258, 270–271, 279–281, 296–297

Ageism 20, 28, 38, 82, 115, 145, 177, 254, 281

Aggression 6, 23, 26, 33, 37, 40, 49, 51, 69, 71, 73, 92, 104, 126, 185, 259, 293

Agitation 6, 37–38, 51, 68–69, 76, 110, 126, 185

Alcohol
    abuse 4, 16, 20, 23–24, 30–31, 33–34, 39, 44, 49, 59, 67–69, 87, 89, 94, 96, 98–99, 101–103, 107, 114, 117, 119, 163, 220, 222, 226, 233, 261–264, 280
    related dementia (see Dementia)

Alienists 5–6

Allandale Hospital, Cessnock 161–162, 219

Almeida, Osvaldo 206, 238

Alt, Augustus 15

Alzheimer, Alois 121–122

Alzheimer's disease (see Dementia)

Alzheimer's Australia (see Dementia Australia)

Alzheimer's Disease International (ADI) 134–135, 201, 289–290

Alzheimer's Disease and Related Disorders Society (ADARDS) (see Dementia Australia)

Amentia 4, 68

American Geriatrics Society 127

American Psychiatric Association 125

Ames, David 174, 196–197, 200, 206, 215

Anderson, William Ferguson 128, 140

Andrews, Emily 8–9, 11

Andrews, Gary 140–141

Andrews, Gavin 226

Antidepressant medication (see Psychotropic medication)

Antipsychotic medication (see Psychotropic medication)

Ararat Mental Hospital (Asylum) 76, 79–80

Arie, Tom 130–132, 148, 194–196, 212, 224, 235

Arie course 131–132, 135, 196–197, 210, 222

Asylums (see Mental hospitals, Benevolent asylums, Hospitals for Aged and Destitute)

*Asylum to Community* 149

Attendants (see Mental hospitals)

Australian Association of Gerontology (AAG) 138–139, 148

Australian National University (ANU) Social Policy Research Unit 253–254

# Acknowledgements

Many people assisted me in researching and writing this book. While I have previously written medical historical articles for medical journals, this is my first foray into broader aspects of history and medical history. Historians Ed Duyker, Hans Pols and Stephen Garton gave me much needed advice and guidance particularly related to the historical aspects of research and presentation. The archival work involved assistance from staff at the Queensland State Archives, State Library Victoria, Public Records Office of Victoria, Libraries Tasmania and the State Records Office of Western Australia, but I am particularly grateful to staff at the State Library of NSW in Sydney and the NSW State Archives and Records at Kingswood where I spent many hours examining medical casebooks and other historical records.

The development of older people's mental health and dementia services is largely a phenomenon of the last 35 years and so many of the key participants were able to provide me insights of their involvement and observations. I interviewed many colleagues who work and research in dementia care and old age mental health about their careers for podcasts that are available on the RANZCP website. Other interviews were conducted by phone or email specifically to address issues for this book. Thank you to David Ames, Elizabeth Beattie, Richard Bonwick, Henry Brodaty, Tony Broe, Gerard Byrne, Ed Chiu, Marianne Cummins, Colleen Doyle, Richard Fleming, Leon Flicker, Meredith Gresham, Kathy Hall, Neville Hills, Mary Ingrames, Kate Jackson, Deborah Koder, Julia Lane, David Lie, Samantha Loi, Jeff Looi, Helen McGowan, John McIntyre, Rod McKay, Duncan McKellar, Shirloney Morgan, Martin Morrissey, Bob Moss, Daniel O'Connor, Jill Pettigrew, Judy Ratajec, Judy Raymond,

Wayne Reid, John Snowdon, Janine Stevenson, Eddie Tan, Stephen Ticehurst and Sid Williams for your willingness to provide me with information and your time. From the UK, Claire Hilton and John Wattis provided information and observations about service development there.

Other colleagues facilitated contacts and information sources. In this regard I thank Maureen Bell, Graham Edwards, Bob Goldney, Peter Shea and Richard White who share my interest in the history of psychiatry and provided assistance. John Condon, Rebecca Graham, Steve Macfarlane helped with contacts and information. A number of people were helpful in providing specific information by way of archival notes, books, chapters, and theses and I thank Rebecca Kippen, Karolina Krysinska, Paul Peng (Prince of Wales Hospital Library), Elizabeth Priestley (NSW Mental Health Association) and Anthea Vreugdenhil. Humphrey Bower assisted with information about his father Herbert Bower, while Dick Steel, Anne McGregor, Judy Owen and Michelle Dawson were helpful in providing information about G. Vernon Davies.

The RANZCP have been helpful throughout this project including facilitating and hosting the podcast interviews. In particular thank you to David Beal, Jon Cullum, Ailish Graham, Kim Keane, Kathryn McGrath, Jackie Mottica, Andrew Peters, Jacqueline Shiel and Susan Yates for the various types of assistance provided.

I was very fortunate to get feedback on earlier drafts of various chapters of the book from Henry Brodaty, Ed Chiu, Ed Duyker, Stephen Garton, Samantha Loi, Kylie Radford, John Snowdon and Stephen Ticehurst. The book only improved with each input and I am extremely grateful. Thank you to Nick Walker, Anna Nechkina and the team at Australian Scholarly Publishing for their assistance.

Thank you to all of my work colleagues at the Eastern Suburbs Older Persons Mental Health Service and the older people that I met during my career as your contributions to my understanding of the issues important in old age mental health and dementia care were integral to this book. Finally, as a 'retirement' project researching and writing this book over the last three years has certainly taken up a lot of time and I thank my wife Debbie for her understanding and patience.

Printed in Australia
Ingram Content Group Australia Pty Ltd
AUHW022326020624
395193AU00003B/27